The Stolen Brain Chip

*

A Tale for Healthcare Professionals

Elisabeth Link, M.D.

First published in the United States of America
by Monasteria Press LLC, San Francisco

Paperback ISBN: 978-1-7372582-3-0
Hardback ISBN: 978-1-7372582-5-4
eBook ISBN: 978-1-7372582-4-7

Library of Congress Control Number (LCCN): 2021950975

Monasteria Press LLC

DEDICATION

For my husband Thomas Link, M.D.

We often block our own blessings because we don't feel inherently good enough or smart enough or pretty enough or worthy enough... You're worthy because you are born and because you are here. You alone are enough.

Oprah Winfrey

CONTENTS

The Stolen Brain Chip

*

A Tale for Healthcare Professionals

Elisabeth Link, M.D.

PROLOGUE

Silicon Valley University of Evolutionary Computation (SUEC) was established in 2025 in a secluded location in the hills above Redwood City, California. SUEC realized a new model of collaboration between major tech giants and the state of California to develop truly cutting-edge technologies within the framework of a research-intensive university. *Evolutionary computation* is an area of computer science that uses principles from biological development processes to solve computational problems. In evolutionary computation, an initial set of solutions is generated and iteratively updated by small random changes until a target performance has been achieved. Many of the tech tools developed and explored at SUEC are years ahead of what is available anywhere else. Therefore, SUEC has attracted the most famous faculty from around the country and the brightest students from around the world, outperforming nearby Stanford University and the University of California in excellence and exclusivity.

To provide convenient medical services, SUEC owns a hospital, which is located in nearby Redwood City. Since the student population at the university is relatively small and in excellent health overall, the hospital is open to the public. The 200-bed university hospital provides medical emergency care, general medical care and a variety of medical specialty services for both adult and pediatric patients.

On May 24, 2032, an incident at SUEC led to a series of events, which resulted in more than fifteen major injuries, five hospitalizations and four deaths. The confidential summary report provided here uncovers the sequence of events that led to these fatalities, based on personal observations by Dr. Lili Pham, radiologist at SUEC hospital, and investigations by the FBI. The investigator team started a race against time to rescue a young student from a ruthless killer, retrieve a national treasure and prevent an implosion of the most eminent university in the world.

- 1 -
Lili
THE THEFT

Monday, May 24, 2032, 8.05 am.

As Lili walked over the perfectly green lawn on the campus of Silicon Valley University of Evolutional Computation (SUEC), she wondered why she had been called to the dean's office. The university system has some similarities with a high school. If you were asked to come to the principal's office for an unscheduled visit, there was a high probability that there was some kind of trouble. But as much as Lili tried to anticipate the problem, she could not imagine what it was.

About five years ago, Lili was recruited to SUEC as one of ten radiologists to provide medical imaging services for the university's brand-new hospital. As a professor at SUEC, she had clinical, research and teaching responsibilities. But she was not high enough in the hierarchy chain to meet the dean on a routine basis. So, it was unclear to her why she had been summoned to the dean's office. As a physician-scientist, she had received both praise and criticism over the course of her twenty-plus years in the academic world. Lili did not count her awards and would not expect the dean to personally thank her for her work. As a female faculty member, she was used to daily microaggressions and stereotype threats. On more than one occasion, she had been called "opinionated" and "difficult." But she was not aware of any current issue that her inclination to ask hard questions and demand an environment of integrity might have caused. To the best of her knowledge, Lili had not annoyed anyone recently. In addition, the students in her team were all doing well. Or had one of them violated the rules?

Lili had passed the lawn at the base of the SUEC campus and walked towards two mirroring C-shaped promenades that led up the hill to the main University building. The octagonal university building sat like a landed spaceship on top of the dark green redwood hills. As a scientist, Lili was always fascinated by the sight of the beautiful and unique construction of the SUEC flagship. The base of the building was cut into the serpentinite top of the largest Redwood-lined hill in the area. About two-thirds of the contemporary steel and limestone building rested on the ground and about one-third overhung the SUEC valley. The building was about 15 meter tall, with a cathedral-like cupola, steel and limestone facade and eight large, multicolored, arched windows, which reflected the golden morning sun. An enormous pedestal supported the part of the building that protruded into the valley. The pedestal used an advanced steel plate shear wall system to resist the lateral loads of earthquakes and high winds. The protruding part of the building was further supported by an array of steel columns and multiple posts around the perimeter of the building provided enhanced strength to withstand even the strongest earthquakes. Lili had never seen a more impressive building.

Lili turned right and walked up the promenade leading to the main entrance. The promenade on the left was reserved for tourists and ended at a terrace. Lili saw several people already walking up and down the hill with their tour guides, taking photos of the octagonal building and the breathtaking 360-degree view over the valley. Between the promenades, on the hillside below the main octagonal building, were several smaller limestone buildings, like little offspring of the main octagon. These buildings housed the lecture hall, several conference rooms, dormitories for the students, an apartment building for faculty, a library, research labs and supporting facilities. At the end of each promenade was a terrace and a café, one for visitors on the left and one for campus personnel on the right of the octagon. As she approached the café on the right, Lili saw people drinking their coffee at bistro tables under the shade of majestic redwood trees. She heard the relaxing sound of water flowing through a nearby fountain and smelled coffee mixed with the aroma of dark red roses, which outlined the entryway to the main building. *What could possibly be wrong in this picture-perfect bubble?*

Lili opened the door to the main SUEC building, where a cool breeze met her along with the mechanical humming sound of the air conditioner. The dean's executive assistant, Stella Pellegrini, was sitting at a large, C-shaped desk in the entrance area, which served as a gate to the main lobby. Stella had been working with Dr. Bennett since the inception of the university, and she was the gatekeeper here. Lili had met her on many occasions in the café next door and they had become well acquainted over the years. But unfortunately, Lili had not much time to chat with Stella today. She was late and had to focus on the security formalities to check in. Lili swiped her ID card, stared into the iris detector and cleared her forehead for the temperature sensor. A beep signaled that the computer had cleared her, and Stella confirmed her entry into the building. Stella looked relieved as she saw Lili walking through the metal detector. "Great to see you, Lili! Thanks for coming over on such short notice. They are waiting for you."

"They?" Lili's anxiety levels were creeping up. *An urgent team meeting?* As casually as possible, she said, "I thought you asked me to come to see Dr. Bennett for a one-on-one? Who else is there?"

Stella looked around and lowered her voice. "I don't know for sure, but I believe they are from the FBI," she whispered. "Looks like some serious business." Her response did not exactly ease Lili's mind.

"Do you know what the topic of the meeting is?" she asked.

"I am afraid I have no idea. But you will find out in an instant." Stella smiled and extended her arm towards the lobby. "You know the way to Dr. Bennett's office, right? I don't have to walk you over? My knee starts hurting if I walk back and forth too often."

"No problem," Lili said. "I am on my way."

Lili stepped into the diamond-shaped main hall of the octagon building. She had seen it many times, but its stunning beauty struck her every time. The pedestal underneath the building extended into a steel and platinum column in the center of the atrium, which rose three stories high to the ceiling where it merged into multiple branches, like a majestic tree. The steel branches supported a gigantic octagonal cupola. The base of the central pillar was lined by an indoor garden of potted orchid plants. The orchids were labeled with little signs for the education of SUEC students and visitors. In the past, Lili had arrived for administrative meetings an hour early to take photos of these amazing plants. There were white *egrets*, dark red *liparis latifolia*, golden *oncidium forbesii*, light pink *miltassia* and blue *phalaenopsis*, among others. But today, there was no time to enjoy the beauty of these flowers. Lili walked by the orchid garden and up the dramatic spiral glass stairway, which led around the central column to the second and third floors of the building. A platform on the second floor provided a great view over the atrium and served as a connection to the executive offices of the university leaders. Lili walked down the hallway to Dr. Bennett's office. The door was closed. As she came closer, she heard at least three voices inside, engaged in a lively discussion. She knocked, opened the door slowly and stuck her head into the room.

"Hello, Dr. Bennett!"

Dr. Bennett, a senior, obese white man with a receding hairline, deep set nose and bright, gray eyes, looked at her with a similar expression to his assistant.

"Lili, there you are! Please come in!"

Lili looked around the spacious office, which featured a large window, green wood parquet, a large glass desk with an ergonomic chair, a modern oval conference table and a large computer monitor at the wall. Dr. Bennett sat at the upper end of the conference table with four other people, who looked up as she was entering. To her right, she saw Dr. Annya Segond, a woman in her mid-forties with shoulder-length, layered red hair and unblinking, pale green eyes. Annya was a SUEC professor and the director of the emergency care services at the hospital. Lili knew her very well from multiple joined clinical services. Annya was the most composed and unflappable person she knew, cool in every situation, a characteristic that served her well in the ER. Beside Annya sat a thin, middle-aged man with short, grayish hair and delicately leaded glasses, who was wearing a lab coat and a university badge — perhaps a research faculty member. He was looking at Lili with an anxious, haunted gaze. On the other side of the table sat two men in expensive looking, perfectly ironed, dark gray suits. One of them was an older white male, perhaps in his late fifties, with stern blue eyes, a Romanesque nose and sparse, gray hair. The other was an attractive younger Black man, perhaps in his late thirties, with clear, hazel eyes and black micro dreads.

Dr. Bennett introduced Lili first. "This is Dr. Lili Pham, our radiologist and physician-scientist. She is an expert in medical imaging, and she knows both clinicians and students at our university."

"Nice to meet you, Dr. Pham," the older man responded with a formal bow of his head.

"Nice to meet you, too," Lili countered politely. After the COVID-19 pandemic, nobody shook hands anymore. That era was over.

Dr. Bennett went on to introduce the rest of the party in his office. He pointed to the older man in gray. "Lili, this is Special Agent Angus Weber, an expert in criminal justice from the FBI," and he pointed to the younger man, "and this is Special Agent Terrel Wright, an expert in forensic psychology."

Lili was thoroughly impressed — and relieved at the same time. Whatever the problem was here, it could not possibly be anything she or any of her team members had caused. Her students had been involved in some of the usual university drama. Using their tech gadgets for non-permitted actions, disputes about authorships on scientific publications, parties on the lawn, etc.... But Lili was pretty sure none of these would spark the interest of the FBI. So, what was going on?

Dr. Bennett continued, "I believe you know Dr. Segond from the clinic."

Lili exchanged a gaze with Annya and nodded.

"And this is Dr. Robert Hill, a professor of neurosciences."
Lili looked at the man in the white coat and nodded again, although she had no clue who he was. The faculty community on campus was relatively small. If you were around long enough, you got to know most of the other faculty, at least by name or by remembering their face from some local event. But this person did not ring a bell. Lili had never seen him before. Perhaps he was new....

Dr. Bennett explained, "The reason why we are coming together today is that important and sensitive research material has been stolen from Dr. Hill's research lab. The chief of our security services at SUEC informed the FBI earlier this morning, which led to agents Weber and Wright's visit here today. Before I continue explaining any details, I need you to sign a confidentiality agreement. What we are about to discuss is a matter of national security and strictly confidential. It cannot be discussed with anyone outside of this room. Is this clear?" Everyone in the room nodded.

Lili's curiosity was sparked.

Dr. Bennett handed each person at the table a form and a pen.

Lili thought she had forgotten her reading glasses but found them on her head. She tried to focus and read the form. Too many thoughts were racing through her brain at the same time. *What am I getting into? Are we in danger? What could possibly be so important in a research lab that it caught the interest of the FBI?*

She signed the form. So did her colleagues. Dr. Bennett collected the forms with an approving nod.

"Let me show you a video from one of our security cameras." Dr. Bennett opened a file on his computer. It showed a research lab, probably from an engineering department, with benches and desks covered with a variety of cables, screws, batteries and other electronic gadgets. The lights were low and there was nobody in the lab although Lili got the impression from the chaos on the benches that this was probably a very busy place. She did not see any windows in the video, and therefore it was difficult to tell what time of the day this was. Then she noticed an electronic clock on one of the computer screens, which showed a time of 4.25 am.

Suddenly, two people entered the scene. Lili could only see their shadows in the twilight. One of them was thin and of medium height. The other was muscular and tall. They were both wearing jeans and black hoodies with the hoods covering their heads. They kept their faces down, avoiding the camera as if they knew where it was. Despite the darkness in the room, they moved rather quickly around chairs and other obstacles towards a desk in the back. One of the shadows reached into their pocket and pulled out two small instruments. Lili saw a small light appearing. One was a flashlight. The first shadow held it towards the lock, inserted the other instrument and turned it back and forth until a drawer opened. The other shadow quickly removed a metallic box from the drawer, and both hurried towards the door. The video ended.

Dr. Bennett clicked on a second video file. "Here is a video from the hallway shortly afterwards.

Lili saw a long, empty, neon-lit hallway with a shiny, apparently freshly waxed floor, white painted walls and a heavy steel door at the end. She tried to recognize the building but had never seen this hallway before. In most research buildings at SUEC, multiple doors along a hallway led to multiple labs. In this case, it seemed like there was only one entrance, one long hallway and one lab at the end. As in the lab, Lili could not make out any windows. The two shadows appeared, keeping their heads down as before. Lili could only see the backs of their hoods. They ran towards the exit.

Suddenly, the first shadow slipped. Lili saw the thief flying through the air, clutching the box in their right hand and landing on the ground. Everything went very quickly. Lili tried to get a little closer to the computer screen, but it was hard to see details. Most surprisingly, a second later, the other person started to slip as well. The shadow person first bent dangerously backwards, trying to regain balance by moving their arms around like a helicopter, then they bent sideways, and ultimately fell forwards on their outstretched right arm and shoulder. The hood of the hoodie was thrown backwards, and Lili saw a long, thick ponytail appearing, held in a delicate, ornamental hair ring – this was likely a woman! There was no sound on the video, but she could almost hear the crash of the accident. Meanwhile, the first shadow slowly sat up, holding their right wrist. The fingers of the right hand did not move. The woman slowly crawled towards the box and grasped it with her left hand, carefully avoiding moving her right arm. She got up as well and the two slowly limped towards the exit. They opened the steel door by leaning against it and disappeared into the early morning dawn.

Lili could not help but think. *Professional thieves would not have been caught on camera, slipped in tandem or lost their cover so easily. The FBI is chasing two amateurs!*

Lili looked back at the others in the room. "The fact that one of the thieves fell seemed to be bad luck. But how could two thieves fall at the same time?"

Dr. Hill smiled proudly and explained, "Our research team invented the floor cover. What looks like wax on the floor is actually a patented adhesive formulation. If you walk with a typical pace of about one meter per second over the tiles, the adhesive will stick to the sole of your shoe. This is because the body weight is evenly spread over the tile, and the adhesive can interact with the sole. But if you start running, the limited contact of your shoe with the ground will prevent this connection and you will slip and fall. We created this as a security measure for our facility. Our lab workers walk at normal pace. Anyone who runs would likely be an uninvited guest."

Lili asked, "What would happen if a fire broke out in the lab?"

"The entire hallway is fireproof," he responded, "and we applied the adhesive to only a short distance. In case of an emergency, we can roll out a carpet that covers the area."

Lili was intrigued. "Where is this lab? I don't remember ever seeing it?"

Dr. Bennett said, "This lab is in a secure underground location, which we cannot disclose. Dr. Hill is working on a new brain chip technology, which can enhance human brain function. While others have developed brain chips in the past, there are major improvements with Dr. Hill's technology. In the past, microchips for brain-computer interfaces had to be implanted on the surface of the brain to achieve the desired interaction with the brain tissue. Dr. Hill's brain chips can be implanted in the soft tissues of the scalp and can communicate with the desired brain area through the bone of the skull. This makes the implantation very easy and does not require a brain surgery. In addition, Dr. Hill's brain chips are not designed to restore the function of an injured brain area. His technology is designed to enhance the function of the normal brain. In other words, his chips can create super-human brain function."

Lili started to understand. "And the thieves stole these new brain chips?"

Dr. Bennett nodded. "There is significant risk if these chips get into the wrong hands. Imagine a thief who can enhance their vision or hearing capacity ten-fold, a terrorist doubling their reflexes, a nation like Russia or China copying this technology…."

Lili asked, "How many chips did they steal?"

Robert Hill, the scientist, answered, "There were five prototype chips in the box. Although we do not know if any were damaged with the fall."

Lili looked at the FBI agents. "And agents Weber and Wright are here to get the chips back?"

Dr. Bennett explained, "Yes, indeed. And this is where you and Dr. Segond come in. We need your help!"

Annya spoke for the first time. "They first consulted me, Lili, and I suggested we add your expertise as well." She turned to Dean

Bennett. "Ben, can you please show us the second video again and slow down the fall of the first person."

Dr. Bennett hovered the mouse to the beginning of the video, then advanced it until it reached the part where the first person slipped. He zoomed in on the right arm and replayed the fall in slow mode. They could see the right hand flexed at the wrist, trying to hold onto the box. The person fell on their flexed wrist. Annya and Lili exchanged glances and Lili summarized. "This is almost certainly a Smith fracture."

Mr. Weber, the older FBI agent, asked, "What is a Smith fracture?"

Lili tried to explain it in general terms. "Well, most people fall on their outstretched hand. This is due to a reflex that tries to protect us from falling on our face. The common fall on an outstretched hand leads to an angulation of the bone of the lower arm (the radius) backwards, away from the palm of the hand. This is called a Colles fracture. However, in our case here, the thief tried to hold on to the box and fell on their flexed wrist. This leads to an angulation of the distal radius, the bone above the wrist joint, in the direction of the palm of the hand. We call this a Smith fracture." Lili took out her notebook and created a quick sketch to show the FBI agents what she meant.

Dr. Bennett exclaimed, "Lili, what a great sketch! I did not know that you are not only a radiologist but also an artist!"

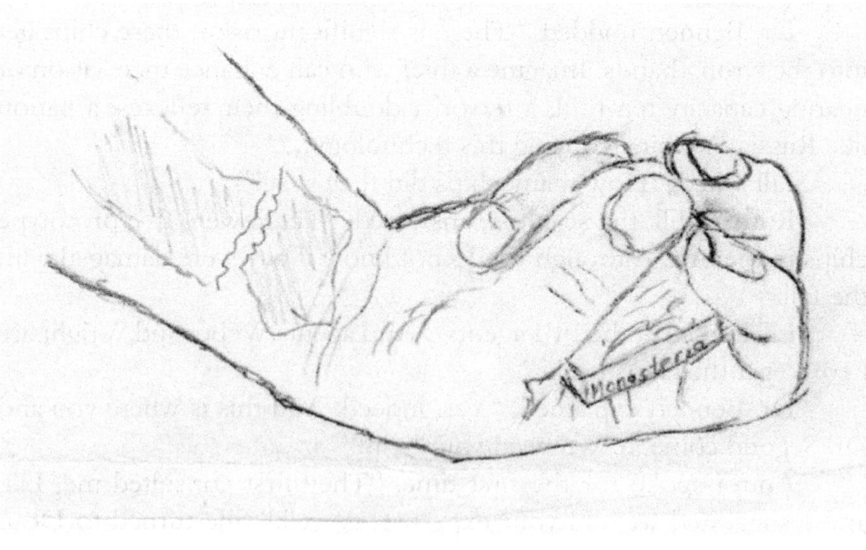

Agent Wright quickly synthesized the information. "So, you are saying that our suspect broke their forearm, and the type of injury is very rare? How do you know they broke their arm at all?"

Annya responded with her usual confident, calm voice. "Of course, we don't know this for sure. But the way the wrist seems deformed on the video, how the thief supports the right wrist with their left hand and the absence of any finger movement of the right hand strongly suggest that he suffered a fracture."

Lili added, "A Smith fracture only happens in less than five per cent of wrist fractures. So, if this person did suffer a fracture and seeks medical care, it should be possible to identify them."

Dr. Bennett smiled. "Let me show you another video."

He clicked on another video file on his computer. This time, they saw the entrance area in front of the emergency room of SUEC hospital. It looked like a quiet morning. A lone security person was standing in front of the door. Not much else was happening. The time stamp on the upper right corner of the video showed 5.18 am.

Then, a person in jeans and a black hoodie entered the scene. They walked through the sliding doors of the ER, holding their right wrist with their left hand. Lili could not believe her eyes. This was almost certainly the same person that they saw earlier in the hallway! She thought, *these people really need a brain enhancement chip!*

Again, the person held their head down so that they could not see their face. Lili did not see the other person anywhere. Apparently, the person with the wrist injury entered the ER alone.

The camera flipped to the ER waiting room. Here, they saw about fifteen people of different ages, genders and races, none of them in jeans or a hoodie.

Dr. Bennett explained, "We found the jeans and hoodie in the men's restroom. They must have changed there. We assume they might have worn a second set of clothes underneath."

"Could these be two of our students?" Annya asked.

"We checked on all of our students this morning," Dr. Bennett responded. "Most of them reported to their morning classes. Two are on vacation and four called in sick. Our security team checked on every single one of them and none of these students had a wrist injury. Three students are unaccounted for. We are in the process of tracking them down and checking them for any injuries."

Agent Weber looked at Lili and Annya. "Based on the information on these videos, we were hoping that you two could help us identify the first suspect."

Annya responded, "That should be possible. However, I must caution you that we see a significant number of patients who come to us with a fake or borrowed ID. We can see what we find out and go from there."

Agent Weber nodded. "Terrel and I will visit the lab with Dr. Hill, to see if we can find additional evidence. In the meantime, can you two please go to the ER and see what you can find there?"

"Wouldn't that violate patient privacy?" Lili asked.

Agent Weber explained, "We certainly respect patient privacy as much as possible. That's why we are asking you to assist us. You can review your patients' files as usual and inform us if you see a fracture that fits the injury to our suspect. The United States government can access information it deems necessary to protect the security of the nation. The Homeland Security Act gives the FBI authority to conduct the investigations necessary to prevent domestic terrorism, and to access the information needed to do so. We can obtain a court order to review a specific patient's file, if needed,."

Lili nodded. "Thanks, I understand. I will be happy to help."

Dr. Bennett added, "There is one more thing. We have a symposium with twelve major donors this coming Thursday. And I really mean *major*! Ten of the donors will give two billion US dollars each, and two of them will donate five billion. That means we expect to receive thirty billion dollars to support research at SUEC over the next decades. If we add that to our existing endowment of thirty billion, SUEC will have a larger endowment fund than any other university in the world!"

For the first time at this meeting, Lili saw Robert Hill's eyes lighting up. He added, "Imagine the impact on our research work! We will exponentially grow and accelerate the development of new technologies!"

Agent Weber nodded. "This investment will secure the leadership of the United States in technology development. At the same time, SUEC will be vulnerable to spy and theft activities, both from domestic and international agents. It seems that the threats have already started. That's why we are here."

Dr. Bennett added, "As you can imagine, we cannot have any negative publicity over the next few days – and hopefully not at all. Two of our donors specifically dedicated their gifts to the development of brain-computer interfaces. If they were to become aware of issues with the security and integrity of our research labs, we could risk losing them and billions of dollars of research funding. Moreover, if two donors pulled out, this could have a domino effect on the others. Therefore, I am committed to doing everything in my power to resolve this brain chip issue as soon as possible. In the meantime, this operation has to be kept absolutely confidential. No word to anyone. We cannot risk losing these funds."

Annya and Lili nodded.

Dr. Bennett closed the meeting. "Okay, we have a plan. I hope we will find the stolen brain chips soon and bring the thieves to justice. Thank you all for your help. We will meet again later this afternoon. I look forward to seeing you again at five pm in my office."

***

What a morning! Lili and Annya got up from their seats and walked towards the door. Agent Weber got up as well and offered to get the door for Annya. She looked at him with a stern gaze. "Thank you, Agent Weber, I'm good!"

He smiled at her. "Oh, I like independent women!"

"Thank you," Annya responded politely. "Yes indeed, I'm pretty self-sufficient. "

"Well, in case you do need assistance, Terrel and I will be here for you. No need to get too independent!"

"Thank you, Agent Weber."

Annya and Lili exchanged blank stares. Then, they left Dr. Bennett's office together, while the men stayed back and discussed a few more items.

As they passed Stella's desk, she looked up in anticipation. "Two women on a secret mission?" she asked with a smile.

"We are just heading back to the clinic," Lili said.

"Of course," Stella responded. "And Dr. Bennett got so interested in your work that he wants to see you again later this afternoon?"

"Exactly!" Annya smiled. It was hard to hide anything from Stella.

"I see." Stella smiled as well and waved them goodbye.

Lili and Annya left the building and walked down the promenade.

Annya looked at Lili from the side. "Did you know that we have a secret research lab here? Or who knows, perhaps we have several."

Lili shook her head. "I had no idea."

Annya stayed silent for a while, apparently processing the information that Dean Bennett had just revealed to them. "Who do you think these thieves were? They seemed to be familiar with the lab."

Lili nodded. "Yes, it looked like they knew their way around. They also knew where the cameras were. But they did not know about the adhesive on the floor."

Annya sighed. "I wondered if they were children, perhaps teenagers."

That made a lot of sense to Lili. "I agree, that would explain the combination of technical savviness, clumsiness and irrational decisions. Who in their right mind would go to the ER next to their robbery site?"

Annya responded, "Perhaps someone in severe pain who is freaked out by the fact that they can't move their fingers?"

Lili nodded. "That is certainly possible. Perhaps we will find out more at the ER."

They had arrived at the parking lot of the university campus. They got into their cars and drove down the hills to the university hospital.

- 2 -
Lili
SMITH FRACTURE

Monday, May 24, 2032, 10.00 am.

"Okay, let's identify patients who came here with a broken wrist. The goal is to find a patient with a Smith fracture." They had arrived at the ER, and Annya was ready to get to work.

Lili nodded. "I will review x-rays of both adults and children taken here today."

As they approached the front desk, they were greeted enthusiastically by Dr. Santiago Lopez, the clinical fellow. "Hello Annya!" he exclaimed. "I've been waiting for you. Can you please have a look at the patient in room three. I would appreciate your opinion."

Annya smiled at him. "Of course! I will be there in a minute."

She turned to Lili. "I will join you as soon as possible. We can check right wrist injuries from today and narrow the field from there."

Lili looked at her. "What if the suspect is still here?"

Annya responded, "Our team here is very efficient. According to the video, the person in the hoodie walked into the ER around five this morning. Now, it is ten am. It does not take that long to take an x-ray and apply a cast. The patient is almost certainly gone by now. But I will let Santiago know that I want to personally see everyone with a wrist fracture who is still here."

"Okay, sounds good!"

Lili walked into the Radiology reading room and started to review the x-rays from the night and early morning. Focusing on right wrist injuries only, she saw eleven radiographs of a right wrist. Four were normal and seven showed wrist fractures. She ordered the list of radiographs by age of the patient and started to look at them one by one, starting with the youngest patient and working towards older patients.

Lili heard someone entering the room behind her. She looked around and recognized Agent Terrel Wright coming towards her with the receptionist Aiko Tanaka at his heels. Aiko was a resolute, wiry elderly lady who took her duty to control the entrance to the ER very seriously. Nobody got past her without her approval.

"Lili," Aiko exclaimed with anger in her voice, pointing at Terrel. "This man claims to be a colleague. He said he needs to see you, but he did not show me his ID."

"That's okay," Lili responded. And lowering her voice, she added, "Mr. Wright is an FBI agent. He wants to review x-rays of a crime suspect with me. He completed HIPAA training, no worries."

Aiko's eyes widened. "An FBI agent!" she exclaimed, visibly impressed.

"My apologies, Mrs. Tanaka," Terrel responded, smiling at Aiko. "I should have told you earlier, but I did not want to stir up any excitement in the waiting room." He showed her his FBI ID. Aiko stared at it. Her jaw dropped. She looked from Terrel to Lili, trying to assess the severity of the situation.

Lili reassured her. "There is no immediate threat here, Aiko. We will just review some images."

The tension in Aiko's face eased and her cheeks flushed. "How exciting!" she exclaimed.

Terrel smiled at her. "Mrs. Tanaka, I would prefer if as few people as possible know about my investigation here. I am on an undercover mission."

"Of course, Agent Wright!" Aiko responded eagerly. "Your secret is safe with me. Let me know if I can be of any assistance!"

"Thank you for your service, Mrs. Tanaka," Terrel responded politely. "I am fine for now. But I will definitely consult your expertise if that will be needed during the course of my investigation."

"I will be available any time, Agent Wright." Aiko slightly bowed. Then she turned around and left in the direction of the reception room.

Terrel turned to Lili. "Thanks for helping me out. I hoped it would be a little less dramatic!"

Lili smiled. "My apologies if I have blown your cover. But nobody gets past Aiko here. Without a really good explanation, she would have just expelled you from the property." Lili pointed to a chair. "Please sit. I actually was surprised to see you as well. I thought you wanted to go with the others to Dr. Hill's lab?"

"We changed plans," Terrel responded. "I wanted to be on site in case the suspect is still here."

"I guess we had similar thoughts," Lili said. "But Annya thinks the suspect has likely left by now. Nevertheless, she will check everyone with a wrist fracture who is still here and let me know if she finds anyone suspicious. At the same time, I will check all recent radiographs for a Smith fracture. With that, we are approaching the problem from both ends and should have a result quickly."

"Good idea!" Terrel responded with a winning smile. "If it's okay with you, I will wait with you in the Radiology reading room, so that I get real time updates."

"Of course!" Lili countered. "Let me know if you have any questions."

Lili went back to work and opened the first radiograph. It was from a nine-year old child with a buckle fracture, which showed a characteristic bulging of the cortex (outer border) of one of the bones of the forearm, the distal radius.

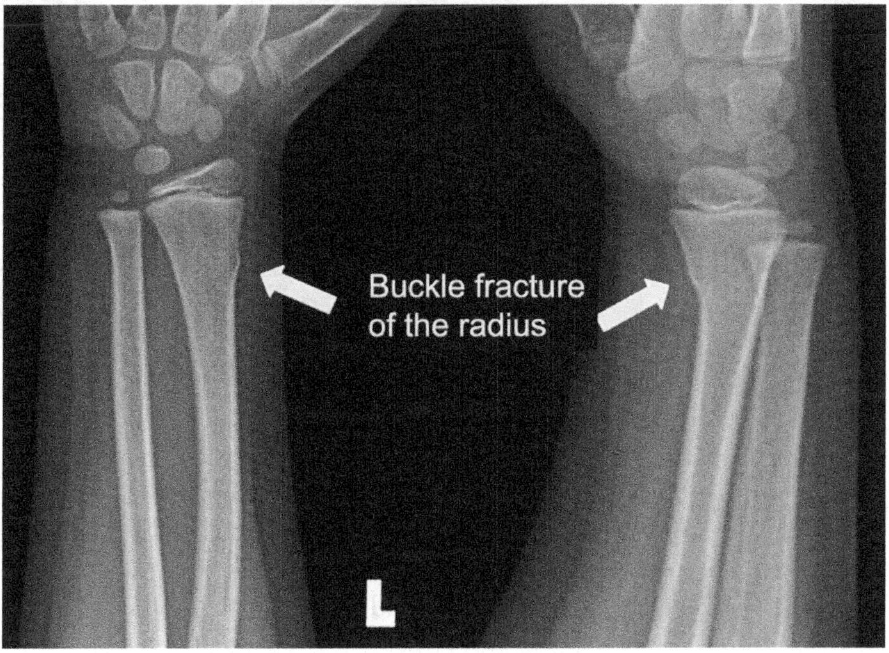

These fractures happen in young children, who have soft, flexible bones. When a child falls on the outstretched hand, the radius is compressed such that one side of the bone buckles upon itself without disrupting the other side. Lili reviewed the radiograph carefully, dictated a brief report and then dropped it from her list. Even though she had not seen the faces of the suspects on the videos, their height and actions suggested someone older.

Next, Lili saw two patients with Salter-Harris fractures. She noticed that Terrel was inspecting the radiographs over her shoulder and explained, "What you see here are fractures through the bones of the forearm, the radius and ulna. These fractures typically occur in teenagers, and we distinguish five types. A Salter Harris type one fracture extends through the growth plate. In this case here, the patient has a Salter Harris type two fracture of both the radius and the ulna."

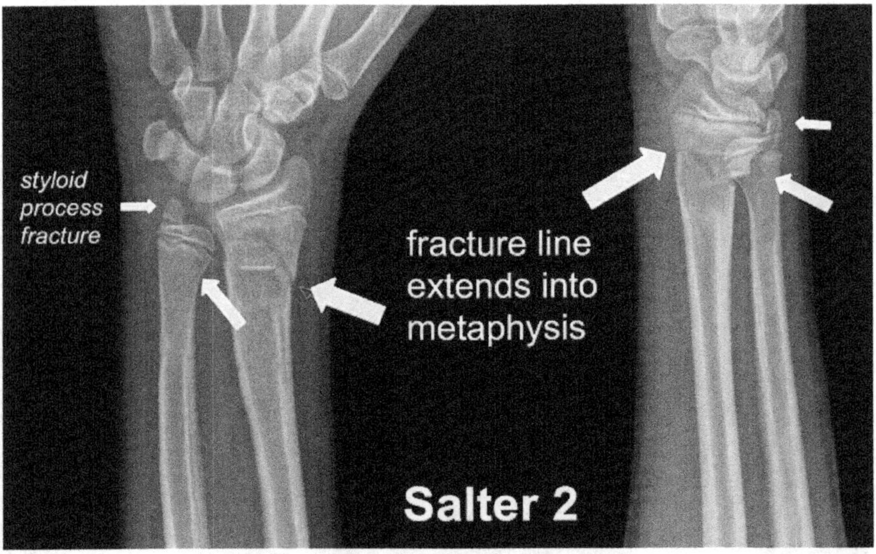

"A type two fracture extends through the growth plate into the metaphysis (or neck portion) of the bone. That means that the fracture line extends from the growth plate away from the joint." Lili showed Terrel the fracture line with her white arrow cursors. She placed a large arrow at the Salter 2 fracture of the radius and a smaller arrow at the

Salter 2 fracture of the ulna. "You can also see that the tip of the ulna, which we call the styloid process, is broken as well. This is a common association and we radiologists always look for this additional fracture in a patient with a wrist injury." Lili pointed at it with her small arrow.

"A Salter three fracture extends through the epiphysial plate into the epiphysis, the lower end of the bone. This fracture is more common in the bones of the ankle but is rarely seen in the wrist."

"Our next patient here has a Salter four fracture of the radius." Lili pointed to the next radiograph. "Here, the fracture extends through the growth plate into the metaphysis *and* the epiphysis." She pointed to the fracture line, which extended into the bone on both sides of the growth plate. "As you can see, this fracture extends into the wrist joint." Lili placed a large arrow at the area where the fracture line extended into the joint.

Terrel leaned forward to see it better. "That is very subtle."

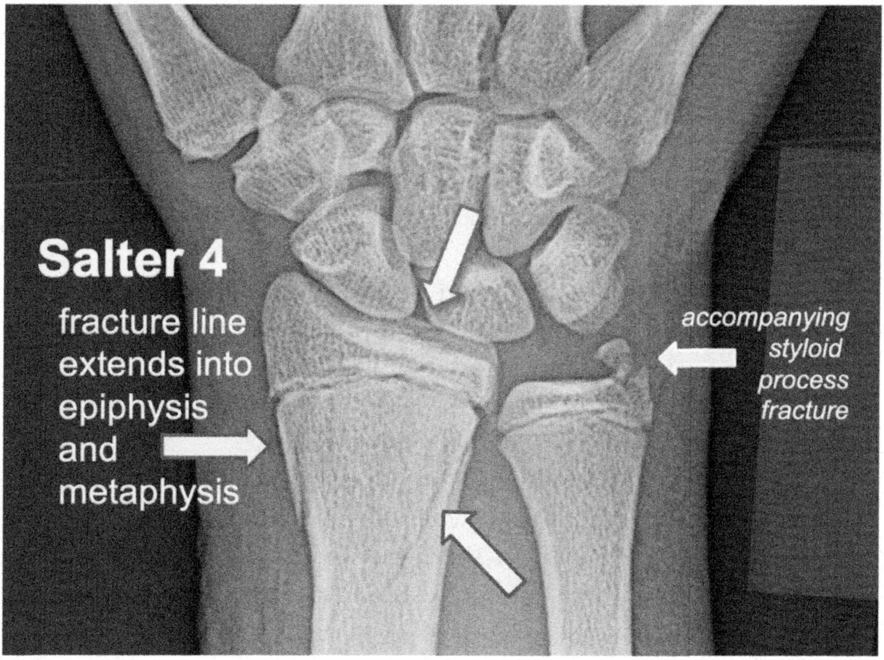

Lili chuckled. "Yes, indeed. That's why we radiologists train in our specialty for four years! Remember, I mentioned that these wrist fractures are often associated with a fracture of the tip of the ulna. So, it is always important to look for that as well. This patient here also had a styloid process fracture of the ulna."

"I remember these Salter Harris fractures from my training," said Terrel, "but I could never memorize the numbers."

Lili raised her eyebrows. "I did not know that FBI agents receive medical training?"

"Well, all special agents begin their career at the FBI Academy in Quantico, Virginia. During their time there, trainees learn about law, behavioral science, forensic science, various intelligence techniques, cybersecurity, weapons of mass destruction, counterterrorism and several other key areas for maintaining our national security. From there, students can specialize. I received specialized training in physical sciences, which includes examinations of whole bones or evidence that is believed to be human bones. One of our teachers gave us a lecture about pediatric fractures. I remember that they mentioned these Salter-Harris fractures, but I do not remember any of the details."

"That is very impressive that you remember the Salter Harris fractures. Many physicians who specialize in other areas and do not see trauma patients don't remember them."

"Well, we do see trauma, even though from a different perspective. And I try to keep up a broad knowledge. You never know when a detail that you learned can suddenly be the key to saving someone's life."

"You are absolutely right! In case of the Salter-Harris fractures, an unrecognized extension of the fracture line into the wrist joint can lead to long-term deformities and disabilities of the hand."

"The Salter-Harris numbers describe this extension within the bone, right? How do you remember the numbers?"

"Well, the injury gets worse with increasing number. A type one fracture extends through the growth plate. A type two fracture extends into the metaphysis (neck) of the bone. It does not extend into the joint space. A type three fracture extends into the epiphysis and the joint space. That is worse compared to an unaltered joint. A type four fracture involves metaphysis, epiphysis *and* joint space. If you like mathematics, you could say. Type two plus type three equals type four. A type five fracture is a crush injury of the growth plate and can impair the growth of the bone."

Terrel inspected the radiographs some more, taking in the information that Lili just provided. "Do you think any of these radiographs belong to our suspect?" he asked.

Lili shrugged. "I cannot completely exclude that. However, the injuries here are typical for teenagers around twelve to fifteen years of age. I would expect that our suspect is a little older. In addition, the typical injury leading to these fractures would involve a fall on an outstretched hand, which was not the case in our suspect."

They looked at the next four radiographs. Three of them demonstrated typical Colles fractures. These are fractures of the distal forearm where the end of the radius is bent backwards, away from the palm of the hand. Two were from young adults and one was from an elderly woman.

Finally, they found what they had been looking for. A Smith fracture.

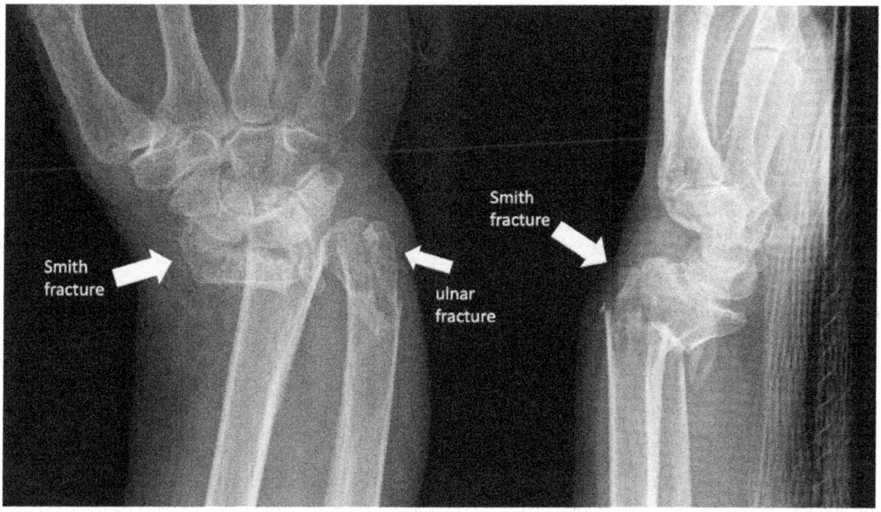

Lili looked at Terrel and pointed at the radiograph. "This would be most consistent with the injury that we saw on the video today. Remember, the thief who held the chip case and fell on their flexed hand. You might remember my drawing."

"Was that the woman with the ponytail?"

"No, the other, taller person. Based on their silhouette and movements, I would have guessed that it was a man. But we did not see their face, so I am not absolutely sure about that."

"So, this could be one of the thieves?"

"Perhaps. This patient has a Smith fracture, the same fracture that the thief in the video this morning likely suffered. But of course, we do not know for sure if this patient here is our suspect. The radiograph could be from someone else. Someone who fell elsewhere this morning and just happened to come to the ER at this unfortunate time."

"Did you see anyone else with a Smith fracture this morning?" Terrel asked.

"No, I did not," Lili responded.

"Then this is our person of interest until proven otherwise. I need to check him out." Terrel opened his notebook and made a note of the name. Dr. Juan Perez.

"A doctor, " he said. "Do you recognize the name?"

Lili shook her head.

"Can you check if he is still here?" he asked.

Lili checked the chart. "No, the fracture was reduced, the patient received a cast, and he was discharged about an hour ago."

"Okay, I will call Dr. Bennett to get Dr. Perez's address and track his cell phone location to pay him a visit," Terrel responded. "In the meantime, please check who else saw the patient. I will send you an artist who will render a phantom image of him. In the meantime, I will visit Dr. Perez and see what I can find out."

Lili nodded in agreement.

Terrel got up and left the reading room.

Annya and Santiago walked in.

"I checked out every patient who is here in the ER right now and did not notice anyone with a Smith fracture," Annya reported. "I had to fill in Santiago that we are looking for a criminal with a Smith fracture."

Lili nodded absentmindedly while still looking through the chart. "Something I do not understand. The note in the chart states that the patient has a height of one hundred and ninety centimeters. Our thief seemed to be shorter."

Lili showed her the radiograph of Dr. Juan Perez.

"This is the radiograph of our suspect today," she said. "We assume that this is the thief from the video that Dr. Bennett showed us earlier today. But the height noted in the chart does not seem to match with the height of the thief on the video. Could someone have taken a wrong measurement?"

Annya shook her head. "We are very thorough here." She looked over Lili's shoulder at the file. "It seems that this measurement was not obtained today," she noted.

"Well, that would be even more peculiar. If the patient was taller in the past, it seems impossible that he shrank since then?"

Santiago pointed at the radiograph. "I saw this patient this morning. He was tall, but not as tall as one-ninety centimeters, probably closer to one-seventy. I remember seeing the name and welcomed him in Spanish. He did not understand me. I did not think much of it at the time. Of course, patients with Hispanic names can have a variety of origins. But considering the mismatch in body measurements, I am getting the feeling that something is not right here. Also, I would think that this patient was too young to have a doctoral degree."

Annya had a thoughtful expression on her face, trying to bring together multiple pieces of information. Suddenly, her gaze brightened. "Perhaps our patient used a fake ID!"

Lili nodded. "That would explain everything!"

- 3 -
Juan
TALO-CALCANEAL COALITION

Monday, May 24, 2032, 10.00 am.

After celebrating the wedding of their neighbors the night before, Juan and Juliana Perez slept in. It had been a wonderful event and they had only returned home at 2 am. Juan had signed up for the afternoon shift in the lab today, which would allow them to enjoy a relaxing morning. Juan woke up first. The sun was sending golden rays through the bedroom window, illuminating Juliana's peaceful face. Juan rolled on his right side, lifted his right forearm to support his head and watched his wife sleeping. Juliana was curled up in a white satin bed sheet, her head facing him, her beautiful long black hair spread in disarray over the pillow, her brilliant dark eyes closed. Her chest was moving with deep and rhythmic breaths. Juan smiled as he remembered the evening before. Wedding celebrations always made him sentimental. The two of them had been married for five years now and he still loved Juliana deeply. Some people said that love would fade away over time, but that had not happened for him. He still loved Juliana as much or perhaps more than on the first day he met her. He gently stroked her hair with his fingertips and playfully moved her loose tresses out of her face. He kissed her gently. Her hair smelled of honey and roses.

Their idyllic moment was abruptly ended by Oscar, their wild and bright goldendoodle, who had managed to open the bedroom door. Oscar raced towards the bed with a delighted bark. As Oscar reached the bed, his four legs took off at the same time. He catapulted himself into the air and a second later, his big paws landed with a smash in the middle of the bed. Juliana's eyes opened abruptly, briefly scanning the situation. She sat up, laughed and embraced Oscar who nuzzled her face. Juan watched his wife, trying to cast an image of her in his mind.

I wished we could stay in this moment forever, he thought.

"Good morning," he whispered into her ear.

"Good morning, darling," Juliana responded, now focusing her attention on him and giving him a long, passionate kiss. "What a wonderful evening last night! I loved the venue!"

"I loved the dessert," Juan said, smiling.

Juliana's arched eyebrows formed a horizontal question mark. "We were full. We didn't have dessert; we hit the dance floor."

"Well, I had one later," he chuckled.

Juliana playfully stroked Juan's cheek, then pulled him closer for another longer kiss. Oscar started barking, trying to insert himself into the situation. Juliana and Juan laughed, got up and took a shower together. Then, Juan and Oscar went to the nearby bakery to buy fresh croissants while Juliana prepared a late breakfast to eat on the terrace.

They settled into comfy chairs. Juliana had prepared perfect Brazilian coffee. Juan loved its unique flavor and delicious, fruity note. He liked his coffee pure and black, while Juliana added a lot of sugar. They started eating their croissants, while Oscar received his favorite treats.

Juliana took a sip of her coffee, leaned back in her chair and looked at Juan. "This place is heaven! We are so lucky to live in this beautiful home!"

Juan nodded, while chewing his croissant. They had moved into this splendid house about two years ago. They had decided that they wanted to start a family and there was not enough space in their previous small apartment. Juliana had found the place, and they had decided to move in, even though it was beyond their budget. Juan had saved some money and used it to subsidize the rent. But his savings were now used up.

"Did your boss give you that raise he promised?" Juliana asked casually.

"Not yet," Juan responded with contempt in his voice. He hated to remember the recent encounter with his supervisor, Dr. Hill. Juan had worked around the clock to develop the brain chip technology. It was due to his hard work that the lab had created the prototype of the brain chip so quickly. The university would make millions of dollars once the chip technology could be marketed. But his supervisor had denied a raise. He had told him that all research staff were paid equally and that he could not pay one employee more than the others. After he had exhausted all options for negotiations, Juan had decided to take things into his own hands. He would provide himself with a much-needed bonus payment.

Juliana watched him through narrowed eyes. "What are you up to?" she asked, leaning back to let a ray of sunshine embrace her tanned face.

Juan was not sure if she meant in general or today. Either way, he was not supposed to talk about his work with anyone outside of the lab. But that rule did not apply to Juliana. She was the most trustworthy person he knew. She was the love of his live and his best friend. Juan was proud of his work with the brain chip technology, and he enjoyed discussing his daily experiences with her. He loved to impress her.

"We will have an important experiment in the lab today," he answered with pride in his voice. "I implanted brain chips into two mice yesterday and will record their behavior today. I will also conduct a functional MRI scan to see which brain areas are activated. The past versions of the chip activated the targeted brain areas, which was a great result. However, we noticed some 'leaking' effects of radiofrequency pulses on adjacent brain areas. This could cause unintended side effects. We are working on improvements to better focus the activity of the brain chip on the targeted area only."

Juliana wondered, "Don't you need more than just two mice in order to generate data that you can analyze with statistical tests?"

"Yes, you are absolutely right," Juan responded. "Ultimately, we will need to test the brain chip in many more mice. However, the chip is incredibly expensive. With an evolutionary approach, we make small adjustments to the chip and test the effects in small numbers of animals. Once we achieve the desired result, we confirm results in many more animals before we can ultimately test its effects in people."

"That is really fascinating! " Juliana said. "I cannot wait for your update tonight! Will you be home in time for dinner? The Smiths sent us an invitation for their grill party next door. I told them we would try to make it."

"Definitely," Juan said. "I have done today's experiments many times and do not expect any delays. I'll look forward to the party."

They finished their breakfast, brought the dishes to the kitchen and loaded the dishwasher. Juan retreated to his study upstairs to check his emails. He opened the SUEC email system and flipped through his inbox. A survey for research staff, a note for his annual laboratory safety training, an invitation for a lecture on implantable brain-chip interfaces and a note from SUEC hospital with a report about his visit to the orthopedic surgery clinic last week. Juan had felt on and off pain in his right foot and finally had taken advantage of the free consultation services for employees at SUEC. The orthopedic surgeon had ordered an x-ray of both of his feet and had diagnosed a tarsal coalition of his right foot, an abnormal union of two bones in the foot. This explained the pain when he walked too fast. The email contained the report and a link to the x-rays that had been taken.

The report stated that the lateral radiograph of the ankle demonstrated the "C sign," which indicated a bony continuity of the inferomedial border of the talus with the calcaneus, two bones of the foot that make up the lower part of the ankle joint. Dr. Lili Pham, a radiologist at SUEC, had marked the C-shaped connection between the two bones with two arrows.

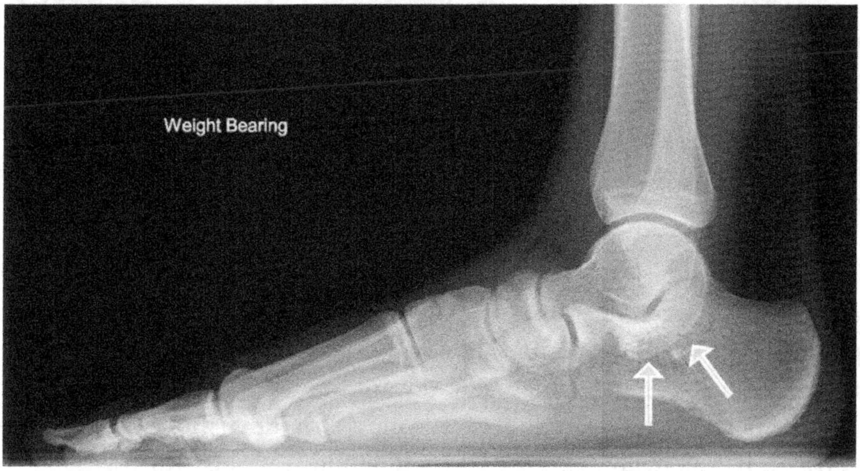

An additional radiograph was obtained in the Harris view to confirm the bony connection. The report explained that for a Harris view, the x-ray camera is placed behind the heel and tilted downwards by approximately forty-five degrees. Juan's Harris view radiograph confirmed the connection between the talus and calcaneus of the foot.

Dr. Pham had marked it with an arrow. An additional CT scan had been also obtained and demonstrated narrowing and sclerosis of the joint space between the talus and calcaneus, which was also marked by an arrow and further specified the diagnosis of a middle subtalar joint coalition. Juan studied the images with great interest. He appreciated the fact that patients at SUEC hospital received a detailed report with marked radiographs that helped them understand the problem at hand.

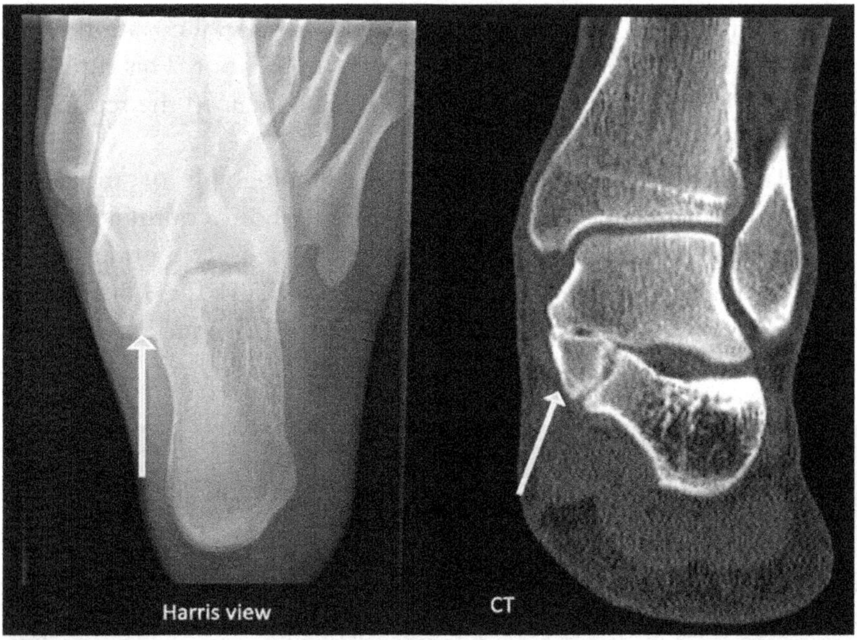

The orthopedic surgeon had suggested conservative treatment for now, advising Juan to walk slowly, which he did anyway because of the pain with faster movements. They had scheduled a follow up visit in a few months to discuss if Juan would want to pursue a surgery to release the connection between the two bones. For now, he did not want surgery. It was really not that bad. He could walk just fine, as long as he didn't run. The only downside that bothered him was that he could not go jogging with Juliana, but she would understand.

Juan continued to check his emails and found a note from Stella Pellegrini, Dean Bennett's executive assistant. He had reported that he lost his lab ID card yesterday and Mrs. Pellegrini had approved a replacement. Dr. Hill's lab required personnel to swipe their ID card at the door when they entered and exited the lab. Juan usually had his ID card clipped to the front pocket of his white coat. He had reported that he left the lab with the ID around 2 pm yesterday, when he went for a late lunch to the hospital cafeteria. When he came back to the lab, he noticed that the ID was missing. He went back to the cafeteria, carefully re-tracing the path he had taken during the noon break. He also asked cafeteria personnel if they had seen it. But he could not find it. Since he was close to the end of his shift anyway, he had decided to go home and reported the lost card via an email to Mrs. Pellegrini. She now responded that SUEC security had approved a replacement. She had remotely de-activated the lost ID card and issued a new ID card for him, which he could pick it up at her desk.

Juan sighed. He had lied. And he felt somewhat bad about it. He had given his ID to Kaleo, a SUEC engineering student. Kaleo had rotated to the lab a few months ago. Juan had served as Kaleo's supervisor and they had instantly connected. Juan even invited Kaleo to his home a few times. Then, a couple of weeks ago, Kaleo had approached him with the idea to steal a brain chip from the lab and sell it on the black market. He had carefully phrased the idea as a hypothetical plan, closely observing Juan's reaction. When it became apparent that Juan would not turn on him and report him to the authorities, Kaleo had become more concrete. Living in Silicon Valley was expensive. Juan's salary as a research associate was not sufficient to cover the costs of living here. He had tried everything else and now felt like he didn't have a choice. The money from the brain chip would solve Juan's financial problems for the next few years.

Kaleo had first asked Juan to just bring him a few of the brain chips. But the chips were in a locked cabinet, and the lab was under camera surveillance at all times. Juan did not want to risk losing his job. So, they agreed that he only had to explain the location of the brain chips to Kaleo and provide his ID card. Kaleo and his girlfriend Susan would take care of everything else. The three of them would split the money. Juan could report that the card went missing and had likely been stolen. Kaleo and Susan would retrieve the brain chips from the lab, and Kaleo assured Juan that nobody would suspect that either of them was involved. That way, Juan would get the needed cash infusion without risking his job – or so he thought. Juan checked his watch. By now, the theft of the brain chips must have been completed. Soon, he would receive a generous share, pay his debts and book a really nice vacation.

While Juan was checking his emails, Juliana went to the bedroom to change into her favorite sports clothes. She worked as an instructor in the nearby Pilates studio and had to get ready for her noon class. *Too bad*, she thought, *this wonderful morning is almost over.* She heard a dog barking on the veranda outside. Was that Oscar? Juliana peeked through the curtains of the bedroom window. The balcony blocked her view of the veranda underneath. Juliana saw a man in a leather jacket walking towards the veranda. Oscar ran towards him. The man reached into his pocket and extended his hand towards the dog. *Had the man just given Oscar something to eat? That was outrageous!* Juliana went down the stairs to the living room and opened the door to the veranda to check out what was going on.

- 4 -
Boris
EVALI

Monday, May 24, 2032, 11.55 am.

Boris Sokolov drove his dark red Tesla Model 3 to the parking lot of the shopping mall two blocks down from Juan Perez's townhome in San Carlos, a town midway between the SUEC campus and San Francisco. It was busy in front of the mall, which was useful for Boris' plan. It was unlikely that anyone would remember him. And just in case they did, he had mounted fake license plates onto his car. The boss had been very clear. *Get the chips and make sure that Juan Perez will not talk.* Boris had the gun ready in the inside pocket of his suit. He adjusted his sunglasses, straightened his suit, opened the door of the car and stepped into the glowing California sun.

The delightful condo complex two blocks down from the mall had a beautiful courtyard at its front, providing a tranquil outdoor area with lush ferns and evergreens. It was hot outside and Boris only noted a few people walking in or out of their homes or passing by on the sidewalk. Nobody seemed to notice him. Boris had carefully studied the location of Juan's townhome at the far-right end of the complex. The condo had a private balcony and private veranda on the opposite side of the courtyard. Boris walked around the house. A roof extended from the house over the veranda, creating a sense of enclosure. The boss had told him that Juan Perez was scheduled for an afternoon shift at work. Therefore, Boris assumed that Juan was likely at home. He quickly walked across the veranda and stepped into the shadow of the outdoor dining area. A beautiful goldendoodle came running towards him, barking and cheerfully wagging his tail. Fortunately, Boris was well prepared. He produced a small salami sausage from his pocket and offered it to the delighted doodle. *Why do people get dogs like this?* he thought. *This pooch is dumb and useless.*

The veranda door swung open and a sassy, long-legged Latina with a perfect hourglass figure came onto the veranda. The woman was probably in her late twenties, wearing a pink polo shirt, white shorts and sneakers, as if she were on her way to a tennis tournament. Her long, curly, black hair outlined a perfectly symmetrical, flawless face with brilliant dark eyes, prominent cheekbones, a small pointy nose and a full-lipped smile. Boris felt as if he had been struck over the head with a brick. He felt anger rising in his chest. He hated arrogant, entitled, flaunting bitches like this.

"Can I help you, sir?" the woman asked with a resolute tone. "Did you get lost? The main entrance is over there." She pointed to the main courtyard.

Boris looked at the woman and thought. *Women who know that they are beautiful think other people are not worth common decency. Women like this have betrayed me, insulted me and laughed at me. This woman will not just brush me off.* He took a deep breath to calm himself down. Then he walked towards her.

"Good morning. I came to see Juan." Boris smiled at her. "I am a colleague from the lab and wanted to inform him about a gas leak that happened in the lab yesterday. I wanted to make sure he is okay."

Boris continued to walk towards the woman who intuitively took a few steps back, into in the frame of the veranda door, blocking the entrance.

"Oh, Juan is fine," she responded lightly, examining him with an uneasy gaze.

"Well, the gas that evaporated does not necessarily cause breathing problems," Boris improvised. "It could affect his mood or behavior. Did you notice him acting in any unusual way today?"

The woman looked at him with skepticism. Clearly, she was not sure what to make of the situation. Boris looked very respectable in his black suit and his demeanor reflected his upper-class heritage. At the same time, his story sounded strange. Boris was prepared for that. He pulled out his iPhone and brought up several images of a CT scan. The scans were indeed his. They had been obtained after he had experienced some breathing problems after vaping.

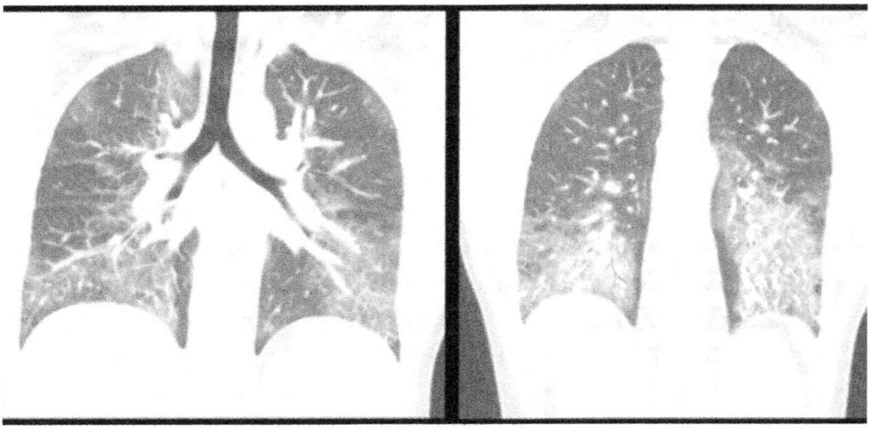

The CT scan showed ground glass and airspace opacities with mild interlobular septal thickening and typical sub-pleural sparing, called EVALI (electronic cigarette or vaping product use-associated lung injury). However, he would sell this as a lab injury to the woman.

"See this?" he asked, scrolling through the images. "This is my lung after the incident. There are major infiltrates in both lungs."

Juliana looked with interest at the CT images. She had worked as a researcher at SUEC hospital for some time and was somewhat familiar with the basics of reading lung scans. The lungs were supposed to be filled with air, which was dark on a radiograph or CT scan. But these lungs here contained white infiltrates. That was concerning.

Boris continued, "Fortunately, I was treated right away with an oxygen inhalation therapy. Easy intervention, just a few breaths via a mask and I was fine. I just want to check on Juan and make sure he is okay."

"Why didn't you just call?" she asked.

Good, Boris thought, *she starts to buy the story. Let's keep talking.*

"I tried to call Juan, but he did not pick up the phone."

"He only responds to callers he knows," Juliana responded with a wry smile.

"I called from a lab phone. Perhaps he didn't recognize the number," Boris responded. "Did you notice him acting in any way unusual today?" The key to his tactic was to find something that she could judge and validate. This would validate him in the process. If questioning someone's behavior, who would not find something abnormal?

She thought for a moment, then decided. "Well, perhaps you can talk with him yourself."

Bingo! She turned around. This was exactly what Boris had been waiting for. He summoned all his angry energy and slammed both arms into her back, pushing her into the room. She flew forwards and her head crashed with a terrible smash against the opposite wall. She fell to the ground, unconscious. Boris quickly turned around and closed the veranda door. He heard a man's voice with an anxious tone. "Honey, are you okay? What happened?"

Steps came slowly closer from the adjacent hallway. Boris had the Glock ready. *This is the slowest man I ever met*, he thought. Juan Perez appeared in the living room entrance. He saw his wife on the ground, her head creating an unusual angle with her body. Juan cried out in horror and jumped to his wife.

"Stop!" Boris said calmly.

Juan looked at Boris with tears in his eyes. It seemed that he only now saw the man in front of him. The gun pointed at Juan's head.

"What have you done?" Juan exclaimed.

"That's what I wanted to ask you," Boris said with a cold voice. "You took something that belongs to us."

The man stared at him.

"Where are the brain chips?" Boris asked.

"I, I don't know," Juan stuttered.

"Wrong answer!" Boris pointed the gun at Juliana.

"I have nothing to do with the theft of the chips!" Juan exclaimed. "I only gave them my ID. That's the truth! Please do not harm her!"

"Who got your ID?" Boris asked.

"Kaleo Kahale and Susan Pellegrini, two students at SUEC. They've got the brain chips. Juliana and I have nothing of value to you!"

Boris memorized the names. But he was disgusted. This guy had no scruples, serving him two students to save his own skin. As Juan looked at Boris, the bullet hit him precisely between the eyes. Juan dropped to the ground, eyes frozen, blood running down his forehead. Boris took the alcohol wipe out of his other pocket, put it on the man's neck and felt the pulse through it without leaving any fingerprints.

Nothing. He was almost done. Boris sent the second shot through the women's right temple. Then, he wiped the gun with a second alcohol wipe and placed the gun into the women's right hand. He collected the wipes in a small plastic bag, put them back into his pocket and turned around to leave through the veranda door.

As he turned towards the terrace, Boris noticed the dog staring at him through the glass window. The dog's head was tilted sideways, his eyes inspecting Boris and his owners on the floor, trying to comprehend the situation. Boris wondered for a moment if he should shoot the dog as well. But he decided against it. A jealous woman might shoot her husband. But who would shoot their dog? Boris turned around and walked towards the hallway. There had to be a front door in this house. He passed by the kitchen, found the entrance door at the other end of the house and left through the front yard. He stopped at a traffic light for pedestrians, crossed the street and walked with long strides towards the mall. He had almost reached the parking lot when he heard a barking sound behind him. He turned around and saw the dog racing towards him from the house. He was almost impressed. He had underestimated that little pooch. Boris started to run to the car, activating the electronic door opening system from a distance. He jumped into the car, smashed the door shut, started the engine, backed out of the lot and left with squeaking tires. A small group of people had stopped their business on the parking lot to watch the spectacle. In the rear mirror, Boris saw the barking dog running after his car. The dog got smaller and smaller as he drove down the street, away from Juan's house and towards the highway. Boris laughed. The dog had lost the chase! He had won! Boris had to stop at a red traffic light before the ramp to the highway. He used this occasion to send a text to the boss. *Mission accomplished!*

- 5 -
Terrel
TWO DEAD BODIES

Monday, May 24, 2032, 12.40 pm.

FBI agent Terrel Wright drove by the mall, noticing a group of people in the parking lot looking down the street in his direction. At first, he thought they were looking at him. This was not unusual when he drove the FBI marked Chevrolet Tahoe. But since he was on an undercover operation today, he was driving an unmarked white Ford. So, no reason for anyone to take any specific notice of him or his car. Then, Terrel noticed a dog running down the street. Apparently, someone had lost their pet. The poor thing seemed to be in major distress. He was barking uncontrollably and seemed exhausted. Terrel wondered what happened. *I hope the dog does not cause an accident*, he thought, as he continued his route and parked on the driveway of the condo complex. Terrel stepped out of the car and walked towards the townhome. The entrance door was wide open. He stopped and rang the bell. Nobody came to the door. Terrel looked around. Perhaps Juan had stepped out? But he could not see anyone. The courtyard was calm and quiet. A mother and a young child, perhaps three years old, were sitting on one of the benches in the far distance, eating ice cream. The pair reminded him of his wife Imani and his three-year-old son Niles, the joy of his life. The little boy waved and Terrel waved back. Then, he stepped into the house.

It was eerily quiet. Terrel shouted "hello" several times into the short, arched hallway. Nobody answered. Terrel looked around. To the right was a stairway that led to the second floor. To the left was the kitchen, a beautiful spherical room with large windows, which faced the courtyard. The room featured sleek white and silver décor and appliances and a breakfast bar. There was nobody in the kitchen. Terrel continued cautiously down the hallway. To the right, behind the staircase, was a closed door. He opened it carefully and found a small bathroom. He moved on to the entrance of the living room. The afternoon sun sent warm rays through the large veranda doors, illuminating the crisp white walls, the limestone fireplace, the grass green sofa, the vintage cocktail table and a Papilio chair. This almost perfect furniture arrangement was in stark contrast to the dead bodies on the wood plank floor. A man was lying on his back, eyes staring at the ceiling, with an obvious gunshot mark on his forehead. His head was surrounded by a lake of blood. Without touching the body, Terrel inspected the man's wrists. No signs of a fracture. Definitely no cast. So, this was not the man who had visited the ER earlier this morning. A dead woman was lying on her right side beside him, facing the man. Her neck was making an unusually steep angle forwards and her head was lying in another lake of blood. Terrel saw a gun in the dead women's right hand. He looked around. The room looked otherwise impeccable. There was no sign of a recent fight and no sign that anyone had searched for brain chips here. Terrel reached for his phone. He took multiple photos of the room and the dead bodies, then he called his colleague, Agent Angus Weber, and 911.

The local police and an ambulance arrived nearly at the same time. Four police officers, three men and a woman, secured the perimeter of the scene with tape. Two officers guarded the scene while the other two started to interview tenants in adjacent townhomes. The crime scene investigators arrived shortly afterwards and started to search for fingerprints, footprints, tire tracks, blood and any other body fluids, hairs or fibers that could provide information about the series of events that led to the death of this couple. Meanwhile, Terrel walked through the rooms of the upper floor to see if he could find any revealing information there. The staircase took a C-shaped upward turn and ended in another short, white-walled hallway, which was narrower than the one downstairs and illuminated by skylights. Four doors led to two bedrooms, a bathroom and a small study. Terrel entered the larger bedroom, which featured a king bed with mismatched bedside tables. A love seat and a potted banana tree were placed in front of French doors that led to a small balcony. He found a wedding photo of the couple on the shelf above the bed. It was painful to look at the photo. They looked so happy. Terrel looked around, but similar to the living room and kitchen, he found no signs of anyone searching the property. He put on a pair of latex gloves, which he always carried in his pocket. He searched the drawers of the walk-in closet and all the furniture in the room for the small metal box that they had seen in the video. Nothing.

Terrel left the main bedroom and entered the study. It contained an L-shaped wooden desk with a computer on it, a black upholstered office chair and a small bookcase. On the desk, to the right of the computer, he found a Valentine's card. The cover showed a big red heart with the question. "You know what I love about you?" Terrel opened the card and read. "Everything!
Dear Juliana, thank you for being in my life! Your Juan"

What a beautiful note. Apparently, the name of Juan's wife was Juliana.

Terrel noted two photos on the desk that showed the couple with a dog. He looked closer. Was that the dog that he had seen on the street earlier today? The dog looked similar, but it could be a coincidence. Terrel looked through the bookshelf and the drawers of the desk. Again, no signs of a prior search and no box with brain chips. He turned on the computer. As expected, it was protected by a password. Terrel tried a few random passwords, using different combinations of Juliana and Juan's initials, first and last names, but none of them worked. *We can deal with this later*, he thought.

Terrel went to the second bedroom, where his search was equally fruitless. He took photos of a few more photos on another bookshelf there. One of the photos showed people of different ages, perhaps family members. Three other photos showed people of similar age to Juliana and Juan, perhaps friends or colleagues. One of the photos showed a group that included Juan, Juliana and Dr. Robert Hill. That was interesting. Terrel made sure to get a good portrait style photo of everyone in this photo. To the right side of the group photo was another photo of the dog. By now, Terrel was quite sure that it was the same dog he had seen earlier on the street. Of course, that made perfect sense. The killer had left the door open and the dog had escaped. The window of the second bedroom faced the driveway of the townhome.

Through the window, Terrel could see his colleague's car approaching. The police guard waved Agent Weber on the property and Terral made his way down to the entrance.

By the time Angus Weber arrived, a small crowd had assembled outside of the house. Angus greeted Terrel briefly at the entrance and instructed him to interview the spectators, to see if he could get any additional information. Terrel wanted to provide Angus with an update about his most recent findings, but Angus shook his head, indicating that he was not ready for a debrief just yet. Instead, he went straight to the living room and greeted the leading crime scene investigator, Mr. Ling Wong. The two leaders retreated to the table on the terrace where Terrel saw them engaged in a lively discussion. Terrel walked back to the main entrance as Angus had asked him, introduced himself to the people in front of the house as a member of the local police and started to engage with them. Most wanted to share that they had seen something, but Terrel found that most of the information was likely not related. Several of them had seen apparently suspicious people in the area a few days earlier. Four of the people in the crowd were neighbors of the Perez couple. They confirmed the impression that Terrel got from his findings in the house, that Juan and Juliana Perez had a loving relationship. They were well-liked neighbors, actively socializing with others and ready to help out if needed. No issues, no drugs, no drama. Two of the spectators had been at the mall earlier. They described the same scene of a distressed dog, that Terrel had seen with his own eyes. In addition, the witnesses both thought that the dog was running after a red car. One of the observers thought it was a Porsche, the other thought it was a Tesla, neither had seen a license plate. Terrel made careful notes about the names of the witnesses and their statements. He saw an arriving van from the San Francisco *Chronicle* and decided to retreat into the house. He did not give his business card to the witnesses in order to maintain the impression that he was a member of the local police. The last thing he needed was a newspaper article or TV report about an FBI investigation of two homicides in the Bay Area.

As Terrel turned back to the house, Angus and Mr. Wong re-entered the living room from the veranda side. Apparently, they had just completed their private discussion and were now heading towards

Terrel and the front porch. The journalists were making their way through the crowd to the front row, as close as possible to the tape line. A cameraman was filming the scene as paramedics were carrying the blanket-covered bodies to the ambulance. The covered heads of the victims and the lack of urgency of the paramedics suggested that they were carrying dead bodies. Mr. Wong stepped forward and talked to the assembled crowd. "Good morning. My name is Ling Wong, and I am leading an investigation into the deaths of two people found in this house earlier today. Mr. Juan Perez and Mrs. Juliana Perez, residents of this home, were both found dead in their living room, with gunshot wounds to their heads. The weapon was found at the scene. This is an ongoing investigation and multiple pieces of evidence still need to be evaluated in the lab. So far, we have no evidence of third-party involvement. We did not find signs of forced entry into the house. Nobody reported a third party, man or woman, entering or exiting the house today. If anyone here saw any suspicious activity or has any other information that may relate to the deaths of these two people, please contact me or my team. We will be around for several more hours and can talk with you in person. We can also provide an email and phone number if you prefer to contact us anonymously. Thank you." He turned around and went back into the house.

Terrel finally got a chance to talk with Angus, debriefing him about his findings. The open door at his arrival, the Valentine card, the happy couple photos. In his opinion, facts thus far did not provide any evidence that the woman had a motivation to kill her husband.

"Well, the gun was found in her hand," Angus countered, "and we have no evidence for a third-party involvement. We do not blame a third party based on an unclear motivation of the people at hand. Who knows what is going on in people's heads?"

"The dog of the owners was seen running after a red car that left the parking lot of a mall a block away from here," Terrel added.

"What does that tell us?" Angus argued. "How do you know it was the owners' dog?"

"I don't know that for sure, but he looked identical to the dog on the photos upstairs, a goldendoodle…."

"Did you check how many goldendoodles are living in this neighborhood?" Angus responded. "That is a very popular breed around here. Do you know if the Perez dog had a collar or microchip?"

"Two witnesses reported that they thought it was the Perez's dog," Terrel said, "but nobody knows where the dog is now. I will check about the microchip."

"Well, people make a lot of assumptions. Would these witnesses be able to confirm in a court hearing that the dog on the street could not have been another dog from a different owner?"

"Probably not," Terrel said.

"That leads us back to square one," Angus responded. "Remember that we are under a lot of scrutiny when investigating a homicide and the stakes are particularly high in this case. We have to rely on hard evidence. As long as we do not have proof that this is a matter of national security, this will be a case for the local police."

"Of course, I understand," Terrel responded. "A hard fact is that someone with Juan Perez's ID checked into the ER this morning after breaking into a science lab and stealing technology of national interest. Now Juan Perez is dead."

"Agreed," Angus responded. "From there, let's not jump to early conclusions. If Juan Perez was one of the thieves, there are no signs of a search in this house. And there are no brain chips either. So, we have to consider that this event here might be unrelated. Perhaps Juan Perez's wife found out about an affair, she got upset, it came to an argument, and she shot him in the process. Who knows? We need more facts before we can reconstruct what really happened here."

"I found a computer in the upstairs study," Terrel responded. "I could not log in. Perhaps we should take it with us to see if it provides more information."

"I already discussed this with Mr. Wong," Angus said. "For now, this is his area of jurisdiction. We do not have any strong argument that the FBI has to be involved. Wong's team will have a look at the contents of the computer and provide us with a report. If there is any evidence that these deaths are linked to the theft at SUEC, then we will take over, of course with utmost discretion. You heard the dean this morning; the stakes are high."

Terrel shrugged. "Your call, boss."

Angus glanced at the clock on his cell phone. "We have to get back to Dr. Bennett's office for our afternoon debriefing with the clinicians. Let's see if we can get any new information them." He walked to his car, opened the door, got in, started the engine and left.

Terrel watched his colleague leave. He was not sure what to think. It seemed obvious to him that these deaths here must be connected to the theft of the brain chips. Or had the FBI an interest in *not* making this connection? Of course, an epic donation would not pair well with two homicides. Whatever the motivation was, if Angus called off the action here, Terrel had to comply.

Terrel walked towards his car. He looked towards the courtyard, where he had seen the woman with the young boy earlier. Was there a pair of eyes under the ferns, trying to make contact? Perhaps his imagination conjured things that were not there? His curiosity won. Terrel backed the car out of the parking lot and slowly drove towards the other end of the courtyard. The eyes seemed to retreat under the ferns. Terrel drove closer and stopped the car beside the ferns. He opened the driver's door of the car, which was facing the ferns. The head of a dog appeared between the green leaves. The goldendoodle. Terrel slowly got out of the car, offering his hand to the doodle, who sniffed it carefully. The dog trembled. Terrel's fingers crawled the chin of the dog, then made their way to the head. Did the dog grin? The two locked eyes. The dog slowly appeared from the greens, now exploring Terrel with increasing confidence. Suddenly, the dog jumped into the car and sat down on the passenger seat.

This is my only witness, Terrel thought. *Perhaps it would be good for us to stick together for a while.* He got back into the car, closed the door and drove towards his home in San Mateo. The dog made himself comfortable on the passenger's seat. Apparently, he was used to car drives such as this. He looked attentively at Terrel, trying to read his expression of kind concern and concentration.

According to the clock on the dashboard, they arrived in San Mateo at 4.05 pm. Terrel stopped in front of his house and got out of the car. The dog followed him. Imani had seen his car approaching through the kitchen window and opened the door, looking in surprise at him and the dog. His son Niles followed, squeaking in delight as he saw the dog.

"Hello, Terrel. What did you bring us here? Did we discuss this?" Imani asked, waving her index finger.

"This is a runaway dog who jumped into my car as I was exploring a crime scene," Terrel explained. "I would like to keep him for a while; he could be my only witness."

"Is he vaccinated? And do you have permission for hosting this dog?" Imani asked.

"I assume he's vaccinated," Terrel responded. "I do not have permission just yet. Both of his owners died today. I was hoping you could make a few phone calls to see if we could foster him until he finds a new home. I would also like to know if he has a microchip."

Imani looked at her husband. He seemed tired. Under normal circumstances, she would have debated this in much more detail. But it looked like her husband had a particularly bad day. She decided to let it go and give him a kiss. She was working part time at a pet clinic and had the needed expertise and connections. "Of course, don't worry about it. I'll take care of it. And he is really cute." They both laughed.

Meanwhile, Niles had embraced the dog and the two had retreated into the house.

"I still have to attend a meeting at SUEC," Terrel explained. "I hope to be back around six."

"Okay, see you soon," Imani responded and kissed him tenderly. Terrel got back into the car and drove towards the SUEC campus for the afternoon briefing in Dr. Bennett's office.

- 6 -
Lili
TEARDROP FRACTURE

Monday, May 24, 2032, 5.05 pm.

Lili was late for the meeting - again. She greeted Stella Pellegrini at the entrance. Stella smiled. "Hello Lili, great to see you again! You know the way, right? My knee still hurts."

"No worries, Stella! I know my way." Lili checked in at the entrance desk and rushed to Dr. Bennett's office.

The others had arrived already. Dr. Bennett welcomed everyone. "Thanks for coming again. I look forward to learning what each of you found out." He looked at Dr. Robert Hill. The scientist was sitting next to him. "Robert, would you like to start?"

"Sure," Robert responded. "Agent Weber and I revisited the lab today. In addition to the box with the microchips that was stolen, I noticed a missing chip gun, which is used to implant the chips under the skin."

Terrel asked, "Does that mean that the person who stole the chip might plan to implant it?"

The scientist nodded. "One would think so and that concerns me quite a bit. The chips have been only tested in animal models so far. We do not know about the functionality or side effects in humans."

Dean Bennett asked, "Did you find any blood or skin abrasions on the floor in the hallway that might allow us to identify the thieves?

Robert responded, "Unfortunately, a lot of people use this hallway. It is our only way in and out of the lab. We looked for bloodstains or any other source of DNA but did not see anything. Agent Weber took swabs from different areas in the lab and the hallway. If we find DNA from somebody who does not work in the lab that will be helpful. But the thieves were wearing disposable gloves. So, there is a low chance of our finding anything."

Annya asked, "Did you remove the adhesive formulation on the floor? It seems really dangerous."

Robert responded, "I am afraid it cannot be easily removed. In addition, it's only thanks to the accident of the thieves in the hallway that we have any leads at all. The adhesive seems to work as intended. I would love to inform our sponsors about that!"

Dr. Bennett looked at the scientist. "As I mentioned earlier today, I am afraid that will not be possible. Our investigations are strictly confidential. The goal is to return the brain chips before our big event on Thursday. Nobody should know that the chips were anywhere other than in the lab. This is crucial for the confidence of our donors in future collaborations with us. Do you understand?"

"Of course!" Robert Hill responded.

Dr. Bennett looked at Annya and Lili. "What did you find in the ER?"

Annya responded, "We found a patient with a Smith fracture who received a cast early this morning."

Dr. Bennett asked, "Could you identify the patient?"

"He checked in as Dr. Juan Perez," Annya said, "but we believe the patient used a stolen or borrowed ID. He was registered in our system, but his height did not match our records. He also seemed to be too young to have a PhD."

Robert Hill exclaimed, "Dr. Juan Perez is one of the researchers in my lab! Juan was scheduled for the afternoon shift in the lab today, but he did not show up."

Angus Weber said, "I am afraid, we have an unfortunate explanation for that, Dr. Hill. I am very sorry to tell you that Dr. Perez and his wife were found dead in their apartment today."

Robert's face turned pale. "Juan is dead?" he asked in a hoarse voice.

Angus responded, "Gunshot to the head. The wife had the gun in her hand and a gunshot entry wound at her right temple."

Robert could hardly speak. "So, someone set this up to make it look like they killed each other or a murder-suicide? Oh my god! This is horrible! Are we all in danger?"

Dr. Bennett asked, "I would caution everyone to not draw any early conclusions. It could have been an unrelated dispute that got out of hand. Jealousy perhaps. If the theft in the lab and Juan's death were related, why did this happen *after* the thieves got what they wanted? That does not make any sense."

Angus suggested, "Perhaps they were arguing over the brain chips and killed each other in the process?"

Annya weighed in. "Actually, I received a copy of the x-ray of the dead woman's cervical spine from the pathologist who did the autopsy. I think Lili should have a look."

Lili looked at her in surprise. Why would the pathologist consult *her* for the interpretation of the radiograph?

Dean Bennett turned to his computer and opened a file, which showed the x-ray.

Lili came closer to inspect the radiograph carefully. "This is a classical teardrop fracture," she concluded.

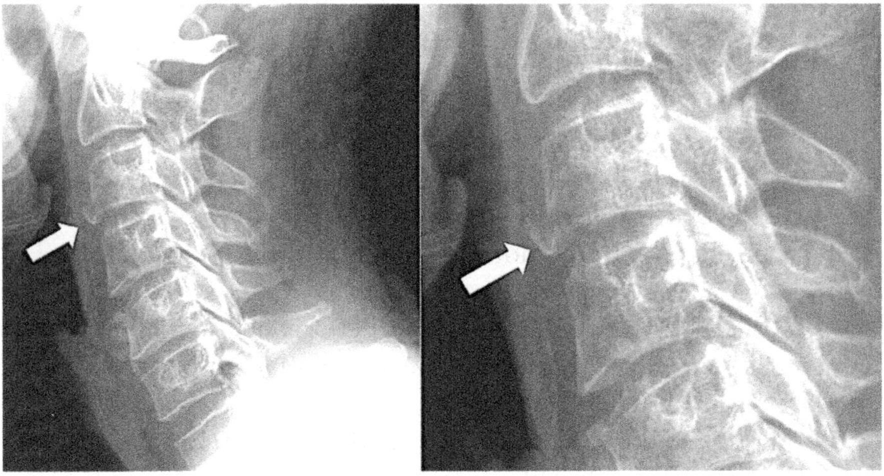

"What does that mean?" Angus asked.

"A teardrop fracture happens if the head hits a solid surface with brute force. An example would be the head hitting the windshield in a car accident or a biker hitting the street headfirst. This leads to a severe compression trauma of the cervical spine. What is most apparent on the radiograph at first sight is a small bone fragment in front of an injured vertebral body. You see it here." Lili pointed to the bone fragment. "We call it the *teardrop*. This bone fragment in itself is not the problem. But it is a sign of a severe injury of the vertebral body, which is often pushed backwards against the spinal cord. If she were still alive, we would do a CT or MRI immediately to evaluate the spinal cord. This injury can lead to a paralysis or worse."

"So, someone smashed her head against the wall or the floor?" Terrel asked.

"Something like that," Lili confirmed. "Or she ran at high speed into the living room, slipped and smashed against the wall. But either way, she likely lost consciousness. I doubt that she shot herself or her husband."

"The reports from the neighbors and the photos in the house suggest a very happy couple," Terrel said.

"I can only confirm that," Robert said. "If this was my team member Juan, then he would never hurt his wife.

"So, someone came to the house and killed the couple in cold blood," Terrel said. "If this was related to the theft of the brain chips, why did they do it *after* they got the chips?"

Annya had been lost in her thoughts. Now her eyes lit up. "What if Juan was not the thief, but he knew the thieves – or at least the one who borrowed his ID. Perhaps the killer wanted to prevent the identification of the thieves."

Terrel looked at her and nodded. "You thought earlier that the thieves were perhaps teenagers or very young people. What if the killer knows them, and he wanted to make sure we don't?"

Annya completed his thought. "That would mean that the thieves are in grave danger. This killer literally walks over dead bodies to achieve their goal. And that might be: Get the chips at any cost."

Angus asked, "So, who was the person in the ER?"

Annya said, "The FBI sent us a composite artist this afternoon. He talked with everyone who had seen the patient and created a facial sketch. Indeed, the witnesses estimated that the patient was around twenty to twenty-five years old."

Terrel nodded. "That's what our forensics team estimated as well, based on the video from the lab. We have to find this guy before the killer does. Did any of you receive the face sketch?"

Angus said, "I haven't got it yet. It usually takes a while to finalize these. We might have to wait until tomorrow."

Annya responded, "I took a photo of the sketch with my cell phone." She opened her phone and passed it around. It showed a handsome young man with dark eyes, prominent cheekbones and wavy black hair, perhaps Polynesian. "I can forward the photo to everyone," she said.

Terrel said, "That should do to get us started. Everyone, please ask casually around, if someone knows this person. But please keep the reason confidential. We do not want to cause mass hysteria." He looked at Robert Hill. "Apparently, Juan knew the thief. So, perhaps other people in the lab know him as well."

Robert nodded. "I will show the photo to everyone in the lab."

Terrel looked at Annya and me. "Apparently, the thieves were familiar with the lab, and they knew the ER was close by. Perhaps they live in the area. Thus, any random person on campus could know them. Can you please show the sketch around? Think of a good story, e.g., you are a hobby artist and are looking for your friend whom you sketched some time ago."

Angus added, "Once we receive the official version, we will also send it through our criminal database and forward it to all police stations in the area. Hopefully, we will find the guy soon."

Dr. Bennett got up from his seat. "That was a very productive meeting. Thank you all for coming! I hope we can return the brain chips to the lab before our symposium. Please remember that we cannot tolerate any negative publicity at this crucial time for our university. You signed a confidentiality agreement. No word to anyone about this! A thirty-billion-dollar donation is at stake!"

I could not help but think. *And the lives of two young people.*

Dr. Bennett concluded, "We will meet again tomorrow afternoon at the same time. Let's bring the chips home! Good luck, everyone!"

- 7 -
Susan
THE BRAIN CHIP

Monday, May 24, 2032, 6.00 pm.

Susan Pellegrini, Kaleo Kahale and Amir Nielsson were sitting on the sofa in Amir's apartment in San Francisco, engaged in a lively discussion about how to best proceed. Amir's apartment was located on the seventh floor of a modern building in the Mission Bay district of San Francisco, close to the waterfront. Susan took a sip from the sparkling cider that Amir had offered them and looked around. The living room featured a paneled white ceiling, abstract floral wallpaper on three sides of the room, a deep-blue leather sofa with a matching chair and a wooden coffee table. Quite chic! The stylish ensemble was facing a large window with a fantastic view on the San Francisco Bay. Kaleo was sitting beside Susan on the sofa. They both enjoyed the view of the dark blue water, speckled with sailboats, yachts and freighters. To their left, the Bay Bridge connected to the shores of the East Bay. Amir brought some snacks and then sat down on the chair. Susan took a few peanuts. Kaleo declined. He placed three pillows under his casted right arm and tried to put his free left arm around Susan. But she flinched when Kaleo touched her shoulder. It hurt! Susan moved to the other end of the couch. Amir looked at her and smiled. They had not seen each other for three years. Meanwhile, she had grown up. Susan was aware that she somehow had an electric effect on men. When she looked in a different direction, she noted from the corner of her eye that Amir was staring at her. He had not done that in the past. Susan casually stroked back her shiny brunette hair and looked into his eyes. Amir looked down. He grabbed some peanuts as well.

"Amir, I am so glad to see you again!" Susan showed her perfectly white teeth. She liked to try different facial expressions during a conversation to test their effects. "I have missed you so much! You are like my brother! How did we lose each other for three long years?"

Amir blushed. It was quite obvious that he did not exactly have brotherly feelings for Susan. Her mesmerizing amber eyes and sensual red lips made him speechless. When they had met at his door earlier today, he was hardly able to speak in full sentences.

"It is so great to see you again, Susan! " Amir responded with a soft voice. "I am sorry that I have been out of touch. I was completely absorbed by my training as a nurse practitioner, but I recently completed my exams."

"Sorry, I should have reached out earlier," Susan responded with a pout. "And congratulations on finishing your exams. That is awesome!"

"It was a hard time. We had to study medicine and take care of patients with chronic health problems after the COVID pandemic. I learned how to take care of patients with lung fibrosis, anosmia, phantosmia, post-traumatic stress disorder, chronic fatigue syndrome and many more."

"That must have been a hard time indeed. I had no idea that chronic health problems would persist until now. I am so sorry I have not been in touch. I promise I will do better from now on. I missed you so much!"

"Well, that is the definition of chronic: The problem does not go away. But it is great to see you again, Susan! And it is great to meet you as well, Kaleo!" Amir added with a polite smile.

"It is great to finally get to know you, Amir!" Kaleo responded, while inspecting Amir carefully. "Susan and I wanted to visit you earlier. But we were also busy at SUEC. You know, SUEC has its own community."

Amir looked from Kaleo to Susan. Susan laughed as if Kaleo had made a joke. She took another sip from her wine. Both young men followed her every move.

Susan pointed at Kaleo. "Kaleo is the captain of the SUEC soccer team!"

"That is impressive!" Amir responded with a sly smile.

Susan looked at Kaleo with pride. She felt special when she was around him. They were like James and Jamie Bond! But Kaleo could also be quite jealous. She had to make clear that Amir was no competition for him. She leaned over to him, kissed his sensual lips and dug the fingers of her uninjured hands into his long dark curly hair.

"Amir lost his parents to a car accident when he was two years old. He grew up with his grandparents in San Mateo, and we lived at the same street."

Kaleo smiled at her and nodded. "I remember, you mentioned that."

Susan sent Kaleo a seductive gaze through her half-lidded eyes. "Kaleo, I am so glad that Amir could help us out today. Amir is my best friend and I really hope that he will become your best friend as well! Amir is incredibly smart, and he could have easily passed the SUEC exam as well."

Kaleo looked at Amir. "Is that so? Did you apply?"

Susan intercepted. "He was too shy to try!"

Amir looked at the ground in embarrassment. "Well, I was just realistic. I believe the SUEC leadership is more interested in extroverted achievers than introverted idealists. And a big part of an academic job is to present at conferences. I have stage fright and would never enjoy that part. I do not enjoy being around large groups of people. I chose to train as a nurse because I love directly interacting with patients. I excel in one-on-one interactions, not on the big stage. I am very happy with my decision. I am doing more good as a nurse than as a student at an elite university. I save lives every day in the hospital."

"I am sure you do," Kaleo responded. His eyes went back and forth between Susan and Amir. Susan turned towards Amir and smiled at him. He smiled back. They clearly had a very strong bond.

Susan turned towards Kaleo and pointed at her right shoulder. "Amir diagnosed my clavicle fracture! And he treated it with a sling figure-eight dressing." She noted the caring look in Amir's eyes and moved a few more inches towards him. She had missed this feeling when they locked eyes and could see each other's thoughts without exchanging a word.

Kaleo casually placed his left hand on Susan's right thigh. "Thank you for helping her, Amir."

Amir looked apprehensively from Kaleo to Susan. "I am happy to finally meet your boyfriend!"

"Kaleo is not only a gifted athlete, but also a graduate student in the engineering department at SUEC," Susan explained with pride in her voice, "He grew up on a farm on the Big Island in Hawaii and moved to California two years ago to attend SUEC. He used to study for his entrance exam at the university café and I often waited there for my mother. That's where we met for the first time."

Kaleo smiled. Susan gave him another kiss, then turned back to Amir. "Kaleo passed the entrance test at SUEC last year. Can you imagine? They get more than ten thousand applications every year from around the world, and they take ten students for the electrical engineering class. I was so impressed!" Susan took Kaleo's hand. He tightened his grip as if giving a Morse signal.

"It was just good luck!" Kaleo said with a goofy smile. "At my parents' home, we did not have easy access to an electrician, and we were always short on supplies when something broke down. So, my entire childhood, I learned how to fix things and make them work even if a critical part was missing. The university leadership wrote in their acceptance letter that they appreciated my ability to design highly functional electronic devices with minimal components. This is an important part of evolutional computation. Removing parts rather than adding them. Making things simpler."

"That is truly impressive," Amir said. There was a short silence. Clearly, the two men did not have a common wavelength. Amir turned back to Susan. "You also wanted to take the SUEC entrance exam?"

Susan exhaled noisily through pursed lips. "Well, I took the SUEC entrance exam two months ago. I am the best in my class and had high expectations. But I received a rejection letter from SUEC with the notification that I had scored *too high* in some areas. Can you believe that? They decided that I was too ambitious, too competitive and too risk-taking."

"I am sorry to hear that," Amir said. "I know how much that meant to you."

Susan's lips tightened and her nostrils flared. "I received the comment that it was concerning to the admissions committee that I sought a leadership role in every situation. During the entrance exam, I allegedly tried to outwit and outperform my rivals. I did not seek the fun of a game; I competed to win!"

Kaleo laughed. "That sounds like my girl!"

Susan looked at him with her eyebrows crunched together. "I do not know why any of that should be held it against me. The letter stated also that I was not caring enough, disregarding the needs of others in favor of my own. That is untrue, insulting and discriminatory! They would never send any of that to a man!" She still felt the anger swell in her chest when she thought about the insulting rejection letter from SUEC.

"Don't take it personally. Thousands of students apply every year and do not get in. Perhaps you could apply again next year," Amir said in a calm voice.

Susan looked at Amir." Well, the comments sent to me were personal. They did not criticize my achievements, they criticized *me*! Why would it be wrong if I want to take charge and make things happen? There is no point in applying again. I won't be a different person next year."

Kaleo shrugged. "You are a smart girl. You could take the test again and give them what they want."

Susan looked at Kaleo. "Why would I have to change who I am? Are you not ambitious? Is it okay for you to aspire to be a leader? Without competitiveness, our civilization would still be in the stone age!"

"You do not need to be a graduate student," Kaleo suggested. "If it is so important to you to be at SUEC, you could work there in a different capacity. We regularly have openings for research managers and administrators. Your mother is the executive administrator of the dean. I'm sure that is a very important position as well."

Susan scoffed. "I do not want to be an administrator. I want to be the dean one day! Here is one key characteristic of highly competitive people. When a setback comes, we don't just sit back and take it. We react!"

"SUEC is not the only university here," Amir weighed in. "Why don't you apply to Stanford or UCSF. I am sure you would be a strong candidate there."

Susan looked from Kaleo to Amir. "I know you both mean well! Thank you for listening! But I don't want to discuss this any further!"

She was upset. But she loved them both. Kaleo was strong, outgoing and adventurous, always ready to explore new things and seizing the opportunities that presented themselves to him. Amir was in many ways the opposite. He was sensitive and composed, always concerned about the wellbeing of the people around him.

Susan clapped her hands together, flashing her charming smile.

"Let's move on and talk about the future. Let's see what we can do with these brain chips!" She spread out the brain chips on the coffee table and gave Amir a summary of the recent events.

His mouth gaped wide open. "You stole new technology from a secured lab at SUEC? Are you out of your mind? You'll have to give these brain chips back immediately!"

"Well, SUEC decided to reject me. I put all of my efforts into their exam. I did not apply anywhere else. Now, I need money to support myself over the next year. I do not want to be a burden for my mother. I can sell the chips, live on the income for a while, study for another entrance exam, apply to other universities and then go on with my life. SUEC has to pay for the chaos that they created in my life. They can easily create new brain chips. So, there's really only a minor inconvenience on their end."

"Susan, you've never done anything like this before. Don't ruin your life! The police are likely already looking for you!" Amir pleaded.

"We are not dumb. We made absolutely sure that nobody could see us," Susan countered. "We knew where the security cameras were, and we made sure that they did not capture our faces. We wore gloves and we discarded our clothes. There are major thefts at department stores every day and the police don't bother."

"Well, you don't want to compare yourself with a thief in a department store. And SUEC is certainly not a department store!" Amir exclaimed. "Breaking into a SUEC lab could be seen as grant theft. You could have the FBI on your heels!"

Kaleo shrugged. "Amir, Susan and I have been through this discussion in the past. I am afraid, if she has a plan in her head, nothing can stop her. And besides, we are already past that point. The theft already happened. Now, we have to move forward."

"So, assuming for a moment that you did not leave a trace and can get away without being arrested. Do you think someone would want these brain chips?"

"Of course! Human desire is bottomless," Kaleo responded. "People always want something new, and we will provide it to them."

"How would you sell the chips?" Amir asked. "You can be pretty sure that the police are already searching for them. If they cannot identify you right away, you will likely get caught when you try to sell them. And then you end up in jail!"

"We did think this through, Amir," Kaleo responded. "There are very sophisticated black markets in San Francisco. A middleman will conduct the entire business for us for a share of the profit."

"If these are criminals, how can you trust them?" Amir asked. "They could just take off with the chips. And how do you find them in the first place?"

"A friend of mine knows a black-market dealer," Kaleo said. "They are professionals. They will want to keep us happy in order to get more of the product."

"And there starts your career as criminals!"

Susan shook her head. "If we sell them, we will have only one encounter with the middleman, get our money and that's the end of the story. Once the chips are sold, nobody can connect them to us anymore. But let's consider all options before we make a final decision."

"Well, we could also create our own business." Kaleo said. "We could take the chips apart, understand how they are designed and then start our own manufacturing process. If we know how to build them, we can found a startup company and sell thousands of them."

Susan nodded. "Perhaps we could do both. We could sell the chips, use the money to emigrate to a place where nobody knows us and then start our own brain chip business under new names."

"The police will surely find you," Amir countered. "Do you want to hide for the rest of your life and never see your mother again?"

"I just want to make the most out of an amazing invention!" Susan said. "A little chip that can enhance your brain! We could demonstrate the greater good for our society. We could implant the chip into blind people and let them see again!"

"First, this is not your brain chip, Susan. Second, I am afraid, that won't work," Amir countered. "You can only see what you have seen. The brain of a blind person does not know how to see, their mind does not know how to see and hence, a chip cannot give them this ability."

"Man, you are so negative!" Kaleo exclaimed.

"I would call it realistic," Amir countered dryly, looking at him with a blank face.

"We could also just use the chips to enhance our own brains." Susan continued the discussion. "Imagine you could triple or quadruple your brain capacity. That could be worth much more than just selling them."

"We do not know if this would be safe," Amir countered. "I have read some of the literature that this group has published thus far. It was actually quite interesting. But to my knowledge, they only have experience in animals, not people. I am concerned about the safety of using it."

"You said that in Sweden, microchips were implanted in thousands of people," Susan said. "So, if the Swedes can do it, why can't we?"

"The Swedes are implanting microchips under the skin of the *hand*," Amir explained. "These chips are sending information to the outside world. For example, with a wave of your hand, you can communicate your ID or your bank account to a computer in order to get access to a building or buy something. These chips are sending information *out* of your body. This is entirely different from implanting a chip that will send signals *inside* your body and change the function of your *brain*. This chip could change who you are!"

"Students at SUEC get tech upgrades every day," Susan said. "It is really not fair that others are excluded from these new developments. I would appreciate an upgrade of my brain software as well."

"You are perfect as you are," Kaleo said, stroking her shiny brunette hair. "You do not need a brain upgrade." He moved closer to Susan on the sofa and kissed her tenderly.

Amir looked at the ground.

Susan turned to Amir. "Amir, I would just like to try it," she said softly. "Maybe, the chip won't work at all. We'd better know that before we ask criminals to pay for it. *That* could be dangerous. If the brain chip works as advertised, then I can demonstrate the capabilities to a buyer. That will bring the price up."

Amir looked very concerned. But Susan knew that she could get him on her side. Amir would do anything for her.

She looked into his eyes with her deep penetrating gaze. "Let me just try," she said tenderly. "You can examine my reaction. If I react weirdly in any way, you can take the chip out at any time.

Amir stayed silent for a while.

Susan added, "If you don't do it, I can find someone else. I just wanted to ask you first."

Amir shook his head and sighed. "Your call, Susan. But I want you to know that this makes me very uncomfortable. If I notice any major side effect, I will remove the chip immediately."

"Excellent!" Susan smiled her irresistible, broad smile. "I have everything here for a sterile implantation." She jumped up from the couch in excitement, walked over to her backpack and unpacked the chip gun.

Amir looked at it with raised eyebrows. "You really thought about everything!"

"Of course, I did!" Susan sat down on a chair at the dining table. She put her hands around her long hair, moved it up to the back of her head and secured it with a hair clip.

Amir got up from his seat and walked out of the room. Susan and Kaleo heard some rushing noise from the bathroom. A few minutes later, Amir came back. He wore medical gloves. He placed a green blanket on the table and spread a number of supplies on it. He put on a second pair of gloves. He then inspected the chip gun and the chip, sterilized both with alcohol wipes and loaded the chip into the chip gun.

He turned to Susan. "Please bend your head forwards so that your chin touches your chest." Susan eagerly complied. Kaleo came closer to watch the procedure.

Amir placed a scrub cap over Susan's head, mostly to keep her long hair out of her neck area, then he removed some hair at the lower end of her hairline with a disposable razor and sterilized the skin of the back of her head. He unpacked a small lidocaine syringe and anesthetized the area. Then, he unpacked a scalpel and created a tiny cut in the skin, to enable entry of the chip. Dark red blobs of blood emerged from the cut.

"I feel nauseated," Kaleo said, fetching the back of another dining chair to steady himself.

Amir looked at him briefly. "Kaleo, I cannot take care of two patients at the same time. Please sit down."

Kaleo walked back to the couch and sat down.

Amir removed a surgical sponge from a sterile package and stopped the bleeding by compression. Then, he placed the end of the chip gun on the incision site and shot the chip under the skin, above the right posterior lower skull. He placed a sterile bandage over the incision site and removed the scrub cap from Susan's head.

"Done," he said, "You can lift your head back up."

Susan looked up, stretching her head to the left and right.

Kaleo looked at her anxiously. "Do you feel anything?" he asked.

"Nothing so far," she responded. "No unusual sensations, on the skin or inside."

"The chip sends very low energy radiofrequency pulses to the brain," Amir explained. "I could imagine that it takes a while until you notice anything."

"I feel great!" Susan laughed. "And I am hungry! Let's order some pizza!"

The rest of the evening was uneventful. The three friends enjoyed a delicious Neapolitan-style pizza from Il Casaro, an authentic Italian North Beach pizzeria. Kaleo had opened an inexpensive but flavorful red wine. Amir constantly looked at Susan, anxiously checking for any unusual behavior. He asked her every few minutes whether she noticed any effects of the chip. She did not. They continued watching Peter Jackson's *The Lord of the Rings*. *The Two Towers*. Amir had a great home theater setup in his living room. He projected movies streamed from his computer with a small projector on a white vinyl roller shade, pulled down in front of the living room window. The three friends had seen the movie several times. But it felt comfortable and reassuring watching the familiar characters overcoming the temptation of the ring and fighting for good in the world. After the movie, they continued discussing the best use of the remaining four chips.

"We could sell the chips to people who suffered a stroke or accident," Susan suggested. "Perhaps we could help them to see or hear better – or even revive a paralyzed arm or leg.

"We still do not know how the chip works exactly," Kaleo countered, "Perhaps the chips are not working at all. They could have been damaged when I fell in the hallway."

Amir cautioned them to be patient. "I read the published reports from the animal experiments and am almost sure there will be an effect," he said. He looked at Susan. "I don't think it is safe for you to go to your room tonight. You might need help when you start noticing the effects of the chip's radiofrequency pulses on your brain."

She shrugged. "I still don't notice anything."

"Let's be careful," Amir said. "You can crash on the couch here if you like. In case you notice any major side effects, I can always remove the chip.

Kaleo looked at Amir with skepticism. "I think we should all stay here," he said. "That will make it easier for us to discuss the next steps tomorrow."

"No problem, I have an inflatable mattress and two blankets in my study next door," Amir responded.

Together, they prepared the couch for the night. It was long and wide enough to make for a comfortable bed for one person. Kaleo inflated the air mattress with a pump. He moved the coffee table to the side and placed the mattress in front of the sofa. Amir brought pillows and blankets from the adjacent bedroom and the three retreated for the night.

- 8 -
Lili
THE FIRST LEAD

Monday, May 24, 2032, 6.15 pm.

Terrel caught up with Lili as she left Dr. Bennett's office. "Hello Lili, can I ask you one more question?"

"Of course," she answered.

"Do you think the patient in the ER with the Smith fracture could have killed Juan Perez?" he asked. "What if he stole Juan's ID and now wanted to conceal his identity? That would be a strong motive?"

"I don't think so," Lili answered. "The killer must have hit the woman with both arms to create a teardrop fracture. She suffered a major blow to her head and spine. I don't think one can do that with a broken wrist. In addition, at the time when Juan Perez's wife suffered her spine injury, our patient had a cast on his right arm. I would imagine that one of the witnesses around the Perez residence would have noticed a person with a big cast?"

"You are right," Terrel responded. "Two witnesses described a man running to his car and racing away in a red sports car. That would likely not be possible with a full arm cast – or at least people would have noticed."

Lili nodded.

"Have a good evening, Lili!"

"You too!"

They had reached the front desk area. Terrel left through the door.

Stella signaled with a hand wave that she wanted to talk with Lili as well. Lili walked over to her desk.

"Hello, Lili. I just saw the news that two people were killed in

San Carlos," Stella said. "One of them was a SUEC researcher. Does this have something to do with your meetings here with the FBI guys?"

"I am afraid I cannot comment on that," Lili said.

"I take that as a *yes*," Stella responded with a serious look. She was always concerned about her own safety and the safety of everyone around her. "You know, I see many people walking in and out here every day. If you are looking for a suspect, perhaps I can help?"

That was a good point and worth a try. The lives of two young people were at stake and it was difficult to hide something from Stella anyways. So, Lili pulled out her cell phone and brought up the sketch from the composite artist.

"Have you seen this man before?" she asked.

Stella's face turned as white as Robert's face earlier.

"Is this the killer?" she whispered.

"I don't think so," Lili responded. "But this man might have important information for us that could help us find out what happened. It is extremely important that we find him as quickly as possible. Do you know him?"

"I think I've seen him before," Stella whispered with fear in her eyes.

"Do you remember where and when that was?" Lili asked.

Susan adjusted her glasses and looked at the sketch again. "I believe it was somewhere on campus, perhaps in the cafeteria. I do not know for sure. But I believe I did see him."

"Please think about it," Lili asked gently. "If you remember any more details, please give me a call." She wrote her cell phone number on a sticky note that she found on the desk and handed it to Stella."

"Of course, I will," Stella responded.

"Thanks for talking with me and offering your help, Stella," Lili said. "I do appreciate it. I really hope we can find this person soon!" Lili looked at the clock on her cell phone. "It is past six pm already. Time to go home!"

"Yes, you're right," Stella responded. "See you tomorrow!"

When Lili made her way to the tree-lined terrace beside the university building, she was surprised to see Terrel waiting outside.

"What was that about?" he asked. "I noticed you and Stella looked tense. Did you discuss something important for our case?"

"She remembers seeing the man in the sketch," Lili responded. Terrel's eyebrows rose in surprise.

"But she does not remember when and where she saw him. So, I am not sure how helpful that is. But anyways, I gave her my phone number in case she remembers any details."

"You would make an excellent detective." Terrel smiled.

"I guess I already am one," Lili responded, smiling back.

"We need people like you in the field," Terrel responded. "Perhaps we can formalize your affiliation with the FBI when this is over.

Lili sighed. "I really enjoy solving mysteries and helping the community," she responded, "but I already do that. I am already one hundred per cent occupied with my work as a radiologist and researcher. Today was a *very* busy day. I am not sure I could do this on a routine basis."

"We could talk with the dean to make sure you have some time reserved for working with the FBI," Terrel said.

"That might be interesting," Lili responded. "I will think about it."

"You are a very talented detective, Lili! Let me know, if you get any additional insights about the suspect," Terrel said and handed her his business card. "You can call me any time. Thanks for working with us on this case. Have a good night!"

"Of course, I will let you know if I find out anything else," she responded. "Good night! "

On her way to the parking lot, Lili called her husband, Mark, to let him know that she was on her way and that she had just received a job offer from the FBI.

"I think you would make an excellent detective," Mark said.

"You sound like the FBI agent!" Lili responded, laughing.

"You are the most inquisitive and honest person I know," Mark said. "You are trained in finding abnormalities. You are smart and diligent. In addition, you have a natural antenna for fraudulence and corruption. I think you would be very valuable for the FBI."

"How would I add anything to my already full plate?" Lili asked.

"Yes, time is definitely your problem. But perhaps you could figure it out," he said. "You work hard, and you are an excellent multitasker! My only concern is that I don't know how the FBI would handle your provocative questions. You make sense out of things by engaging people in intellectual debates. That works in the university environment, but the FBI might have a more hierarchical approach."

Lili chuckled. She loved Mark's pointed insights and reflections. They had met thirty years before at a social event for gifted students and engaged in a conversation that went on for hours, forgetting everyone and everything around them, only realizing that they had to leave when somebody came to remove the chairs on which they were sitting. They had married a few years later and their conversations had continued ever since. Mark *was* a true intellectual. Every day, Lili looked forwards to discussing the events of the day with him. He was the smartest man she knew. He supported her when she faced difficulties, he kept her grounded in times of success and he made her laugh about small-mindedness and political interference.

"Are you still there?" Mark asked.

"Sorry, I got lost in my thoughts. I'm at my car. I will be home in about an hour."

"I ordered Thai food for dinner," Mark said. "It should arrive at the same time as you."

"That sounds fantastic," she responded. "I had a really long day today."

"Me too. Drive safely," he responded. "And see you soon!"

Lili got into her X3 BMW and drove down the I-280 to San Francisco, where they lived. The I-280 is one of the most beautiful highways in the world. Lili loved this time of the day when the sun was starting to set over the hills of South San Francisco, adding radiant colors to the magnificent California scenery. From a distance, she could see the fog coming into the city from the ocean. She loved the feeling of diving into the cool, slightly salty evening air there. Mark called it their *champagne air*.

The long ride also provided an opportunity to reflect on the events of the day. They got the information that the stolen brain chips could enhance the function of the brain. But how did these chips work exactly? This was important to understand if the thieves planned to use them. Lili made a mental note to ask Dr. Hill about this at their next meeting. The two FBI agents were very different. Agent Angus Weber was a cool and reserved leader, collecting information, not really actively contributing anything. Agent Terrel Wright was very sociable, inquisitive, rationalizing, adding critical insights that drove the investigation forward. Lili wondered, how Angus had become the superior and Terrel the second person in line. Perhaps it was a matter of experience because Angus had surely been longer on the job than Terrel. Or perhaps there were other factors involved. Her thoughts continued to wander to the events of last evening. What if Stella knew more than she admitted? She seemed almost shocked when she saw the drawing of the thief. Was she hiding something? Lili's thoughts were interrupted as she reached her home in San Francisco, a two-story Victorian-style house in the Sunset district. She activated the automatic garage door opener and drove into the garage. Home at last!

- 9 -
Susan
TRIQUETRUM FRACTURE

Tuesday, May 25, 2032, 6.00 am.

Susan woke up and tried to orient herself. There was little light in the room, coming from an LED nightlight in a plug in the wall to her left. She was not at home or in her new apartment in San Francisco. She remembered the events of the past day. She was snuggled under a blanket on the couch in Amir's living room, lying on her left side to avoid any pressure on her right shoulder, which was hurting. Kaleo was lying on the air mattress beside the sofa. She could hear his rhythmic breathing sounds, calm and reassuring. The room looked different than yesterday, larger and deeper. She looked around. The rolling shades were still down. She noticed the outline of the wooden coffee table, which had been moved in front of the fireplace to her left to make space for Kaleo's air mattress. Between the sofa and the coffee table was a skinny potted palm tree. Susan had not noticed it yesterday. Even though slightly dehydrated and crinkled, the leaves of the palm tree looked beautiful. She felt a strange sensation of happiness just by looking at this plant. Was there a spider making its way over the palm leaves towards her? As she tried to look at it closer in the dim light, it almost seemed like the moving spider left a stream of static copies behind it, like a multiple-exposure stroboscopic photograph. That was weird. Was this the chip in action or just her sleepy mind playing with her in a room that was half-dark and unfamiliar? She got up, carefully tiptoeing around Kaleo's mattress towards the window. She removed the shades in front of the window and was struck by a magnificent view on the San Francisco Bay. In front of her was the most spectacular sunrise she had ever seen in her life! The outlines of the buildings and the water of the bay were bathed in brilliant rays of red light, which slowly turned to different shades of orange and yellow.

She saw the sun appearing as an orange half disk on the horizon, then rising to become a golden disk on the cloudless sky, sending millions of glittering sparkles over the water. As the sun rose over the bay, parked sailboats, freighters and tankers were illuminated by different shades of red, orange and yellow. Close to the Mission beach park, she saw two seals playing in the water. She felt a wave of pure and utter joy.

Susan heard a mild short cough behind her. She turned around and saw Kaleo's sweet hazel eyes blinking at her. She had woken him up by opening the shade in front of the window. The incoming early morning sun illuminated Kaleo's face. Susan was captured by the three-dimensional beauty of his soulful eyes, as if she were seeing them for the first time. Kaleo's irises sparkled in multiple fascinating colors, from gold to chocolate. His dark pupil enlarged as he looked at her. He reached for her with his uninjured left arm, pulled her close and kissed her.

Susan toppled forwards and had to steady herself on her free left arm to avoid falling on her injured shoulder or Kaleo's cast. They both laughed.

"Isn't this an amazing sunrise?" she asked.

"Well, it is pretty, indeed," Kaleo responded with a gentle smile. "But it is also six in the morning. Getting up too early just ruins the whole day. I would like to get a little more sleep. Would you like to join me here on the mattress?" He patted the space beside him and looked at her with a longing gaze.

"Maybe later!" Susan whispered. She got up and Kaleo turned around on his air mattress, carefully repositioning his casted arm. He pulled the blanket over his head. Susan watched him for a moment, a little undecided what to do. Then she heard rhythmic breathing from under the blanket. Kaleo had fallen asleep again.

Susan had slept in a T-shirt that she always carried in her backpack for occasions such as this. She grabbed her jeans and shirt from yesterday, which were neatly folded on a chair in Amir's study, went into the bathroom and dressed. She did not feel tired at all. The impression of the beautiful sunrise had energized her. She put the T-shirt in her backpack. She really needed some fresh clothes. Her rented room was only four blocks away. Perhaps she would stroll over there.

She grabbed her jacket and backpack and went towards the door. She passed by the kitchen and saw Amir preparing toast for breakfast on the granite kitchen counter. The smell of fresh coffee came from a roaring, old-style coffee machine. Amir looked up in surprise.

"Hello, Susan. You're an early bird," he said.

"Same to you," she responded, smiling. Amir's emerald-green eyes looked as interesting as Kaleo's had a few minutes ago. Amir's eyes seemed to have a new level of depth and fascinating vivid multifaceted pattern. They reminded her of fresh green leaves adorned with little specks of gold, like glistening sunlight in the dense forests of the Sierra mountains.

Amir blushed. "What's up? I have to get up early to be on time for my morning shift in the hospital, but you could sleep a little more."

"I was captivated by the stunning sunrise this morning," Susan responded. "You have an amazing view from your living room."

"Yes, I loved the view from the moment I first walked into the apartment, and I still enjoy it every time I come home," Amir said. "It almost broke my budget to buy the apartment, but I managed to afford it by cutting down on other expenses."

"You own this place?" Susan said, impressed.

"Yes and no," Amir responded. "The bank owns it and I managed to afford the monthly loan payments. If I continue doing that for the next thirty years, I will own it shortly before I retire."

"How old are you now?" Susan asked. Of course, she knew. She merely wanted to make conversation so she could just look a little longer into those fascinating eyes. She and Amir had been friends since they were children. So, really, no awkwardness here.

"You don't remember? I am six years older than you, so twenty-three now," Amir responded, looking at her attentively.

"Well, perhaps you can accelerate your business plan when we sell the chips." Susan thought out loud. "It would be my great pleasure to compensate you for helping us.

"That would be nice," Amir smiled. "But I prefer to stay on the legal path. I will be always there to help you, Susan. But I do not want to get involved in any illegal activities. I really wish you would give the brain chips back!" He looked at her again with this intense gaze.

"Thank you, Amir. I appreciate your help!" Susan brushed her hair behind her ear. "I guess it is a little late for that now. How would

I explain that one is missing?"

Amir nodded. "Yes, I know. I just hope you'll get out of this without ending up in jail or a hospital, or both."

"You know I can take care of myself. I'll be fine." Susan smiled at him.

Amir sighed. "Would you like a coffee?"

"No thanks," she responded. "I want to swing by my apartment and grab some new clothes. There's a Starbucks on the way."

"It is possible that the police are looking for you and Kaleo," Amir said. "I believe it would be safer for you both to stay here for a while, not to mention the uncertain effects of the brain chip. Why don't you enjoy a lazy morning? I should be back in the early afternoon, and we can plan the next steps then. It seems like you are feeling okay right now. Or do you notice any side effects from the chip?"

"I couldn't feel better," Susan responded, smiling. "We did not look into the surveillance cameras when we were in the SUEC lab. Therefore, it should take the police some time to identify any suspects – and hopefully, they will not get to us at all. So, I would think that we should be okay, at least for now. I will make sure to take as little time as possible over there."

"Alright. You are a grown-up now. Take good care of yourself," Amir responded.

Susan waived goodbye, opened the apartment door, went down the stairs and left the building. As she stepped on the sidewalk, she felt an overwhelming flash sensation. The morning light was so bright. Susan put her hand over her eyebrows to create some shade. The street was huge! She realized that the field of view that her eyes were capturing had doubled – or perhaps tripled. The colors of the cars, street signs, trees and houses had intensified as if someone had dialed up the color saturation button on a computer program. But what was most peculiar, and fascinating, were the moving objects. Similar to the spider that she had observed earlier in the living room, moving cars and people seemed to produce a series of discrete, stationary images along their paths. Multiple copies of an old woman were passing her on the sidewalk from the right to the left, as if the woman were leaving a visual trail. Multiple imprints of a dark green BMW came into her view from the left, like a beautiful shiny caterpillar, stopping at a traffic light. The static images faded away after a few seconds and were replaced by new trails of stroboscopic images from new moving objects entering Susan's field of view. Susan watched the graceful wingbeats of a white dove above her and the trail of identical copies following it. Based on the arc of the dove's trail, Susan could project the bird's flight path and foresee the tree branch on which it was going to land. And there it landed. *Amazing!* she thought. *I can see time!* Susan took her new vision in with awe. She felt a genuine, deep connection to the stunning world around her. Ignoring the pain in her right shoulder, Susan extended both arms to embrace it all. *What a wonderful world!*

But the fairytale sensations did not last long. Susan was literally thrown out of her daydream. A powerful physical force hit the back of her right arm and hand. She was thrown around, heard a loud crash and hit the ground. Susan felt a sudden sharp pain in her right arm and heard someone's voice yelling at her. The dove looked scared and flew away. Susan tried to focus on the situation in front of her. A young man on a small black motorcycle had veered into her space. Or perhaps she had veered into his space. Who knew? She was on the ground. The man was standing above her, looking down at her with a very angry face, yelling profanities. Susan realized that they had collided. She mumbled an excuse.

Amir had just stepped out of the door on his way to his morning shift at the San Francisco General hospital. He looked at the approaching motorcycle as Susan smiled at the sky, extended her arms and stepped into the bike lane. Amir rushed towards her but arrived two seconds too late. A motorcycle driver had already crashed into her and hit the ground. The motorcycle driver jumped up and was yelling at her with a raised, clenched fist. Amir stepped in quickly to de-escalate the situation. He introduced himself as a nurse practitioner and asked the motorcyclist if he was injured. He was not. But he was not sure about his motorcycle. Amir's composed and matter-of-fact demeanor calmed him down. He got up and exchanged business cards with Amir. Fortunately, he did not want to call the police. After talking with Amir for a few minutes, he politely asked Susan if she was okay. She confirmed she was and apologized. He picked up his motorcycle, started it successfully and left. Susan was still holding her arm, looking at Amir with squeezed-shut eyes and clenched teeth.

"I'm sorry for the trouble," she said. "I didn't see him coming."

"Clearly you did not," Amir responded. "Does your arm hurt?"

"I'm not sure if it's my shoulder or my hand," she said. "Perhaps both."

"I think you should see a doctor," Amir decided. "You can come with me to the hospital."

"It's too risky," she whispered.

"I will make sure you're in and out in no time," he responded.

Susan sighed and gave in. Amir helped her up. He usually walked the few blocks to the hospital, but due to Susan's condition, he called a cab. The car came immediately. Susan missed the car door handle by reaching to the left of it. She adjusted her grip and looked relieved to find the handle. They both got in. Amir gave the driver directions to the hospital, and they took off.

"Do you have problems with your vision?" Amir whispered to Susan on the back seat.

"I wouldn't call it problems," she responded. "It feels more like an upgrade. I can see more than I used to see. I guess I have to learn how to process the incoming new information."

"Well, the *new information* got you injured," Amir said with anger in his voice. "I would like to take the chip out right now!"

"Psst," she whispered. "You can't right now, and my arm is more important at the moment. I can see just fine. I just have to get used to my new vision. I will be more careful, I promise!"

The car arrived at the entrance to the hospital. They got out.

"Do you think you can walk in on your own from here without causing another collision?" Amir asked.

Susan nodded. "Of course! I walked around in your apartment and down the hallway without any issues, remember? The motorcycle accident was just an unfortunate coincidence."

Amir hugged her gently without touching her right arm. "Be careful. We should probably avoid being seen together. That will keep you safe at my home. I'll ask a friend in the ER to make sure you are seen as promptly as possible."

"Thank you!" she smiled. "I feel better already."

Amir looked at her, thoughtfully. "They have a metal detector at the entrance to the ER," he said. " If it beeps, you need to explain why.

You could tell them that you had an injury as a child and that you have a small metal plate at the back of your skull."

"Okay, will do!" Susan said. She waved goodbye to the three versions of Amir in front of her, turned around and walk towards the ER entrance.

The security person at the entrance welcomed her. She looked back at Amir. He sent her a shy wave and walked in the opposite direction, towards the personnel entrance at the east side of the building. Fortunately, the cab ride had helped him to catch up some of the time he had spent attending to the accident. He would not be late for the morning report.

Susan was directed to a patient care room where an ER resident examined her right hand and shoulder. Both hurt quite a bit. The resident looked in her eyes for such a long time that she almost wanted to tell him that this was becoming inappropriate. He made some notes into a computer file and sent her to the x-ray room, where a technician obtained x-rays of her right shoulder, right arm and right hand. A nurse practitioner led her back to the examination room. Nothing happened for a while. Susan sat down on a chair, waiting for the physician to come back. She closed her eyes for a moment. Perhaps she should have stayed with Kaleo in the flat. Or if they had gone to her apartment together, perhaps this would not have happened. Her thoughts were interrupted by a pinging sound from her phone. Susan took her phone out of her backpack and noted a series of missed calls and texts from her mother. She sighed. Her mother had found out that she had called in sick at work.

Susan texted back. *Hi Mom. I am fine. I have a flu and need some sleep. Will call you tomorrow!* She added a red heart.

A physician in a white lab coat came in.

"Hello, I am Dr. Williams," he said. "How are you doing?"

"Hello," Susan responded. "I collided with a motorcycle this morning and now my arm hurts."

"Yes, I can imagine that," Dr. Williams said. He went to a computer on the right side of the examination room and opened a computer file, which displayed an x-ray.

"This is your right shoulder," he explained, "and here is a fracture of your mid clavicle, the collar bone. This is the most common location for a clavicle fracture after the accident that you described. As you can see, there is also a small fracture fragment along the fracture line. Fortunately, the connection between the clavicle and the scapula (shoulder blade) is intact. We call it the acromioclavicolar (AC) joint. The AC distance is normal. It is usually less than thirteen millimeters, with less than five millimeters asymmetry compared to the contralateral side."

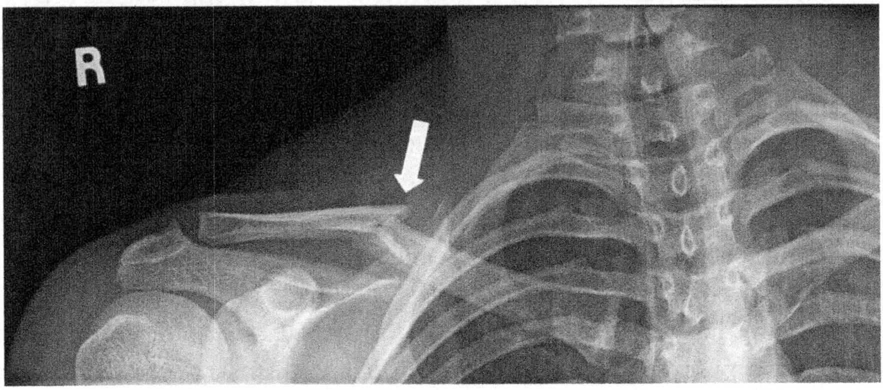

"So, you are saying that I broke my collar bone, but the rest of my shoulder is fine?" Susan tried to understand.

"Yes, correct," he responded, "but I have a question for you."

"Sure, what is that?"

"How come you already had a figure-eight dressing on when you came into the hospital? Did someone already take care of you?"

"My father is a paramedic," Susan lied. "He saw me in front of my home and wanted to make sure the shoulder is stabilized."

"Why did he not come with you to the ER?" Dr. Williams asked.

"He had an urgent case to attend to," Susan lied again. "He checked my vital signs to make sure I am okay, brought me to the ER entrance and then asked me to walk in by myself." That was close to the truth, although she was talking about Amir, not her father. Susan sincerely wished that her father was here with her today. But the bitter truth was that he had died of cancer five years ago.

Dr. Williams looked at her with skepticism. But he did not press the matter further. He pulled up the radiograph of her right hand.

"This is your right hand." He pointed to the lateral radiograph of the hand. "Can you see the small bone flakes here at the dorsum of the hand?"

Susan shook her head.

"You have a dorsal avulsion fracture of the triquetrum, a small bone at the base of your hand," he explained.

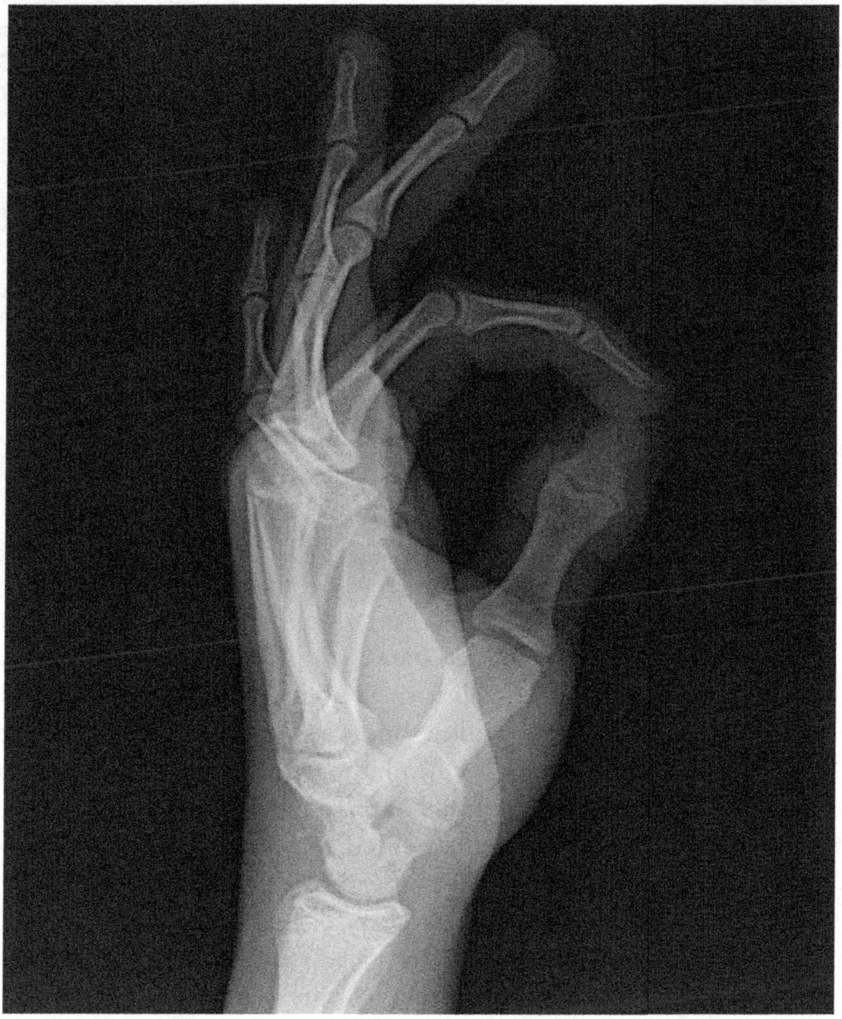

He magnified the image and pointed to the bone fragments.

Susan looked at the radiograph, fascinated. Now she saw it! The more she looked at it, the more three-dimensional it appeared. It almost seemed as if the radiograph were alive and breathing!

Susan laughed. "It looks like a pooping duck!"

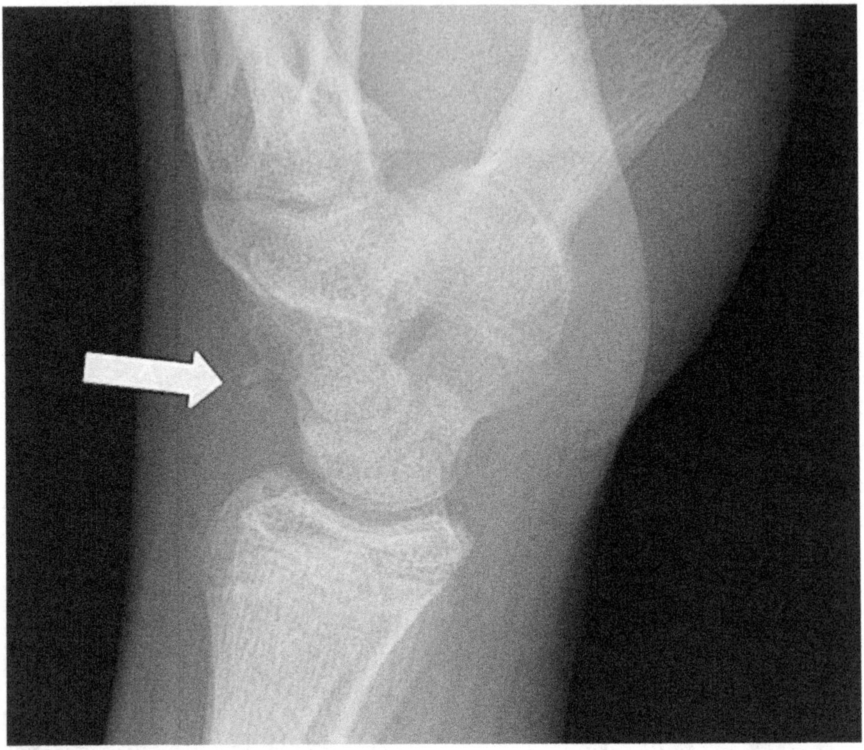

"Well, this is your injured hand, young lady," Dr. Williams said. "But some people indeed call it the pooping duck sign. The duck is created by the overlying shadow of three bones of the carpal bones. The scaphoid bone creates the head; the lunate bone creates the body, and the triquetrum creates the tail of the duck. If the triquetrum breaks, then there are bone fragments behind the duck, which some people call the pooping duck sign. So, this means that you have a triquetrum fracture, which will require a cast to heal. I will prescribe a lower arm cast and a new dressing for your clavicle fracture."

"I am glad I came to see you," Susan said.

Dr. Williams did not answer for a while. He looked at her with a serious expression. Then, he said. "There is one more thing I need to ask you."

"Yes?"

"What drugs did you take?"

"I did not take any drugs," Susan said, shaking her head.

"Well, you have the largest pupils I have ever seen. If you did not take any drugs, then I will order a CT scan of your brain to check for any intracranial abnormality. Perhaps you suffered a brain trauma with your accident today."

Susan swallowed. She had to avoid a CT scan at all costs. That would reveal the brain chip. She looked at the ER physician. "Well, we had a party last night and it is possible that somebody slipped something into my drink. I did feel weird yesterday, but I'm feeling much better now."

Dr. Williams looked at her. "The effect of the drug might have caused your accident," he said. "I don't think it's safe for you to walk home alone, even if it's not far away. Can somebody pick you up?"

"Yes, of course," Susan responded politely. "I will call my brother."

"Okay, that sounds like a plan," Dr. Williams responded. "Call your brother. Meanwhile, Jim Ho, our orthopedic nurse practitioner here will prepare the cast for you and fit it on after your call. Jim will walk you to the ER reception afterwards and confirm that a family member will accompany you home."

"That sounds good!" Susan said with her most charming smile.

As soon as Dr. Williams had left the exam room, she texted Kaleo.

Am at the ER, need to be picked up by my brother.

It was not easy to hold the phone and write with her hurting hand. But fortunately, her thumbs were okay.

He responded right away. *You do not have a brother.*

She replied. *My brother is Kaleo.*

WTF, who will buy that? Perhaps half-brother?

Works for me! Susan typed.

Okay, am on my way! I will wait outside. Text me when you are ready.

Will do! Thank you!

A few minutes later, Jim Ho picked her up in the examination room and led her to another room, where the cast material had been prepared. Susan was delighted that she could pick a color for her cast. She chose red, which looked very pretty. Jim carefully padded the right hand and lower arm and then applied the red cast. An x-ray technician took another x-ray, to make sure the arm was positioned well in the cast. Jim then exchanged the figure-8 dressing, which had been overstretched and displaced during the fall, with a right arm sling. He explained that this would keep the clavicle (collar bone) and hand calm, while allowing some movement of the shoulder joint. Jim then led her to the ER reception. Susan texted Kaleo, who entered the ER. Jim immediately noted Kaleo's cast.

"Was he involved in your accident as well?" he asked Susan.

"No, he had a separate accident recently," Susan responded.

"What a co-incidence," Jim laughed. "A couple with two arms in a cast! Make sure you have shoes without laces available!"

"Together, we have two healthy arms," Kaleo responded with a grin. "No worries, we will be fine!"

Nobody asked any questions regarding their obvious dissimilarity as claimed brother and sister. They were both exceptionally good-looking. That was enough to link them as family. Everyone at the reception was captured by the double cast duo. The receptionist asked if she could take a photo, but Susan politely declined. Kaleo claimed that he forgot his ID and signed the exit form as Kai Pellegrini. Susan beamed at him. She felt an overwhelming sense of love and gratitude as they walked out of the ER.

- 10 -
Lili
PELLEGRINI STIEDA LESION

Tuesday, May 25, 2032, 6.00 am.

Mark and Lili were blessed with a deep, long and undisturbed sleep. Since they were both physicians, one of them was on call almost every other night. Therefore, an entirely calm and undisturbed night was a rare luxury for them. On Tuesday morning, they were woken up by the ring tone of Lili's iPhone. It was Annya. "Guess who is here in the ER?" she asked.

"The other thief?" Lili asked.

"Close enough," Annya responded. "Dr. Bennett's administrative assistant!"

"Stella?" Lili asked in surprise.

"That's the one."

"Is she there as a patient?"

"You know I can't comment on that," Annya said. "But I have a feeling that her visit might be related to the FBI investigation. Therefore, as the FBI folks explained, national security overwrites patient privacy. I noticed your conversation with her last night, when I walked out, and I thought I'd let you know. I don't think a medical emergency brought her here to the ER. She is sitting in the waiting room, chatting with our ER personnel. You know her better than I. Perhaps you can talk with her, to find out what is really going on."

"As you know, I am coming from San Francisco," Lili responded. "I will be there around 7.30 am."

"That will be perfect timing."

Lili arrived at SUEC hospital as planned, checked in at the entrance with her hospital ID and walked directly to the patient waiting area. It was packed with people. There was an elderly man on a stretcher being checked in by a nurse practitioner. Several people were standing in line at the entrance desk. Almost all the seats were taken by people of all ages, some visibly ill, holding their belly or a limb, others less obviously unwell, checking their phones or chatting with companions. Multiple members of the ER team were rushing in and out of the waiting room, inviting patients to the patient care area, updating waiting family members or escorting treated patients to the exit. It was busy. Lili looked around but did not see Stella anywhere. She walked along the ER hallway and found her in one of the examination rooms. Stella sat on a stretcher and was checking her phone. The door was open and nobody else was there at the moment. So, Lili stepped into the room. "Hello Stella, what are you doing here?"

Stella looked up and her face brightened as she saw Lili walking in. "Hello, Lili, it is so good to see you! Perhaps I got too excited last night. My knee started to hurt again overnight, and I decided to consult Dr. Segond in the ER this morning. Since we know each other, I was hoping for a quick visit, just to make sure there's nothing serious. But I have been waiting for quite some time. Dr. Segond told me that she cannot make exceptions based on personal acquaintances. I was here first, but she took care of somebody else who arrived after me."

Annya stepped into the room. "Yes, indeed," she said with a resolute tone and polite smile. "I am sorry for the unexpected waiting time, Stella. Unfortunately, the ER does not operate like a restaurant. We cannot serve patients on a first come first serve basis. We have to take care of the sickest patients first. I had to attend to another patient who had a life-threatening emergency. I hope you can understand."

"Of course," Stella responded, "no problem at all."

"I actually just reviewed your radiographs with the radiology resident," Stella continued. "Based on your physical examination and the radiograph, I can tell you that we did not find any acute problem. You have osteoarthritis, degenerative changes of the bones of your knee joint. In addition, there's an older injury. Either of these may cause your pain. I wrote you a prescription for motion exercises with a physiotherapist. You can also take some over the counter pain medication, if needed. But I would hope that you would try physiotherapy first. If Lili has some time, perhaps she can show you the radiograph, so that you can see what causes the pain."

"Thank you, Dr. Segond," Stella responded. "I will try the

physiotherapy first. That sounds good to me. I would also be interested to see the culprit on the radiographs."

"I will be happy to show the radiograph to you, Stella," Lili said.

"Thank you, Lili!" Annya looked at Lili with gratitude. Through the half open door, they could see two paramedics with a patient on a gurney passing by. Annya turned to Stella. "I wish you all the best!" She bowed her head slightly and rushed out of the room.

Lili showed Stella the way to the radiology reading room. She opened the picture archiving computer system and brought up the frontal radiograph of Stella's knee joint. It showed degenerative changes and a curvilinear lesion at the medial lower end of the thigh bone (femur).

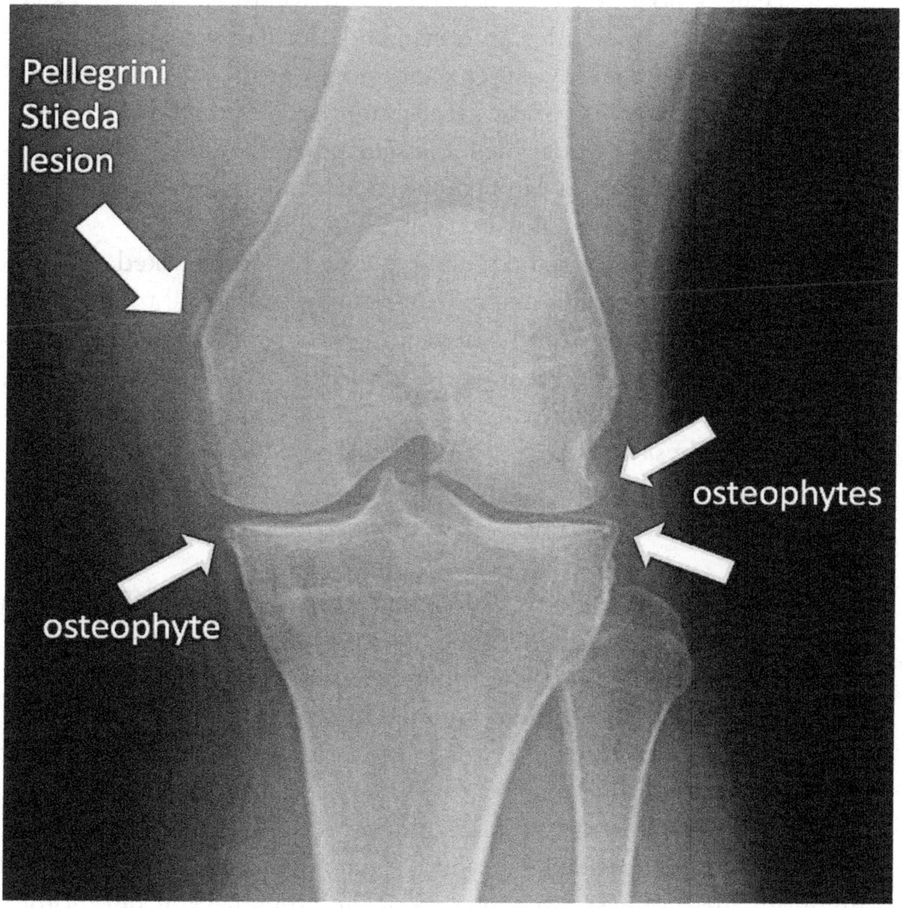

""“You have osteoarthritis,” Lili explained. “There are osteophytes on your femur, the upper thigh bone, and your tibia, the lower thigh bone.”

What are osteophytes?”

“Osteophytes are bone spurs — smooth, bony lumps that grow off a bone.” Lili showed her the abnormality. “In addition, you have a Pellegrini-Stieda lesion.” Lili pointed to the small bone fragment.

“What is that?” Stella asked.

“In technical terms, it is an old avulsion injury at the medial femoral condyle, which led to a calcification of the medial femoral collateral ligament,” Lili explained.

“How funny, is has my name!” Stella exclaimed.

“Yeah, I do not have an explanation for that.” Lili chuckled. “The lesion was named after an Italian and German surgeon.”

“Oh, I know that my father’s ancestors were physicians in Italy,” Stella said. “Perhaps one of my great-grandparents created the name.”

“That is certainly possible,” Lili said, while scrolling through two additional radiographs, a lateral view and a sunrise view, to see if anything else was abnormal. Everything was fine.

“I still don’t understand what it is exactly,” Stella asked.

“In non-technical terms, it is an injury of the distal thigh after a prior trauma, probably months or years ago. In most instances, it does not cause any pain. But if it does, it can be treated with exercise, medical treatment or even surgery. As Annya said, since your pain is intermittent, physiotherapy is probably the best first step.”

“Okay, thank you for explaining this to me,” Stella responded, looking at the radiograph with great interest.

Lili thought they were done and turned to her computer. The screen showed a long list of radiographs that were waiting for her review. But Stella made no signs of leaving. There was a moment of silence.

Then, Stella sighed and continued the conversation. “Lili, since I am here, could you have a quick look, if you can find a recent radiograph of my daughter?”

Lili was surprised. “Your daughter?”

“Well, I believe she fell yesterday and might have sought medical attention. She is only seventeen years old and therefore, as her mother, I should be able to check that she is okay, right? I am very worried.”

Lili saw tears swelling in her eyes.

"I am not sure I understand," she responded. "What exactly happened? Why are you not asking your daughter yourself how she's doing?"

"Well, that is not currently possible. I cannot find her at the moment. Can you please keep this confidential?"

Lili tried to understand the situation. "If you want to share information about your daughter, I will do my best to keep it confidential. However, if this is needed for her safety, it is possible that I will have to share it. What happened?"

"Susan was scheduled to start a summer internship this week with Twitter in San Francisco. I rented a room for her there so that she would not have to commute. Yesterday, I found out that she did not appear for her first day. She called in sick. I tried to reach her, but she does not answer her phone. I called one of my friends in San Francisco last night, to check on her in person, but Susan was not home."

"So, she's missing? Lili asked, "Did you call the police?"

"You know, they usually ask to wait for at least twenty-four hours. Those twenty-four hours are not over yet. So, I do not know for sure. Perhaps she was at the gym or meeting a friend and I am just overreacting. But she called in sick and therefore, she should have been in her room?"

"So, your daughter does not answer her phone," Lili summarized, "and now you're asking me to check her medical file here in the ER? I still don't understand?"

"Well, I got very concerned when you showed me the facial sketch yesterday," Stella explained. "First I did not know why I had this reaction. But then, I realized that the guy on the sketch is a friend of my daughter Susan. He came to our house several times."

That was some news! "Why did you not mention this yesterday?" Lili asked.

"It took me some time to bring the pieces together," Stella responded, tears now running down her cheeks. "I remembered that I had seen this guy before. But I did not remember right away where it was. Then, we were at a dinner last night with Aiko, the ER receptionist, and she mentioned that a police officer had generated a facial composite drawing of a patient in the ER earlier that day. Aiko thought that she had seen that guy before on campus, perhaps he was a SUEC student. Suddenly, I realized the connection. There was a crime suspect in the ER and I knew him because he was a friend of my daughter Susan. The guy was injured, and Susan called in sick and does not answer her phone. Perhaps this is just a silly coincidence. But what if there is more to it? What if she is injured as well? I just want to make sure she is safe!"

Lili decided that there was enough evidence to connect the daughter to the FBI case and it would warrant checking her x-rays.

"To my knowledge, the man on the sketch did not come to the ER with a young woman," she responded. "But let's double check if we find anything about your daughter. Can you spell her full name please?"

"S-u-s-a-n P-e-l-l-e-g-r-i-n-i," Stella spelled the name.

Lili entered the name into the computer system.

"The last entry was from about two years ago. No recent x-ray or other consultation about a trauma," she told the visibly distressed mother, "But I would like you to talk with Terrel Wright, one of the men who met with us yesterday.

"Why would I want to talk with him?" Now, Stella was confused.

"I am also not sure, but I believe he might have some information about this guy and your daughter," Lili responded.

"Okay, if he can help me find her, let's talk with him as quickly as possible!" Stella exclaimed.

Lili pulled Terrel's business card from her purse and called his cell phone number. Terrel responded right away. Lili explained the situation. He listened carefully. At the end, he said that he was on campus and could come to see them around ten. Fortunately, Dr. Bennett had requested backup clinical coverage for Lili this week so that she could attend to this situation. She was not officially assigned to cover any clinical services, although she had planned to help her colleagues as much as possible. So, Stella got a coffee and Lili reviewed and dictated a pile of medical imaging studies that had come in from the ER. At ten am, Terrel, Stella and Lili met in front of the hospital. They spotted a table under the large pine trees to the right of the entrance area, which provided both shade and privacy.

"Thank you for sharing your concerns with us, Stella." Terrel opened the conversation. "When did you last try to contact Susan?"

"Just now, while we were waiting for you," Stella responded with a trembling voice. "This is quite unusual for her. She sometimes does not respond right away. But when I contact her, she always calls back after a few hours at most."

"That is concerning indeed. I believe there might be a connection to a case that we are investigating. I would like to show you a video," Terrel said, "however, I need your affirmation that you will keep this absolutely confidential."

Stella nodded eagerly. "Of course, Agent Wright. I already signed a confidentiality statement with Dr. Bennett yesterday. And if this will help me to find Susan, I certainly promise anything you want!"

Terrel pulled an iPad from his briefcase and adjusted the screen so that it avoided the sunlight. "I may be completely wrong here, but I want to check with you, if this video might show your daughter."

He double clicked the video file of the theft in the lab, the one they had seen yesterday. Stella watched it carefully. At the scene where the woman fell, the hoodie fell backwards and the ponytail appeared, Stella clutched both hands to her mouth. "That is Susan," she exclaimed. "I gave her the little metal circle ponytail ring for her birthday!"

"Are you sure it is her?" Terrel asked. "It could be some other girl with the same hair ring?"

"Well, I do not see her face," Stella responded. "But this woman has the same body height and shape as my daughter. She also has the same hair, the same ponytail ring and her movements look familiar. I believe it's her. What did she get herself into? Is she in danger?"

"I do not know that," Terrel responded. "But it is very helpful that we now know who to look for. I will start a search right away and will keep you updated as soon as we find her. In the meantime, please keep contacting her. If she responds, please call me right away." He handed her his business card.

"I'm so afraid!" Stella said. "Please bring her back to me!"

"I will do everything I can to make that happen," Terrel responded. He put the iPad back into his briefcase, got up, said goodbye, pulled his cell phone and walked away with long strides, talking on the phone.

- 11 -
Kaleo
THE CONNECTION

Tuesday, May 25, 2032, 10.30 am.

"How about a coffee?" Kaleo asked as they were walking down the street in front of the General Hospital.

"That would be amazing," Susan answered. She realized that she hadn't had breakfast yet. She saw a cozy little corner café three blocks away, where people were sitting outside. "Let's go there." She pointed to the café.

Kaleo squinted. "Are you sure there's a café?" he asked.

"Yes, of course, silly!" Susan laughed. "They have cappuccino and croissants and sandwiches, all we need for a great start into a happy day!"

"Have you been there before?" Kaleo looked confused.

"No, I see it on their plates!" Susan laughed.

Kaleo looked at her in amazement. "So, the brain chip is enhancing your vision?"

"Yes!" she beamed at him. "It works! My vision has been unlocked. I see so much more than I used to see. I can see a larger area than before; I can see much further into the distance, and I see much more detail as well. I can read the menu at the café which is now two blocks away. I can see the eyes of a man in a car across the street looking at us and I can see a four-leaf clover in the grass right beside us."

To prove her point, Susan reached down to the front lawn of a house they were passing by, picked up a four-leaf clover and gave it to Kaleo.

He laughed with her. "Here is our lucky charm for the day!"

She looked at him with a softness that he had not noted before. "It is absolutely amazing, Kaleo. I wished I could turn it over to you like rosy sunglasses. All the colors appear more intense, as if someone had switched on a color button. I feel like I had previously only known their faded versions."

"It sounds as if you are high?" Kaleo asked.

"I don't think this describes it accurately," she said. "I do not feel tipsy or drowsy at all. I rather feel a sense of absolute sobriety. My mind has become exponentially clearer. Most importantly, I feel *good*! I feel connected with everything around me, connected with *you*!" She tried to squeeze his fingers that were sticking out of the cast.

Kaleo smiled. He liked Susan's transformation.

They had arrived at the café. They found a vacant bistro table, sat down and ordered two cappuccinos, a chocolate croissant for Susan and a cheese sandwich for Kaleo. The warm California morning sun and the smell of the freshly brewed coffee embraced them. After enjoying her delicious croissant, Susan leaned back and closed her eyes. Kaleo opened his cell phone and scrolled though the news of the day.

"Oh my god!" he suddenly exclaimed.

Susan looked at him, irritated. "Shush." She put her index finger in front of her mouth. "The people at the other tables are looking at us!"

Kaleo composed himself and lowered his voice. "The article here says that Dr. Juan Perez and his wife have been murdered!"

"Your friend at the university?" Susan leaned over to him and looked at the online newspaper in disbelief. "It must be a misunderstanding. They probably mean a different person with the same name."

"I don't think this is a misunderstanding," Kaleo responded. "They say here that he was a researcher at SUEC!"

Susan shook her head. "Why would anyone kill a researcher at SUEC? Perhaps a rejected student wanted to open a spot?"

Kaleo shook his head. "Susan, this is not funny! I have never heard of someone killing a person in order to get a spot at a university. First, that is no reason to kill anyone. There are plenty of other universities out there! Second, the odds of the killer's getting the spot would be far too low."

"Perhaps that's true – unless you know you are the next on the waiting. list." Susan smiled at him.

"Susan, don't say such a horrible thing. Remember, I got access to the lab with a university ID that I got from a friend. That friend was Juan Perez. I used his university ID to open the door to the lab. And later, I used his ID to identify myself as Juan Perez in the ER."

Susan stared at him. "Do you think Juan was killed because somebody thought he had the brain chips?"

"That's exactly what I'm thinking," Kaleo whispered, tears swelling in his eyes. "Susan, this is my fault. Juan was killed because of me."

"We do not know that at all," Susan countered with a resolute voice. "The article states here that both he and his wife have been killed. You certainly do not have anything to do with the wife." Susan looked at Kaleo. "Or do you? She is very pretty?"

Kaleo scoffed, "Don't be ridiculous!"

"Who knows why these people have been killed? Perhaps they were dealing drugs. Perhaps they got involved with the wrong people. Perhaps they killed each other."

"The article states that the wife had the gun in her hand." Kaleo read out loud. …the man had a gunshot to his forehead and the woman had a gunshot to her right temple."

"See, they probably killed each other," Susan tried to reassure him. "Love and jealousy are the most common reasons for murder."

Kaleo shook his head. "I don't like this, Susan. This is too much of a coincidence. If they were killed because someone was searching for the brain chips, then that person did not find what they were searching for. They could come for us next!"

"Nobody knows we were involved," Susan responded. "And we have to make sure it stays this way. We better sell the chips fast."

"Your idea to stay with Amir was really smart," Kaleo said. "Nobody will look for us at his apartment. Let's go back there." He pulled out a few bills from his wallet and placed them on the small tablet with the bill. He got up and extended his free left arm to her.

Susan took his hand and got up as well. "I really need some fresh clothes." She pointed to her right side. "See, my entire right side is dirty from the fall this morning."

Kaleo shook his head. "I think it's too dangerous. We should get back to Amir's place. You can wear one of his T-shirts. We can sell the brain chips on the black market tonight and head home before anyone suspects us of being involved."

"I need fresh clothes!" Susan insisted. "If you are afraid to go there, I can just go quickly by myself. It will only take a few minutes. We can meet at Amir's apartment in half an hour or so."

Kaleo sighed. "I will not leave you alone. Remember, when you walked on the street by yourself this morning, you ended up in the hospital! If you think it's absolutely necessary, we will stop at your place. But let's make this as quick as possible."

"Of course, honey!" Susan gave him a long kiss. "Thank you!" They left the café and walked towards Susan's apartment, which was only four blocks away.

***

Boris had parked on a small lot across the street and observed the couple from a distance. Now he saw them walking towards Third Street. Did they plan to go to Susan's rented room? This would be his opportunity. Boris got out of the car and followed them, carefully seeking the cover of the shadows of the buildings.

- 12 -
Lili
HILL-SACHS DEFECT

Tuesday, May 25, 2032, 10.30 am.

After meeting with Stella Pellegrini and Terrel Wright, Lili went back to the hospital. She had just reached the entrance when she heard a woman's voice calling her name. She turned around and saw Stella running after her, waving. Lili stopped. Stella reached her, catching her breath.

"I just received a text from Susan!" she exclaimed. "She said she is sick with the flu and will call me tomorrow."

"That is great news! You should inform Terrel so that he does not issue a search for a missing person," Lili responded.

"I am not sure about that. Susan didn't tell me where she is, and she still did not answer her phone when I called her. I have a bad feeling about this. I still think it would be helpful if Terrel searches for her. She could be in grave danger. Juan Perez and his wife were killed!"

"What do you want me to do?" Lili asked.

"I will drive to San Francisco and check if Susan is at her new room as she said she is. I wondered if you would accompany me?"

"I am sorry, I have to check a few cases in the hospital," Lili responded. "You have seen how swamped my colleagues are. I cannot leave them right now, but I could join you later this afternoon?"

"I cannot wait a minute longer," Stella responded with a trembling voice. "I have to see my daughter and make sure she is okay. I also want to be with her when the FBI questions her about the theft of the brain chip. Hopefully, her young age will be considered in her favor. That was really a very stupid mistake. I don't know what she was thinking."

"Okay, why don't you see if you can find her at her apartment in San Francisco," Lili responded. "Please keep me updated. I cannot join you right now. But as you know, I live in San Francisco and will drive home later this afternoon. I can stop by Susan's apartment to see you both then."

"Of course, that sounds good," Stella responded. "Please keep your fingers crossed that I find Susan in her apartment!"

"I hope that will be the case!" Lili patted her back. "Please keep me posted."

"I will!" Stella turned around and left in the direction of the parking lot.

***

Lili entered the hospital and went back to the Radiology reading room, where her colleague Matthew Holmes was busy reviewing imaging studies that had piled up. Annya was walking by in the hallway. She saw Lili in the reading room and came in to catch up. "It is still very busy in the ER at the moment."

"Any life-threatening emergencies that we should prioritize?" Lili asked.

"Not at the moment," Annya said. " I just referred a patient with a new cardiac infarction to our cardiology clinic. Two other patients with appendicitis are on their way to the operating room. Matthew already provided the Radiology reports for them. Several others may have bone fractures. It would be great if you could help diagnosing them quickly. One patient in the waiting room said that if we do not come to see her in the next ten minutes, she will be leaving. I don't know why she thinks this is a threat to us…." Annya smiled. She looked tired, her energy getting drained in the peak of the morning rush. While Lili worked both as a physician and scientist, Annya focused entirely on her clinical work. She worked literally around the clock in the emergency room.

"You saved multiple lives this morning," Lili said. "You are awesome, and we know it!" She smiled at Annya. Even the strongest woman needed some reassurance sometimes. "Let Aiko talk with the impatient woman. We will make sure that there will be no backlog from the Radiology side."

"I am so glad that you are my colleague," Annya said, smiling again. "I know you will always have my back."

"Of course, I will. We are all honored to work with you!" Despite its fast pace, Lili liked the environment of the emergency room. For the most part, values were simple and clear here. Preserving health and fighting death. The academic environment was much more complex, multifaceted and political.

Lili started to review the radiographs of three patients with fractures of the humerus (the main bone of the upper arm). All three were elderly patients, one man and two women, and all fracture lines went through the surgical neck (just inferior to the tubercles, where the shaft of the bone begins). The anatomical neck is represented by the closed growth plate in adults and much more rarely affected. Lili prepared reports for these x-rays, referring to the Neer classification, which considers four anatomical parts of the humerus. The surgical neck, the greater tuberosity, the anatomical neck and the lesser tuberosity.

After a while of uninterrupted image reviews, Annya came into the reading room again. "Lili, you won't believe this!" she exclaimed. "Dr. Robert Hill just arrived with a dislocated shoulder! Can you please show me his radiographs?"

"How did that happen?" Lili asked in surprise.

"He said he found another intruder in the lab when he came in this morning. It came to a fight. Dr. Hill was pushed backwards and fell directly on his left shoulder."

"Well, let me have a look," Lili pulled up Dr. Hill's radiograph.

The radiograph demonstrated caudal (lower) and medial displacement of the left humeral head.

"Indeed, this is an anterior shoulder dislocation," Lili explained. "In addition, there is a classical Hill-Sachs defect in the posterolateral humeral head due to a depression fracture from the impaction with the anterior glenoid rim. There is also a Bankart lesion in the anteroinferior glenoid fossa."

Agent Angus Weber entered the reading room. "Good morning, ladies. I was informed that there was an incident that involved Dr. Hill and his lab?"

"That is correct," Annya responded. "We were just reviewing his radiograph."

"Did he suffer an injury?" Angus Weber asked.

"Yes," Annya nodded and turned to Lili. "Lili, can you please explain the findings on the radiograph?"

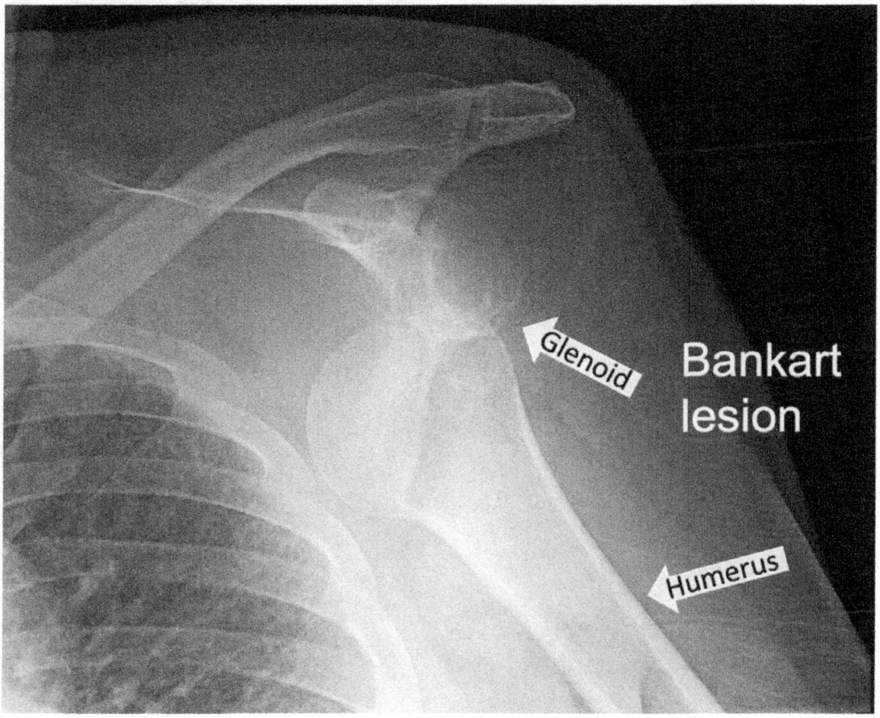

"Of course!" Lili showed them the radiograph. "The ball-like head of his upper arm bone, the humerus, popped out of his shoulder socket, the glenoid. This is usually caused by a violent, high pressure external rotation with the arm in an elevated position."

Annya looked at the radiograph. "Can you tell if the humerus bone was displaced anteriorly and not posteriorly?" she asked.

"Well, when the humeral head is displaced medially and overlies the glenoid, the dislocation is anterior," Lili explained. "In a posterior dislocation, the humeral head does not move medially.

"Why do you need to know that?" Agent Weber asked.

"It is important to clarify if the humerus dislocated anteriorly or posteriorly because this tells the ER physician whether to push the bone forwards or backwards to place it back into the shoulder socket."

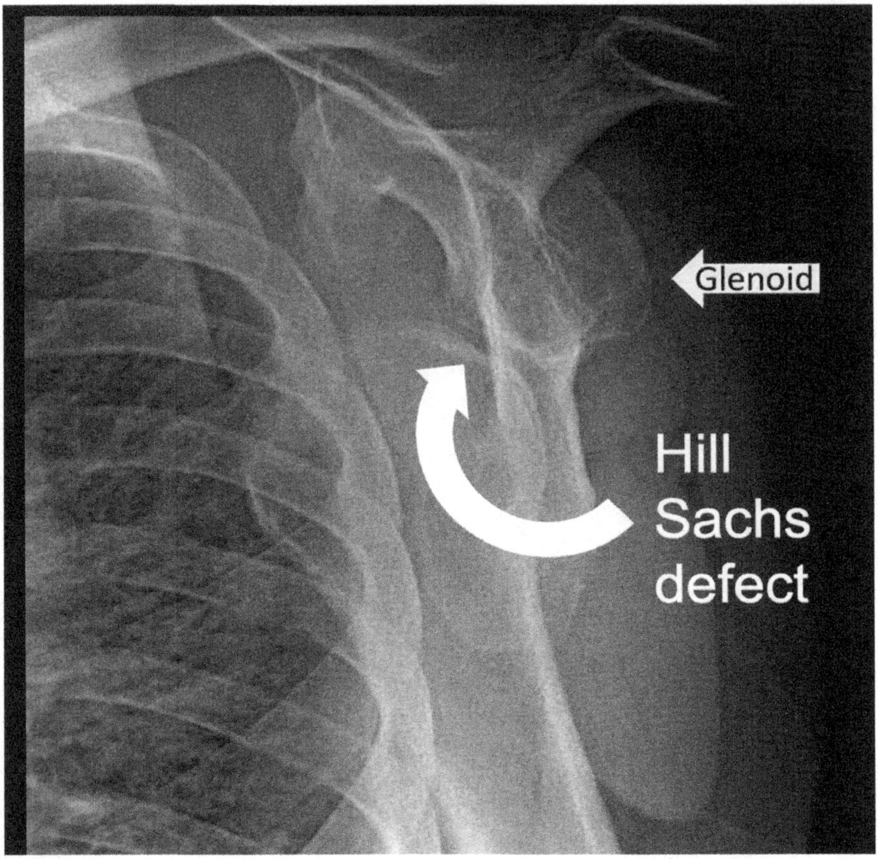

Lili pointed to the lateral view radiograph. "We usually take a second view from a different angle to confirm the direction of the dislocation. We did this here as well."

Lili looked through her list of radiographs and pulled up a shoulder x-ray from another patient. She clicked the button to remove the patient information in order to show de-identified images for educational purposes.

"See, this radiograph of one of our patients earlier today looks different," she explained. "There is a loss of the normal half-moon overlap sign between the head of the humerus and the glenoid. In addition, there is a fixed internal rotation of the humeral head with a rounded appearance, the so-called light bulb sign. We obtained an additional axial radiograph. As you can see, the humerus dislocated posteriorly and there is an impaction fracture of the anterior humeral head, also called a reverse Hill Sachs defect."

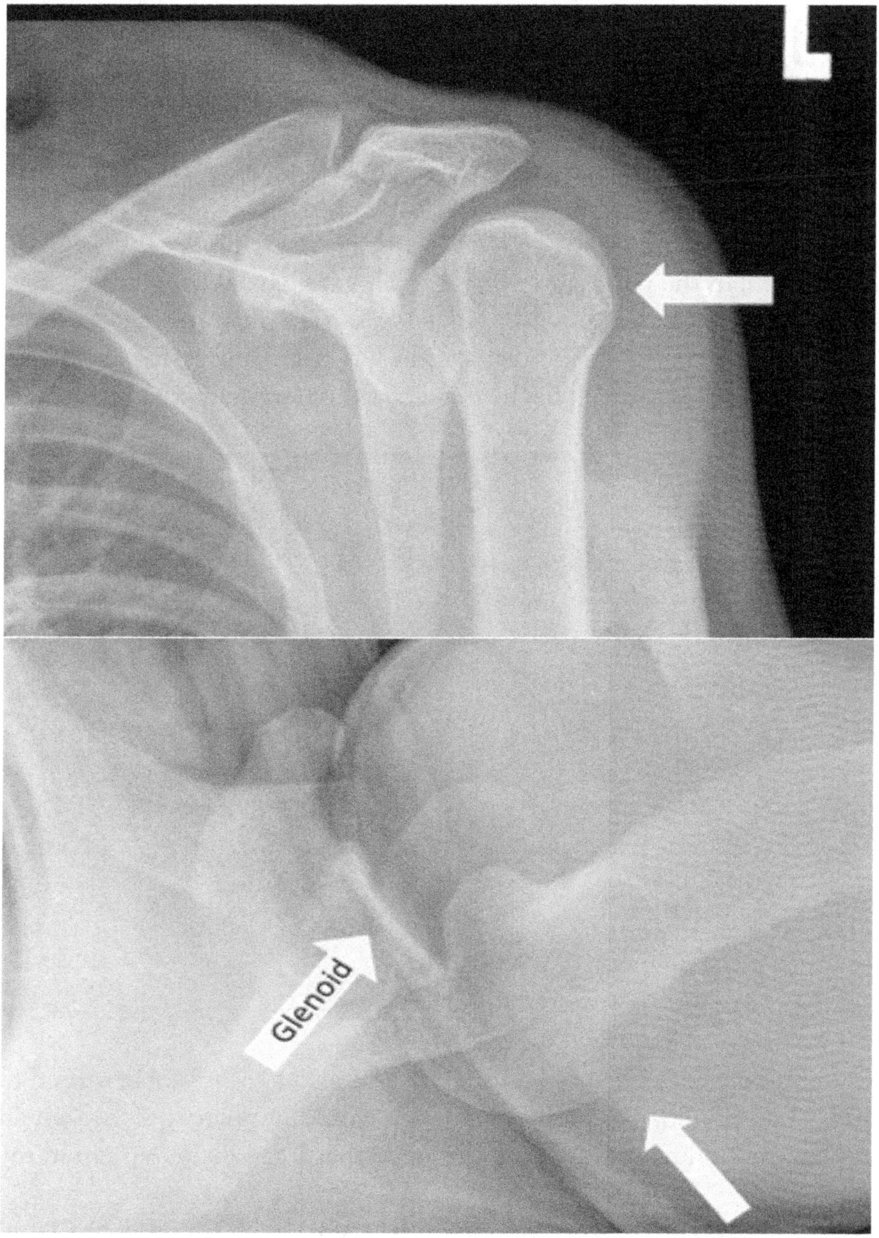

"Thanks for explaining that to us," Annya said.

"So, Dr. Hill received a blow to the shoulder that pushed the bone of his arm forward. Do you know details of Dr. Hill's incident? Can I see him to ask him a few questions?" Angus asked.

"He did not tell me much," Annya responded. "He was in pain, and I tried to help him out as quickly as possible. Our orthopedic surgery colleagues were in the ER to see another patient. I asked them to consult on Dr. Hill as well. They went to see him right away and presumably have reduced the dislocation by now." Annya turned to Lili. "Lili, can you check, if you can find a post-reduction image?"

"Yes, here is a post reduction image of Dr. Hill," Lili said and showed them the radiograph that was obtained just a few minutes ago. "As you can see, the surgeon has successfully put the humeral head back into the glenoid. The dislocation has been successfully reduced. You can still see the Hill Sachs defect of the humeral head."

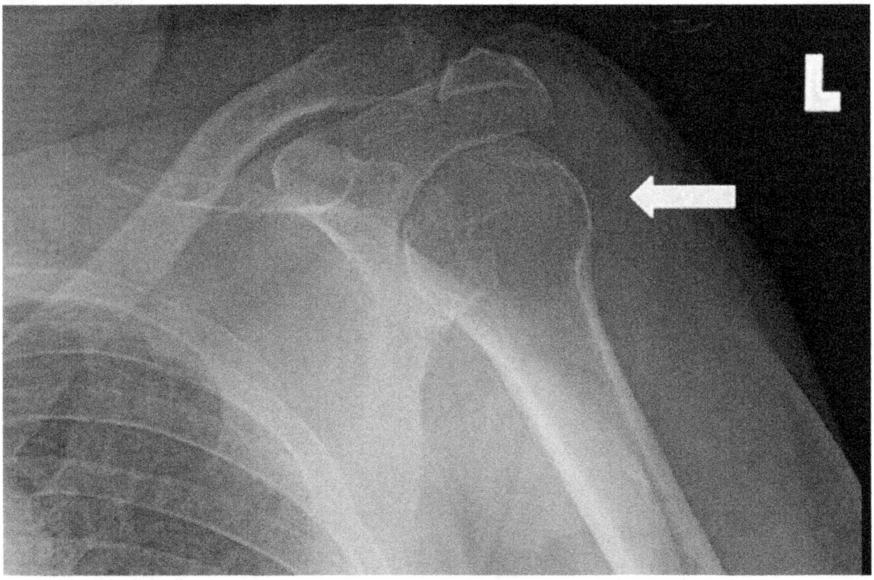

"Okay, let's go and see him." Angus said to Annya. He turned to Lili. "Lili, would you please join us. I would appreciate if you could repeat the findings of the radiograph so that I can include them in my report."

"Of course," Lili responded, and went up to follow Annya and Angus to the patient room.

Robert Hill was sitting on a stretcher, visibly distressed. His right arm was stabilized in a sling.

"Annya, you brought the whole team!" he exclaimed.

"Yes, I did," she responded with her usual calm, melodic voice. "Do you feel better, Dr. Hill?"

"Yes, I feel much better after the surgeons put the shoulder back in place," he said.

"I am glad to hear that," Annya said. "Will it be okay with you if Agent Weber asks you a few questions?"

"Of course!" Robert Hill invited the FBI agent to come closer with a waving gesture of his good arm. "What would you like to know?"

"Thank you for your time, Dr. Hill," Angus said. "Can you please describe what happened? Please provide as much detail as possible."

"Well, I came into the lab this morning and to my surprise, I saw another intruder in the lab."

"When was that approximately?" Angus asked.

"I believe it was around eight forty-five am," Robert Hill responded. "I thought I was the first in the lab. Most of our researchers arrive around nine am."

"But you were not the first?"

"No, there was a man sitting at my desk, whom I did not know. He wore black clothes, black gloves and a black ski mask. He had broken into the cabinet behind my desk and taken out the folder with the description of the brain chip. You might remember, I showed you yesterday that I keep the patent files and technical concept plans as hard copies in my cabinet. The man held a small camera in his hand. I assume he wanted to take photos. I am not sure if he already had."

"How do you know it was a man and not a woman?"

"I grabbed him by his ragged, long-sleeved shirt and uncovered a muscular, hairy forearm. It was definitely a man, a white man."

"What happened next?"

"The man jumped up, grabbed his camera and tried to escape. I grabbed his arm and we started to struggle. He then gave me a forceful push, which threw me backwards into the cabinet. I felt a blow to my right shoulder and an immediate excruciating pain. I saw the guy running towards the door. He slowed down as he entered the hallway, as if he knew about our floor adhesive. He walked with long strokes out of my field of view, and I heard the metal door squeak and shut."

"Did you follow him?" Angus asked.

"No, I needed all my energy to hold on to my consciousness. I nearly passed out due to the pain. I just closed my eyes for a while and tried to catch my breath. Then, I took all my strength to put the folder back into the cabinet and close it. After that, I called a cab and went straight to the ER."

"Do you have any idea who the intruder might have been?"

"I have no idea. I don't think it was any of my lab members. But it was strange that this person knew where to find the brain chip files. Even most of my team members do not know where I keep them. "

"That is peculiar indeed." Angus made a note in his notebook. "I would like to inspect the crime scene. Are any of your team members there right now? Could they let me in?"

"I asked my lab manager to personally supervise the lab to prevent another incident like this. She can certainly let you in. I would also be happy to accompany you."

"I don't think that is a good idea," Annya protested. "You need some rest. I am ready to discharge you, but only if you promise that you will go home."

Robert Hill looked at Annya. "Dr. Segond, I know you mean well. But these thefts can ruin my career. I must get the chips back and bring these criminals to justice as soon as possible."

"The FBI is here to help with that, Dr. Hill," Agent Weber said. "I agree with Annya. Please go home and take care of yourself. You cannot do much anyways while my team is inspecting the scene. I will keep you updated as soon as I find anything new. I will also contact you if I have any further questions or need help."

Robert Hill sighed. "Of course, it seems that I have no say in the matter." He smiled at us. "That's okay. I understand. My husband is already on his way to the ER. He will pick me up and take me home."

The conversation seemed to be officially over. But Lili thought this encounter might be an opportunity for her to learn a little more about the brain chip and the threat that it could pose. She had waited in the back of the room and now stepped closer. "Dr. Hill, can I also ask you a few brief questions?"

Robert Hill looked at her with a polite smile. "Of course, Lili. What would you like to know? Also, most faculty here at SUEC address each other by their first names. You can call me Robert if you like."

"Okay, sure! Robert, can you please explain to me, how the brain chip works exactly?"

Lili saw delight in his eyes. Despite the pain in his shoulder, this was clearly his favorite subject to talk about. He adjusted the sling around his arm.

"Well, I cannot disclose the technical specifications to you for confidentiality reasons, but I can describe the effects on the mammal brain. When implanted under the skin over a specific area of the brain or spinal cord, the chip can enhance the function of that area by sending low level radiofrequency pulses to that area. For example, when implanted under the skin behind the ear, the chip can stimulate the auditory cortex and provide enhanced hearing capabilities. When implanted under the skin of the lower posterior skull, the chip can stimulate the visual cortex and provide enhanced visual capabilities."

"That sounds pretty amazing."

"It is! This chip technology is the result of many years of hard work. However, we are still in early phases of *in vivo* testing in animal models. The brain chip is not ready for prime time just yet."

"Why is that? Are there side effects?"

"Thus far, we mostly studied the effects in rodents and guinea pigs. We got short term experience in monkeys and one test in a human volunteer thus far."

"Who would agree to be a first human volunteer?" Lili wondered.

"Actually, I was the human volunteer," Dr. Hill responded with pride in his voice. He seemed to have forgotten the pain in his shoulder and was clearly energized by the conversation.

Lili was impressed. That was a level of commitment that she would personally not approve. "What did you find when you tested the brain chip?"

"I actually have a slightly impaired hearing capacity and so I tried an implantation over the temporal lobe." He pointed to the area above his right ear. "I experienced a remarkably enhanced hearing ability. In addition, I encountered episodes of synesthesia!"

"What is synesthesia?" Lili asked.

"Synesthesia is a neurological condition in which information meant to stimulate one of your senses stimulates several other senses. In my case, I could see music and I smelled certain words. For example, I smelled my lab when someone called my name and I smelled pine trees when someone said the word *pine tree*."

Lili tried to imagine the experience of smelling words. "Did you find that useful?" she asked.

"Well, I did hear much better and that was certainly useful," Robert Hill responded. "But I would say the value of the bran chip was more of a revelation of an entirely new human experience. I felt like my brain was unlocked. You might have heard that humans only use a small portion of their actual brain capacity. It felt like this chip enhanced my *consciousness*. I felt a fundamentally new experience of connecting to my surroundings. I lost any concern about myself, which caused a feeling of immense joy and serenity. This effect was likely due to increased blood flow to the brain area close to the chip and reduced blood flow to the default mode network."

"*The default mode network*." This rang an alarm bell in Lili's head. She tried to remember where she heard this before. "Wait, I believe this reminds me of something I learned in medical school." Lili tried to retrieve the information from her memory. "Can drugs cause this same effect that you just mentioned, reduced blood flow to the default mode network?"

"Well, psychedelic drugs such as LSD can cause similar experiences," Robert explained with a shrug.

"That is interesting. But a drug is slowly metabolized and excreted from the body while a brain chip remains and provides a more permanent effect. One might not want to be in a constant state of such altered brain activity?" Lili thought out loud.

"Yes, of course," Robert responded. "You might remember that this brain chip is under development and was not yet ready for deployment to the public. We were working on decoupling the neurostimulator effects on natural senses from effects on self-perception, mood and consciousness."

"How far did you get with those improvements?" Lili asked.

"Well, we just got started to modify the chip technology to provide more localized effects," Robert Hill explained. "The brain chips that were stolen have the same effects as the one I studied on myself."

"In other words, the stolen chips could induce some sort of hallucinations or altered perceptions? I really hope we will get the chips back before anyone implants them!" And another concern came to Lili's mind. "LSD can also cause horror trips, right?"

"We call them bad trips," Robert corrected defensively. "We have not encountered a bad trip with our chip. But you are right. The chip could in theory induce a bad trip. We did consider this. The chance of a bad trip increases the longer a subject is exposed to the electromagnetic waves emitted from the chip. As a safeguard, we added a 'turn off' option to the chip. If you push it with your finger or thumb and hold it down against the skull for thirty seconds, then it is turned off."

"And what if the chip is not turned off?" Lili wondered.

Robert Hill cleared his throat. "Well, if a subject were to encounter a bad trip – and I have to say that this is purely hypothetical. We have not come across this scenario thus far – I would strongly recommend turning off the brain chip as quickly as possible. If the affected brain area continues to be stimulated, the chip could lead to permanent damage of the brain and induce permanent bad trip experiences."

Lili shuddered. "You mean somebody would be locked in a nightmare?"

Robert Hill nodded. "The experience would likely be much worse than just a nightmare. It would be much more vivid, much more realistic, and much more frightening."

Annya had calmly worked beside them at her computer, writing her report about Dr. Hill's shoulder injury. Now, she turned towards them. "I am afraid we have to end this conversation now," she said. "This is the ER and not a chat room. Plus, I am not sure a discussion about worst nightmares is the right conversation for my patient. I would like to start the discharge procedure now so that we can vacate this room for the next patient. The ER is full, and I need to keep things moving!"

"Of course, I understand." Lili got up and turned to Robert Hill. "I wish you a good recovery, Robert!"

He smiled at her. "It was great talking with you, Lili. I will be happy to connect again at a later time and talk about science!"

"I would love that! Have a good day!"

Lili left the exam room and met Agent Weber in the hallway. Apparently, he had been waiting for her.

"Hello Lili, could I have a quick word with you? I would like to document your interpretation of the x-ray of Mrs. Perez's cervical spine and Dr. Hill's shoulder injury.

"Of course, Agent Weber!"

Agent Weber waved her towards the small break room next-door, where Lili provided him with a detailed report of the x-ray findings for his records. Lili observed him closely during their conversation. She was not quite sure yet what to make of him. Was he a friend or not? Agent Weber appeared very self-assured, disciplined and reserved, perhaps a bit rigid. He did not show any sign of emotion as she explained the findings on Robert Hill's x-rays. He then asked her to show him the x-rays of the suspect again and diligently made notes as she explained the teardrop fracture of Juliana Perez in more detail. Even though they talked for quite some time, they did not connect on a personal level. The interaction felt more like an interrogation to Lili. When they were done with the formal part, Lili tried to break the ice and learn a little more about him.

"Agent Weber, have you and Terrel worked together for a long time?" she asked, although she already guessed from their independence that this was probably not the case.

"No, Terrel only joined my unit recently," Angus responded. "My previous partner was injured in a shooting incident last year. She was not able to do this job anymore and retired."

"I am very sorry to hear that," Lili said, while thinking. *Sometimes, a brief conversation can clarify why people are the way they are.* Agent Weber's reserved and inquisitive nature suddenly made sense to her.

"I don't really want to talk about it," Angus said, focusing his gaze on his notebook.

"I completely understand," Lili responded. An awkward silence followed. *There is so much pain in the world that we are not aware of.*

"Well, I guess we are done here." Agent Weber got up abruptly from his seat. "I will see you later this afternoon in Dr. Bennett's office!"

"Of course, see you later this afternoon!" Lili got up as well.

They parted in different directions. Lili walked back to the Radiology reading room. Agent Weber left to inspect the research lab. When Lili passed the waiting area, she saw an anxious looking young Indian man rushing into the ER, embracing Robert Hill and inspecting his injured arm. They both engaged in a lively conversation. Robert noticed her curious look and waved at her to come closer. "Hello Lili, would you like to meet my partner?"

Lili stepped towards them and shook the man's hand. He was at least ten years younger than Robert and very handsome. Robert pointed at his companion. "This is my partner Dr. Atharv Patel. He is an expert on artificial intelligence research at SUEC. Atharv, this is Dr. Lili Pham, a radiologist and physician-scientist at SUEC."

Atharv smiled at her, flashing two rows of perfectly white teeth. "Great to meet you in person, Lili! Robert spoke very highly of you!"

Lili looked at both men. "Thank you! I am flattered to hear that. I was also very impressed how Robert defended his lab."

Atharv padded Robert's back. "The lab is everything to him!"

Robert looked at Atharv. "Well, you certainly come first, Atharv!"

Atharv laughed. "I don't want to challenge that statement, honey!"

Lili saw Annya greeting her next patient in the distance. She briefly looked over to them. Lili had to get back to the reading room as well. She turned to Atharv. "I hope you will keep an eye on Robert. He needs some rest now!"

"I sure will! It was great to meet you, Lili." Atharv put his arm around Robert and they both walked towards the exit of the ER.

Robert looked over his shoulder. "Thank you for all your help, Lili!"

"My pleasure! I wish you a speedy recovery!" Lili turned around and left towards the Radiology reading room.

- 13 -
Susan
THE BRAIN CHIP

Tuesday, May 25, 2032, 12.00 pm.

After leaving the café, Susan and Kaleo walked down Third Street in San Francisco with the plan to pick up some fresh clothes from her apartment. Susan had already forgotten the article about the Perez family. But Kaleo was visibly nervous. Juan and Juliana Perez had been killed. Perhaps they had a fight that had nothing to do with the brain chips. Or Juan and his wife were killed because of the brain chips. And Kaleo and Susan had them now. Kaleo trembled. He was physically strong, but he was not brave. He liked adventures such as trekking through the Sierra or wild water rafting, but he did not like conflict, let alone violence. In fact, he strived for peace and harmony in every situation. One exception was Susan's safety. He loved her with all of his heart, and he would do everything to keep her safe.

Meanwhile, Susan was enjoying the effects of the brain chip. She looked around. *I am superwoman!* she thought. *I can see better than anyone on the planet!* It felt good to be special, especially after the SUEC consortium had rejected her. In essence, the SUEC letter had told her that it was bad that she desired to be a leader. But for Kaleo, it was expected. Susan was still upset about this injustice. But she reminded herself to hold her head high and not dwell in self-pity. There were lots of miserable people in the world and she would not be one of them. She would not become bitter because of some rigged system. Everybody else at SUEC had started ahead of her. Now, she would take charge and catch up. She would accelerate her career by herself. She would learn how to use the brain chip and then demonstrate her new abilities to the press. She would present the implantation of the chip in her head as a SUEC experiment. When the SUEC leaders read about her new abilities in the *New York Times*, they would not know what hit them. She, Susan, would be celebrated as the pioneer of a new era of brain-computer interfaces. And they had missed her talent!

Susan felt an urge to share her amazing experience with everyone around her, and especially with the arrogant SUEC leaders. But she also knew that she had to be patient and keep quiet for the time being. Susan squeezed Kaleo's hand and looked at him fondly. He looked back at her and smiled. Even if the others did not know about her superior abilities yet – it was sufficient for her and Kaleo to explore it together. She did love him dearly.

Susan continued to explore her new visual abilities and the new world around her. Everything she saw looked different now, more beautiful and more radiant. As she and Kaleo walked by a house with an assortment of flowers in the front garden, Susan stopped to admire the unnaturally bright and intense colors of orange bottlebrush trees, blue violet lavender bushes and scarlet hibiscus plants. A delightful ruby-throated hummingbird was feeding on a yellow trumpet vine. Susan watched the continuous movement of the hummingbird with her newly discovered ability to generate a series of discrete snapshots.

"Kaleo!" Susan exclaimed in excitement. "Look at this dainty little hummingbird. It can fly backwards!"

"That is cute indeed!" Kaleo responded, amused. How many times had they passed by hummingbirds? Susan was looking at this little bird as if she had just seen one for the first time. "If these birds impress you, you should see the honeycreepers when you come to Hawaii with me next summer!" he said, stroking the back of her head and resting his hand on her neck.

"I really look forward to that," she said softly, turning towards him and locking eyes with him. She got overwhelmed by a supreme feeling of genuine and unlimited love for Kaleo. She felt a deep gratitude for Kaleo's existence and leaned over to give him a long and passionate kiss.

Kaleo blushed. *That chip creates a waking dream!* he thought. *Perhaps we should mass-produce the chip and give it to everyone on earth! Love for the world!*

He kissed Susan back and whispered into her ear, "I love you!"

"I know!" she whispered. "I love you, too!"

The couple continued to stroll down the street. Susan stopped at every building, every flower and every butterfly, carefully observing and admiring every detail, squeezing Kaleo's fingers that poked out of his cast and kissing him softly at regular intervals. Kaleo enjoyed every part of Susan's enhanced affection. But he also started to get concerned that they might not reach the apartment before nightfall at this pace. He gently put his left hand on the small of her back and tried to propel her forwards.

Susan looked straight ahead at the sidewalk. The pavement seemed to undulate. "Look," she said to Kaleo, "the sidewalk is breathing!"

"I am not sure what you mean," Kaleo responded. "I hope you do not see the first signs of an earthquake with your enhanced vision."

Susan focused on the surface in front of her. Multicolored rays of sunlight seemed to mix with the breathing pavement, causing multiple blobs of color that were floating around in front of her. A squirrel crossed in front of them and vanished in a blue lake of color. Susan gasped, pointing ahead. "Did you see that?" she exclaimed. "That little squirrel just vanished!"

"Susan, the squirrel went up that tree," Kaleo responded, pointing to a tree to their right.

Susan looked at the tree. The squirrel was gone. The sun behind the tree sent bright bolts of light through the leaves, creating a billion sparkles in front of her eyes. She squinted and noticed that the branches of the tree began to reach out to her. She extended her arms to acknowledge their connection and lost her balance, slipping forwards. Kaleo caught the back of her T-shirt and pulled her back with his non-casted left arm.

"No more accidents today, please!" he said.

"Oops," Susan exclaimed, laughing. She was not irritated by these new sensations, but rather immensely fascinated. But she did notice the concern in Kaleo's eyes.

"Perhaps we should just sit down for a moment," she suggested, pointing to a small bench at the sidewalk in front of them. Kaleo nodded and they both sat down. She gave him another long, amorous kiss.

"Don't get me wrong," he said, grinning. "I appreciate the ambrosial effects of this brain chip!" His look became more serious.

"But I am afraid it might interfere with your safety. Just this morning, you ran into a motorcycle, you cannot walk to your apartment on your own and you just nearly fell into someone's garden. Imagine if this had been the street!"

"Well, we had a few complications," Susan responded. "This is because no human ever tested the chip. It is an amazing experience. I feel like my brain is unlocked. I just need to learn how to handle my new abilities. It may be like learning to ride a bicycle or walking around with new glasses. There will be a few falls until I have figured it out."

"Susan, I cannot watch you at all times. I am really concerned. You could get seriously hurt!" Kaleo exclaimed.

"Shush," Susan interrupted him, tapping her left index finger on his lips. "Don't move or say anything for a minute," she whispered. "Let's pretend we are just sitting here, enjoying the sun."

What was this about now? Kaleo got more and more concerned about Susan's erratic behavior. But he complied. They sat on the bench in silence for about two minutes. Then she leaned over to him and whispered into his right ear.

"Do you see the guy in the black leather jacket, who just passed us?"

"I see his jacket and blue jeans," Kaleo responded. "What about him?"

"I saw him outside of the hospital when you picked me up today. Then, I saw him again in a parked car across the street from our table in the café. Now, it seems as if he is following us."

"Are you sure you saw the same guy three times?" Kaleo asked. "Or perhaps the chip lets you imagine things?"

"I am sure it is the same guy. My perception has definitely changed. I feel connected with everything, as if a boundary has dissolved that separates me from the rest of the world. It is amazing, and I can see more things at once than previously. I can see more intense colors and I can see more details, near and far. But I do not hallucinate. Everything I see is present in the real world, I just see it differently. My newly enhanced vision allowed me to recognize that this man is present wherever I go. This man is observing us!"

Kaleo looked at Susan. "Okay, let's assume for a moment that you are right. What would you like to do about it?"

"The guy looked me right in the eyes," Susan responded. "I

believe he knows me. He disappeared around the corner. Let's walk in the opposite direction."

"But we wanted to pick up your stuff at your apartment?" Kaleo said.

"I think we should lose this guy first," Susan responded. "We can walk one block back and take a little stroll along the waterfront. It is a beautiful day, and we need some time to think about our next move anyways."

They got up from the bench and quickly walked into the opposite direction. When Susan looked over her shoulder, she did not see the man again.

- 14 -
Boris
PATELLA FRACTURE

Tuesday, May 25, 2032, 12.00 pm.

Boris followed Susan and Kaleo from a distance. He watched them carefully, trying to find out as much as possible about them. The guy was broad-shouldered and athletic. Boris was muscular himself and trained in Russian martial arts since he could walk. But it was probably best to avoid physical confrontation. The girl was slim and coltish, an easy target. She was exceptionally beautiful. Her long brunette hair, her even features and alluring smile reminded him of Inessa, his first girlfriend. Inessa had left him for another guy and Boris hated every girl who looked like her. His favorite memory now was the bullet that he had put into the bitch's head. After Inessa, he had Anastasia, a beautiful redhead. She had been almost perfect for about a year until she started to flirt with the bartender in their favorite restaurant. How cheap! This was the second woman Boris had to execute for bad behavior. Still optimistic, he found Sasha, the classiest Russian woman he had ever met. He had been completely enchanted by her perfect figure, her long, wavy blonde hair, her sparkling light-blue eyes and her soft, sexy lips. She had looked like an angel. And how she walked in heels! Like she was born in them. He had been madly in love with her – until she started to make out with his friend Carl. One afternoon, Boris came home early and found them in his bed. He remembered his disgust. And their horrified look at his gun. Boris had felt such relief when he saw the bullets penetrating their skulls. They got what they deserved.

Being in love and being betrayed once was bizarre. Twice was a coincidence. And three times was a pattern. These pretty bitches caused nothing but pain. They lured good, honest men like him and then choked them. He had been so naïve, letting them trample on his feelings. He had given them everything. And these bitches had never cared about his needs or his longing for someone who would love him back. He was still *angry*. He would never let anybody disrespect him like that again! He hated cheaters and traitors….

Fortunately, Boris had always been an optimist, a glass half-full kind of guy. Boris was proud of always making the best of every situation. He had been betrayed by three women in a row, but he had discovered his talent in shooting shitheads. And he had evolved into a stronger man. Before Sasha, he had been aroused by the movements of a sexy woman. Sasha waving at him from a distance, Sasha walking towards him, Sasha's hand gliding down his body. Since Sasha's death, he felt aroused by the tone of his semiautomatic pistol and the sight of a dead doll. He had perfected his shooting skills and found a profitable profession. Boris now worked as a professional killer for one of the largest underground agencies at the West Coast. He taught traitors respect. He was famous now! And every time he put a bullet into someone's head, he fondly remembered Sasha and Carl.

Boris saw Susan and Kaleo walking towards the apartment on Third Street. The boss had sent him the address and the couple was clearly heading in that direction. But they were moving slowly. The girl was stopping every few meters, pointing to who knew what, discussing the matter with the guy, moving on and stopping again two meters later. The guy had his left hand on her back, gently talking to her and trying to lead her forwards. But of course, the bitch did not listen. Boris felt hate encircling his chest, sending a rush of adrenaline to his head, making him dizzy. He took a big deep breath to clear up his mind. *Focus!* he told himself. *This will soon be over.*

The couple sat down on a bench at the sidewalk, talking with each other. Boris strolled closer, trying to catch any parts of the conversation. Perhaps this would give him a clue, what the two were up to. Suddenly, the girl looked him straight in the eye. Boris felt caught and struck by her penetrating gaze. For a moment, their eyes locked. Boris focused all his energy on staying calm and composed. The girl could not possibly know him. He unfocused his eyes from hers, looking past her with a blank face, pulling his cell phone out of his pocket and pretending to answer a call, slowly moving his gaze towards the other side of the street, away from her. He passed the couple and walked around the next corner. Here, he took a deep breath and waited under the shade of the trees along the sidewalk, watching out for them.

A young couple stopped and asked him for the way to the museum of modern art. *Did he look like the tourist information office?* Boris faked a smile and pointed in the opposite direction of the museum. The couple took off. His anger boiled up again. He knew that he had to keep his emotions in check if he wanted to stay unnoticed. Boris pulled up his medical image gallery on his iPhone. This always helped him to calm down his emotions. Before Sasha, he had worked as a physician assistant in an acute care clinic in Southern California. He had been fascinated by medical images of fractures and had taken photos of them. Over time, he had assembled an impressive collection. How inspiring it was! After Sasha, he had collected at least one new image every week and reviewed it after work. He particularly enjoyed remembering the distressed faces of beautiful women when they looked at the image of their broken bones. The cheaters! He remembered their agonizing pain and fantasized about inflicting similar injuries on them. After Sasha, Boris had used his image gallery as a "hands on" guide to causing pain in his victims, when his task was to scare someone or extract information, rather than killing them right away. All along, reviewing his collection brought him a deep sense of control and satisfaction. Boris opened his folder and pulled up x-rays from a woman who suffered from fractures of the patella (kneecap).

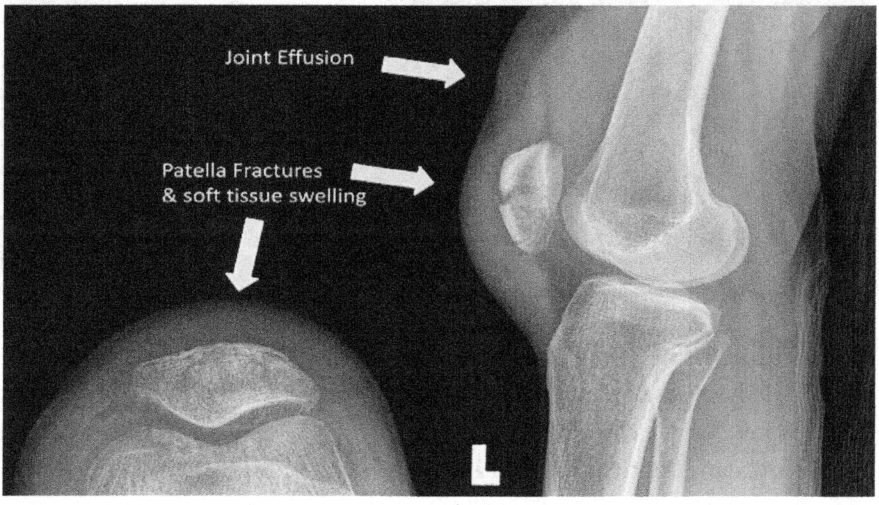

The fracture lines were clearly visible on the sunrise view and the lateral radiograph of the left knee joint. The sunrise view is taken with the knee flexed and shows the patella as if it were rising over the horizon of the knee joint. The radiograph is taken with the x-ray beam tangential to the patella and parallel to the long axis of the lower extremity. In this particular patient, there was also a massive soft tissue swelling over the patella and there was a large joint effusion, which led to an opacification (white shadow) of the suprapatellar recesses of the knee joint. The patient had been involved in a car accident, where her knee had been slammed against the dashboard. Boris followed the fracture lines on the radiograph with his index finger and recollected the pained expression on the woman's face. He felt energized.

Boris looked at another case, which showed air in the right knee joint, seen as dark bubbles on the radiograph. This patient had suffered a stab wound to the knee joint. *Fascinating!* Boris remembered how he had learned to recognize the air on the radiograph.

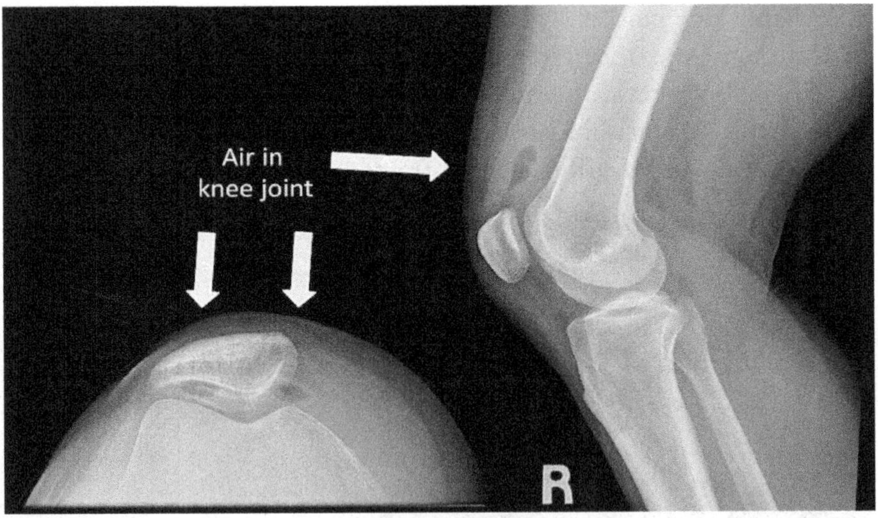

Finally, he came to his favorite case. A bilateral luxation of the patella! The patella normally sits on the groove of the femur (thighbone), in front of the knee joint. A trauma or congenital condition can shift the patella sideways out of alignment, which was the case in this patient here. The patella was not seen in front of the femur, but to either side of the femur.

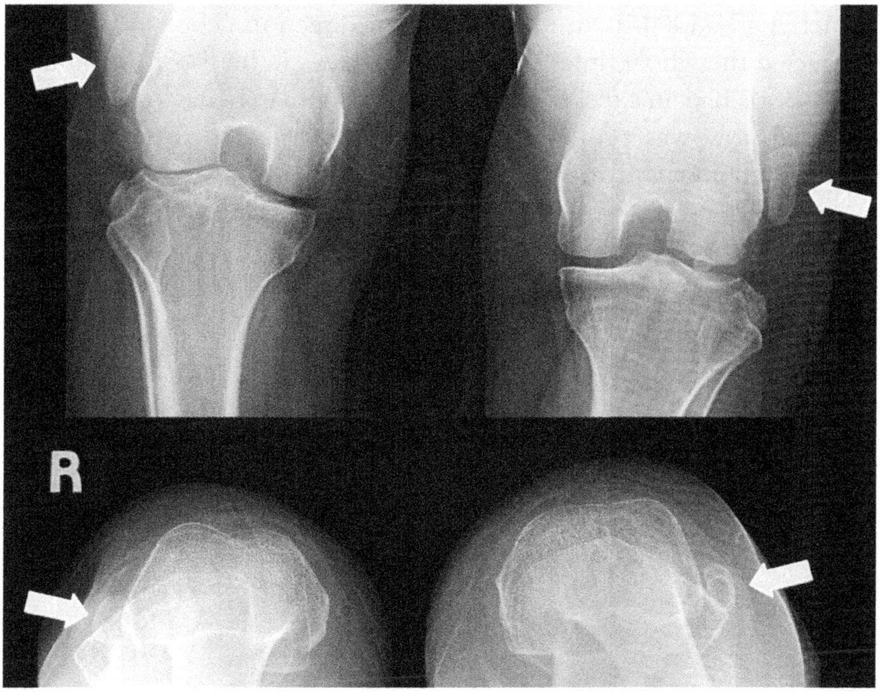

Boris scrolled through his image collection while waiting under the trees. Every few seconds, he scanned the cross street for Susan and Kaleo. He suppressed his urge to peek around the corner of the building that was hiding him from the couple. He did not want to risk being seen again. But finally, his impatience succeeded, and he did walk to the corner of the street and took a quick look towards the bench. *Damn – the bench was empty! The couple was gone! How could he have missed them?* Boris walked towards the bench, searching for the couple in all directions. Then he circled around the block, but he did not spot them anywhere. His anger returned and boiled into rage. His burner phone made a buzzing sound, indicating an incoming text message. He always carried a second phone for confidential communications with the boss. He saw his note *Did you get her?*

He texted back *Not yet. WIP.*

Another buzz sound. *LMK*

He responded. *2nite*

The phone went silent. Boris thought about his recent encounter. The couple had been clearly heading towards the apartment. Then, something had led them into a different direction. The girl had been distracted the whole time. Perhaps some flaws in her soon-to-be-dead head. Boris had an excellent sixth sense for human behavior. Whatever they did now was probably just a detour. He decided to go to the apartment and wait for them there.

- 15 -
Terrel
ACUTE CHEST SYNDROME

Tuesday, May 25, 2032, 12.00 pm.

Terrel had submitted an emergency warrant to track the location of Susan Pellegrini's cell phone. A standard operator can find the location of a cell phone within a distance of about 1000 meters. The exact accuracy is dependent on many factors, most notably the number of cell towers in the area. Conditions in San Francisco were good, and the IT team of the FBI could localize Susan's cell phone precisely, assigning it to specific buildings in the Mission Bay district. Unfortunately, by the time Terrel had arrived in San Francisco, the signal of Susan's cell phone had vanished. Presumably, the battery had died. Terrel asked the IT team to send him the most recent history data of the phone's locations. He planned to work his way backwards from there.

Apparently, Susan had visited the San Francisco General Hospital in the morning and a café close by shortly before noon. With little hope of still finding her there, Terrel went to the café first. He walked around the patio in front of the café and then through the small interior seating area. As expected, he did not see Susan or the suspect from the composite photo. Terrel decided to question the staff of the café. Fortunately, there were only two waiters on service. Terrel discreetly showed them his FBI ID. They were quite impressed and led him to a quiet corner, where Terrel explained that he was searching for two people of interest to the FBI. He showed them Susan's photo and the phantom image of the second thief. One of the waiters remembered Susan. He was not sure about the second person. He did remember that she had been with a young man. The other waiter also remembered Susan and reported that both customers had casts around an arm. He had never seen a couple cast and had wondered what accident had caused it. Terrel made a note. Unfortunately, the waiters did not remember much more. Terrel left the café. On his way out, he felt a sharp pain in his chest. He stopped and grasped for air. One of the waiters came looking after him and asked if he needed anything else. Terrel declined. The pain was slowly getting better. He left.

Terrel next went to Susan's apartment. He rang the bell, but nobody answered. He tried again, unsuccessfully. He always had a lockpick in his pocket and now he used it to open the main entrance door. He saw a long corridor with about five doors on each side, presumably multiple small apartments. Some doors had name signs, others did not. Terrel did not find Susan's name. A staircase led to the second floor and an almost identical corridor. Terrel checked the doors upstairs as well. He was lucky. He found a name tag with Susan's name on the third door on the right. Terrel knocked on the door, but nobody answered. He used the lockpick to open this door as well. He entered a sparsely furnished room, which showed little signs of anybody living in it. The apartment was a living room/dining room combination in an L-shape, featuring two upholstered chairs and an ottoman close to the entrance, which faced a small bookcase with a TV monitor on top. At the corner of the L was a high racetrack dining table with two highchairs, placed like a dining bar in front of a small kitchenette. The other part of the L-shaped room was separated by a dark-blue silk curtain and contained a freshly made queen bed, a nightstand and a small wardrobe, which was placed against the curtain to serve as a room divider. A door led to an adjacent small bathroom. Terrel checked the bathroom and kitchenette. No signs of recent use. The chest pain came back. He bent forwards in agony and sat down on one of the highchairs, resting his forearms on the table. He took a deep breath and waited. The pain slowly ebbed away. Terrel took a pen and a business card out of his pocket and wrote on the back of the card. *Susan Pellegrini. Please call me when you get this. This is an emergency.* He placed the card on the table and left.

Terrel's next stop was the San Francisco General Hospital, where Susan had apparently been earlier that morning. The waiter in the cafe had reported that Susan had a cast around her right arm. Perhaps she had received the cast in the ER here. Terrel walked towards the ER entrance to talk with the security guard. The guard looked him up and down, suspicion flickering in his face, a look that Terrel was used to as a Black man. Terrel showed his FBI badge and introduced himself. After seeing the badge, the guard became much friendlier and eagerly offered to help. Terrel showed him the photo of Susan and the phantom sketch as well. The guard did not remember when Susan had entered the ER. But he did remember that she and a young Asian man came out of the ER around 10.30 am, both wearing casts. That was surely memorable! The guard also remembered that the couple walked away on foot, but he did not remember in which direction exactly. Terrel thought that this information was promising and consistent with Susan's' sighting in the café. Hopefully, the couple was not far away. Terrel thanked the guard and entered the ER.

At the ER reception, Terrel showed his badge again and a photo of Susan. Fortunately, the receptionist also remembered Susan and brought Terrel to the ER physician who had taken care of her. Dr. Calvin Williams was a tall Black man in his late forties, who greeted him with a warm smile. "Hello, Agent Wright, it is great to meet you. I will be happy to talk with you. I am just afraid I have to take care of an emergency first before we can speak."

"Of course, I understand," Terrel responded.

"Please come this way." Dr. Williams led him to a small windowless office, which contained a large desk, a desk chair and two chairs in front of it, presumably for visitors. He invited Terrel to take a seat and rushed towards the hallway. Terrel sat down and looked around. He saw the back of a computer screen and a pile of letters, journals and papers on the desk. Multiple framed certificates were hanging on the wall behind the desk. Apparently, Dr. Williams was a highly accomplished physician with multiple honors and awards. Different people were rushing by the half-open office door. Terrel appreciated a little break. The chest pain had come back, and he was having trouble breathing. He closed his eyes for a moment. After about twenty minutes, Dr. Williams came back and sat down on the desk chair, facing him. Terrel tried to ignore the pain and focus on the interview. He asked about the encounter with Susan this morning, and Dr. Williams described his findings in detail, including the fact that he had thought she had taken some kind of drug. *This was alarming!* Terrel made careful notes. While they were talking, Terrel felt Dr. Williams's observing gaze. After a while, an expression of concern appeared on Dr. Williams's face.

"Mr. Wright," he asked, "do you feel all right?"

"Well, I have had some chest pain all morning," Terrel responded.

"You look like you are in distress," Dr. Williams diagnosed, "and you are taking many shallow breaths, perhaps to avoid pain with deep inspiration. Do you have any known lung problem?"

"I was diagnosed with sickle cell disease as a child."

"Well, that could explain your current symptoms," Dr. Williams said. "I would suggest that you get a chest x-ray right away. That could show us if you have a pneumonia or an acute chest syndrome related to your sickle cell disease."

"I have to find a missing girl as soon as possible," Terrel responded. "She could be in grave danger."

"Well, you cannot help anybody if you collapse on the street," Dr. Williams pointed out. "We are an emergency room here. We can get you an x-ray fairly quickly and you can decide the next best step from there."

Terrel sighed. "You may be right. Let's get the chest x-ray."

Dr. Williams made a phone call, and a nurse practitioner came in, who introduced himself as Kurt. He entered Terrel's information into the computer system and then brought him to the Radiology suite, where an x-ray technician obtained an an x-ray of his chest. From there, Kurt led Terrel to an examination room, where he asked him to lie down on the stretcher. *Ahh, it felt good to lie down!*

Terrel's cell phone rang. He saw Stella Pellegrini's name on the display.

"This is Terrel Wright."

"Hello, Agent Wright," she responded. "I am sorry to bother you. I just arrived at my daughter's apartment. She's not here, but I found your card on the table."

"Mrs. Pellegrini, good to hear from you!" Terrel responded. "I am at the San Francisco General Hospital. Susan visited the ER here just a few hours ago."

"Oh, was she injured?" Stella exclaimed. "Is she still there?"

"I am afraid, she left already," Terrel explained, "but it seemed that she was okay overall, apart from a broken clavicle and broken bone in her hand. These fractures have been taken care off by the ER staff. She received a cast and a sling to support the broken arm. Susan walked away someone who claimed to be her brother. I assume that she is not very far from us. Unfortunately, the battery of her cell phone went off and I cannot track her location right now."

"Susan does not have a brother!" Stella exclaimed.

"I know. It was almost certainly her boyfriend."

"Should I come over to meet you at the General Hospital?" Stella asked.

"I don't think there is much more to do here," Terrel responded. "It would be most helpful if you could wait for Susan in her apartment. Please call me as soon as she gets there."

"I am so worried!" Susan said. "I wished I could speed up the time and fast forwards to the moment when I can talk with her!"

"Sit tight," Terrel responded. "Susan left the ER by foot and the apartment is only a few blocks away. I assume she will get there eventually."

"Thank you for your encouragement, Mr. Wright! Talk to you soon!"

Terrel hung up the phone. They had to wait for Susan to show up at her apartment. So, it was probably okay to use some time to take care of his health. He called Angus Weber and informed him that he would take a break from his duties. Angus approved.

A few minutes later, Dr. Williams came into the examination room. He opened a file on his computer and brought up a radiograph.

"Mr. Wright, please have a look," he said. "Here is your chest x-ray."

Terrel had taken courses on x-ray interpretation as part of his FBI training. He looked at the x-ray with great interest.

"Looks like there is no pneumonia or infiltrate in the lungs," he concluded.

"Correct," Dr. Williams responded. "I do not see any infiltrate in the lungs. That is good news. However, your bones are affected. They are overall quite dense. In addition, the lateral radiograph shows a depression of the upper and lower endplate of the vertebral bodies. This leads to H-shaped vertebrae, a characteristic finding in Sickle Cell disease." He pointed to the H-shaped vertebral bodies.

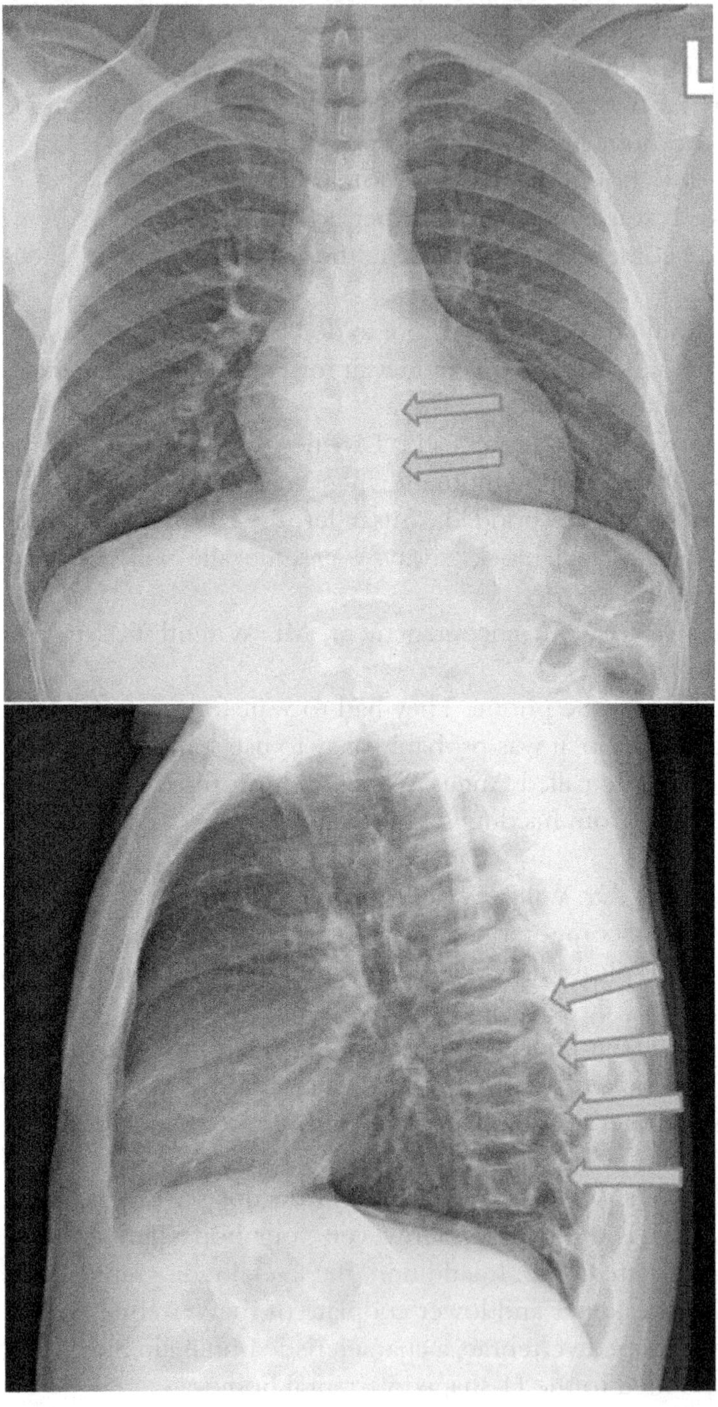
L

"How did the vertebral bodies get to this shape?" Terrel asked.

Dr. Williams explained. "Normally, red blood cells are smooth and round. Under certain conditions, such as stress, an infection or dehydration, some of the red blood cells in patients with sickle cell disease can turn into crescent-shaped cells which look like sickles, hence the name. The sickle-shaped cells can block the blood flow in small blood vessels. When the sickle cells obstruct vessels in the bones, they can cause bone infarctions. This can lead to bone pain, an impression of the upper and lower endplate and H-shape of the vertebral bodies, as seen on your x-ray. When the sickle cells obstruct vessels in the lungs, it can lead to breathing problems, and a condition called the acute chest syndrome."

"Can you treat it?" Terrel asked.

"We will first measure the oxygen level in your blood and take a blood sample to see if you have an anemia or signs of an infection," Dr. Williams explained. "I presume your symptoms are relatively mild, but I want to confirm that. In the meantime, we will give you some fluid via an intravenous line, medication against the pain and some oxygen via a mask if you need it. If we find a severe anemia, then you would need a blood transfusion. But I don't think that will be necessary."

"Remember, I am on duty. I have limited time for this," Terrel said.

"You might just have to invest a little more time to take care of your health," Dr. Williams responded with a compassionate smile. "Of course, you can sign paperwork that you want to leave at your own discretion at any time."

Terrel thought about it for a moment. He knew that it was important for him to remain hydrated. He probably had forgotten to drink enough fluid in the midst of the brain chip case. Dr. Williams was right that he could not chase a thief or murderer in his current condition. He had to get better first.

"Okay," he leaned back on the stretcher and Kurt stepped in to prepare his intravenous line.

- 16 -
Stella
THE APARTMENT

Tuesday, May 25, 2032, 1.00 pm.

Stella was a bit relieved. At least Susan was well enough that she was walking around in the city! *What on earth was she thinking, stealing these brain chips?* Ever since her father died, Susan had become so tense, so focused on achieving something. Stella wiped away a tear in the corner of her eye. Susan was studying around the clock, collecting honors and awards like others collected stamps. As her mother, Stella knew that Susan was just longing for approval and acceptance. But no matter what she accomplished; nothing could fill the gap that the death of her father had caused. Stella had tried very hard, but she could not provide for their expenses and fill the roles of two parents at the same time. She felt drained and exhausted. Why would Susan steal from anyone, let alone SUEC University? Did she not understand that the university provided for both of their living? What if Stella lost her job because of her daughter's stupid actions? Not to mention the consequences for Susan's future! Stella's emotions undulated between concern and anger. She would *make* Susan apologize and give the brain chips back immediately! Stella looked around Susan's empty apartment. She felt such an urgency to talk to her daughter! But Susan was not here. Right now, there was nothing Stella could do but wait. Stella sat down on Susan's bed. This morning had been exhausting! Why not lie down for a moment? Stella took off her shoes, made herself comfortable on Susan's bed and instantly fell into a deep sleep.

***

Stella woke up at the sound of a key turning in the lock of the door. She jumped to her feet and rushed to the entrance to embrace her daughter. But she froze at the sight of a man in a black leather jacket, who entered the apartment. *Was this the suspect from the sketch that Lili had shown her?* No, she decided, the man on the phantom image was Polynesian and had curly dark hair. This man in front of her had Slavic features with light brown hair and short sideburns. The man looked different. He had a pointy chin, flat cheeks and a longer forehead. This was someone else. Stella noted a brief hint of surprise on the man's face as he saw her, which changed quickly into a solemn expression. Keeping his eyes on her, the man stepped into the room and slowly closed the door behind him. Stella instinctively sensed inescapable danger. Her heart started racing and little pearls of sweat formed on her temples. She felt like a little rabbit in front of a hunting wolf. Stella did not move. The man looked at her with his deep dark eyes, silent. She heard the door lock click – it was shut. The man reached with his right hand into the inner pocket of his leather jacket and his hand came out with a weapon. Stella gasped. The man pointed a gun at her.

"Babushka," he said with a calm, friendly voice, "would you please take a seat on the chair over there." He pointed to one of the highchairs.

Stella looked at him with wide, fearful eyes. "What do you want?" she asked with a trembling voice. "If you want money, my purse is over there." She pointed to the bedroom.

"That is very kind of you, to offer me money," the man smiled at her. "But I am here for something else. I am sure you can help me out later."

Stella's thoughts were racing. The man stood between her and the door. There was no escape. But this was an apartment building. The other tenants would surely be around. Perhaps she should scream for help.

As if he had read her thoughts, the man said calmly, "Do you see my gun here?"

Stella nodded.

"One tone out of your mouth and you will be dead."

Stella nodded again, trembling. She sat down on the chair.

The man came closer, pointing the gun at her. He pulled two plastic ties out of his pocket, handed them to Stella and asked her to tie her ankles to the legs of the chair. Susan complied. The man then put the gun on the table and tied her wrists to the chair as well. Stella looked at the gun in terror, tears running down her face. Finally, the man grabbed a small towel from the kitchenette, rolled it to a tight bun and shoved it into Stella's mouth. Stella grasped for air. She thought she might faint.

The man looked at her. Was there pity in his gaze?

"I just need your assistance," he said calmly. "If you cooperate, nothing will happen to you."

Stella stared at him with wide open eyes.

The man looked around, searching for something. He finally found some duct tape in one of the drawers of the kitchenette. He rolled it over Stella's head and mouth to secure the bun in her mouth.

Then he put his gun back into his jacket and sat down on the other chair.

Stella looked at him. He was waiting for something. Or someone.

Susan! Stella started to tremble uncontrollably, wringing her wrists under the plastic ties. But that only caused her skin to break, adding physical pain to the horrendous agony she felt inside.

- 17 -
Lili
THE MOLE

Tuesday, May 25, 2032, 3.00 pm.

The medical team at SUEC hospital got really busy in the ER and time flew by. The rest of the afternoon was uneventful with regards to the brain chip case. Lili checked her phone a few times but did not receive any update from Stella in San Francisco. Hopefully, everything was all right there.

At 3 pm she ordered a family-size pizza from the hospital cafeteria. The hospital leadership had noted that healthcare personnel often did not have the time to walk to the cafeteria during the lunch hour. To address this problem, the cafeteria had created a delivery service for personnel in the hospital, which was very popular. The pizza arrived right away. Lili placed it in the break room and invited Annya, Santiago and Matthew to join her. To ensure continuous clinical services, Santiago and Matthew went to eat first, while Annya continued to see patients and Lili created reports for their radiographs. Then they switched. Santiago and Matthew went back to work and Annya and Lili met in the break room.

"How are you keeping up?" Annya asked, "These have been two very stressful days. One could think we are part of a movie."

"Yes, indeed!" Lili responded. "This morning, Stella told me that the suspect who received a cast here may be a friend of her daughter, Susan. If that isn't shocking enough, Terrel showed her the video from the lab and Stella thought that the second thief with the long black ponytail might be Susan!"

"Wow, that would put her daughter in true danger!" Annya said. "I bet that Juan Perez was killed because of the stolen brain chip."

"And Robert Hill was attacked," Lili added.

"Well, he took on the thief, which was very brave," Annya said.

"If I saw a masked criminal in my ER, I would probably call 911!"

"Same here," Lili said. "But I got the impression that these brain chips are like his babies. I believe he will defend them with everything he's got."

"I am sure you are right," Annya chuckled. "Micro-computers are taking over the world!"

"Do you think *we* are in danger?" Lili asked.

Annya shook her head. "Who would care about us? I don't think we are in any danger. We don't have the chips."

"I hope you are right." Lili had felt uneasy all morning. *What if they were in danger?*

Annya lowered her voice. "Can you keep a secret?"

"Of course!"

"I can protect us if needed," she whispered. "I was harassed and attacked as a young woman. Fortunately, I got away. But I experienced a post-traumatic stress disorder afterwards and I took self-defense classes to ease my symptoms."

Lili looked at Annya in surprise. She had known her for several years now and Annya had never mentioned this. Lili had always envied her for her good looks. Harassment. Perhaps this was an explanation for Annya's preference to be single and her deep passion to help traumatized people.

"Since the incident, I have learned a lot," Annya explained further. "I hold a black belt and am a legal concealed gun carrier."

"Wow!" Lili exclaimed. "Does Dr. Bennett know this?"

Annya smiled. "I did not tell him that. I did not want to smell like trouble. But I am pretty sure the FBI guys will have checked us all out and they might know."

Lili saw an entirely new person in front of her. Annya had always been very uptight about her past. Lili did not know anything about her family or where she had worked or lived previously. *It often takes a strong trigger to reveal traumatizing events from the past,* she thought. *Even though Annya appears calm and composed, the death of Juan Perez and his wife might have shaken her quite a bit. I will keep an eye on her, to make sure she is okay.*

Lili smiled at Annya. "Well, I am honored to have a warrior as my friend!"

Annya smiled back, but her lips tightened. "I do my best to stay away from any confrontations. But if someone attacks me or any of my friends, I will not be an easy victim again!"

The door of the break room flung open, and Aiko's head appeared. As the most senior woman in the ER, she clearly saw Lili and Annya – and any younger woman for that matter – in her chain of command. "Hello ladies, your break is over, we have an incoming polytrauma!"

Lili and Annya jumped to their feet and followed Aiko to the trauma emergency room.

***

At 4:40 pm, Lili made her way to the dean's office for the scheduled afternoon meeting. She asked Annya if she wanted to join, but Annya said that she was too busy in the ER and her shift was not yet over. She had informed Dr. Bennett that she would not be able to come. So, Lili left alone. It took her about ten minutes to drive up to the SUEC campus and another fifteen minutes to walk up the promenade to the octagon building. She would be late – again. Lili entered the SUEC building. There were few people in the lobby and Stella's desk was empty. Lili checked herself in at the ID scanner and iris detector and walked past Stella's desk into the octagon lobby, past the beautiful orchid garden, up the rainbow stairs and towards Dr. Bennett's office. The door was closed. Lili knocked and heard Dr. Bennett calling "come in." She opened the door and saw Dr. Bennett and Agent Weber sitting at the conference table. They both looked at her with serious expressions on their faces. Lili got a funny feeling. She did not know what it was exactly, but the situation in the room felt cold and unfriendly.

"Lili, please come in," Dr. Bennett said with a calm voice.

Lili walked into the room and took a seat at the table.

"Are the others coming as well?" she asked.

"Actually, we wanted to talk with you alone," Dr. Bennett explained.

"Oh?" she said, surprised.

Angus Weber took over the conversation. "I am afraid, there is an issue."

"What kind of issue?" Lili asked.

Dr. Bennett interjected, "Lili, can you please let Mr. Weber finish his sentence. Stop talking back for a moment, would you?"

"I am not talking back," she responded. "I am trying to understand what is going on."

"Well," Dr. Bennett said with distress in his eyes, "we are concerned that there might be someone in our team, who provided the thieves – perhaps also the murderer – with inside information,"

"Why would you think that?" Lili asked, confused.

Angus Weber explained, "We have reviewed all the evidence thus far. Only our core team knew that the thieves had encountered a fracture and that Juan Perez visited the ER. Yet, about an hour after we became aware of Juan's visit to the ER, he was killed. Similarly, only our core team knew about the stolen brain chips. Yet, this morning, someone broke into the lab and tried to steal the concept files. If the thieves had been interested in the concept paper, they would have stolen them with their first visit. Someone in our team is leaking information, knowingly or unknowingly."

"Who could that be?" Lili still did not understand.

"If we go by exclusion," Angus Weber said, "then, Dr. Bennett here cannot be the suspect since he had meetings with various people all day long. In addition, we recorded all his phone calls, texts and emails for security reasons. Annya Segond cannot be the suspect since she worked all day long in the ER. Witnesses can confirm that she did not make any private phone calls between our initial meeting and the Perez killing. You, however, had multiple interactions that influenced our case. You might have — advertently or inadvertently — shared sensitive information with others that informed the criminals that we are trying to track them down. "

"I did not share any information!" Lili responded, outraged about this startling accusation.

"Well, you shared information with my assistant," Dr. Bennett responded. "As a result, she has called in sick. I called her this afternoon to see how she's doing. But she does not answer her phone and she does not seem to be at home. We do not know where she is right now, and I am getting very concerned that she might be in danger!"

"You asked me to show the phantom photo around!" Lili exclaimed, raising her voice.

"We wanted to identify the person in the ER," Angus responded.

"The theft of the chip should have been kept confidential."

"Well, Stella helped us to identify her daughter Susan as one of the thieves!" Lili exclaimed. "And by the way, your colleague Terrel showed the video to Stella and her input significantly informed his mission too...."

"You should not distract from your own indiscretion by accusing an FBI agent," Angus responded with a calm, icy voice. "Terrel was just doing his job."

"So, what are you accusing me of exactly?" Lili asked, holding his hostile gaze.

Dr. Bennett tried to intervene. "Lili, we understand that you might mean well. But we believe that your inquisitive nature might have somehow informed these criminals. Perhaps someone overheard your discussion with Stella – or Terrel – or Dr. Hill. Do you realize that you have had many sensitive conversations in public lately?"

"No, I do not realize that," Lili said angrily. She did not know Agent Weber or his intentions. But she had thought she knew Dean Bennett. She would have expected his support in this conversation. "All conversations that I had were with members of our core team and occurred in closed rooms."

"Well, just as a precaution, we would ask you to not engage any further in your own detective work," Angus said. "Please focus on your clinical work as a radiologist. To preserve the confidentiality of this mission, Dr. Bennett will check in separately with you, Dr. Segond and Dr. Hill and report any relevant observations to me."

"Lili, we are in a very delicate situation here. Please remember that this is a strictly confidential mission," Dr. Bennett added. "You are not authorized to discuss this matter with anyone, enter a crime scene or do any investigations of your own. Is this understood?"

"Of course," Lili responded, her teeth clenched.

Lili turned around and left Dr. Bennett's office. She felt crushed. She had diagnosed the Smith fracture, she had identified the suspect in the ER, she had diagnosed the spine fracture that revealed a homicide and she had uncovered that Susan's daughter was involved. And now these two men were accusing her of being a *problem* to their case? This situation was not "complicated." Two men abused their power to beat a woman down with fabricated arguments. Did they actually believe what they just told her? Or were they just following some undisclosed agenda? Either way, Lili did not deserve to be treated this way! Her input had helped to identify the suspects! Fighting down welling tears in her eyes, she walked down the hallway, stomped down the opulent stairs and out of the lobby.

To ease her mind, Lili called her husband Mark as she walked to the parking lot, telling him about her most recent encounters. As a radiologist and physician-scientist himself, Mark was intimately familiar with the challenges that women faculty were still facing in the field of medicine. His unshakable support and no-nonsense attitude kept Lili sane and grounded. His first response was, "What is wrong with these guys?"

"I don't know," Lili said. "How can they treat me this way?"

"The FBI agent does not know you. So, we give him some slack," Mark responded. "But Dr. Bennett should have stood up for you!"

Whatever was thrown her way, Mark always managed to bring a smile back on Lili's face.

"I know! I was so baffled that he did not have my back!"

"Remember, at the core, this is not about you. This is about them. These guys are overwhelmed by the situation and need to blame someone. I am sorry it was you."

"What baffles me is this horrendous ignorance. They would not have a clue who stole the chips if I had not identified the thieves. Now, they are accusing me? This is really too much!"

"They do have a point that, apparently, somebody is leaking information to the criminals," Mark said in his matter-of-fact tone. "Dr. Perez' name is revealed in the ER and shortly afterwards, he is killed. It could be a coincidence. But it is strange. If we assume that somebody is leaking information and it was not you, who else could it have been?"

"I am not sure," Lili responded, thinking.

"Could it have been the young FBI officer? He was in the ER when you identified Juan Perez?"

"I don't think so," Lili said decisively. "Terrel is rock solid. He is an FBI agent. I assume he went through a very thorough background check before he was trained and started his position. In addition, from my interactions with him, I think he is absolutely straight-up."

"Well, that's a great disguise for a serial killer!" Mark said.

"I am sure, it was not Terrel," Lili said. "Let's not stoop to the same low level. Biases are the stories we make up about people before we know them."

"Just be careful," Mark said. "There is always a true core to annoyances like this. Someone may be out there, extracting information from your team."

"Perhaps someone placed a bugging device in Dr. Bennett's office," Lili thought out loud.

"…or in your reading room," Mark said. "For all we know, somebody could be listening in on our conversation right now!"

Mark made her laugh again. "Okay, I better get going. I just wanted to let you know that I will briefly stop over at Susan Pellegrini's place. Stella went there earlier today, and I want to make sure she's fine. She did not call or text me at all."

"So much for 'do not get involved.'" Mark laughed as well. "Nobody tames my rebellious wife. Do you remember that we have a date for dinner?"

"Of course! I might only be a little late."

Lili and Mark both had very busy jobs. But they always tried to be home for their dinner around 8 pm. This was their daily extension of their first date dinner and continued to be relaxing and rejuvenating for both of them. They sometimes dined out or invited family and friends. But for the most part, they enjoyed this routine for the majority of their evenings.

"I'm just checking on Stella and her daughter. I will text you when I leave Susan's place."

"Okay, sounds good!" Mark said. "Take care!"

"I love you!" Lili send him a mental kiss and a wonderful warm feeling filled her heart. She thought, *I have the best husband in the world!*

- 18 -
Boris
MAISONNEUVE FRACTURE

Tuesday, May 25, 2032, 3.30 pm.

After Boris and Stella had waited in Susan's apartment what felt like an eternity, they heard a key in the lock of the door. Boris jumped from his highchair. The chair crashed to the ground. Stella tried to scream but released only a muffled noise. Boris gave her a stern look, pulled his gun and pointed it on her head. Stella went silent. The door flung open, and Susan entered with a young man. Stella saw the usual innocent, cheerful expression on her daughter's face as she entered the room. She also noted the more mature, alert, protective gaze of her companion as he looked around. *This was the young man from the FBI sketch! My god – they both had casts! Susan was hurt!* Yet they both seemed to be in good spirits. Susan and her friend were completely self-absorbed, chatting with each other as they entered the room. Then they noticed the noise of the fallen chair. The young man looked up and stared at the gun, which pointed at Susan.

Susan saw the gun as well. Her jaw dropped down, and she let out a scream.

"Close the door," Boris said in a low voice.

Susan reached for the door handle, missed it, reached for it again, then shut the door with a bang.

"Are you drunk?" Boris said. "No more noise — or you will hear my gun.

Susan looked at him with an intense, deep gaze. Stella inspected her daughter. Her eyes had changed somehow. Was she really drunk?

Boris looked at Susan. "Give me the chips," he said.

"I'm sorry, they are not here," Susan responded with a tense low voice. "They are in a safe place."

"Show me your purse," Boris pointed at her shoulder bag.

Stella shook her head. *No, no, no!* She tried to tell her daughter to stay away from the man, no matter the consequences. But only a croaking sound came out of her clogged mouth.

Boris looked at her. "Shut up!"

Susan approached the man. "It's okay," she said in a calm voice. "Leave my mother alone. She has nothing to do with this."

"I did not know she's your mother!" Boris said, apparently pleased that Susan complied. "No worries, I respect baboolya." He padded Stella's back. "I would be happy to trade her for you." He stretched out his arms in a gesture of victory.

Susan walked towards him with a resolute look on her face. She offered her purse with an outstretched hand.

"Toss it around," Boris demanded. He liked the control that he had over the young woman.

Susan turned the purse around. Multiple items fell to the ground. Her iPhone, a lipstick, tissue papers, a pen, a few pennies.

"Give it to me" Boris asked, pointing at the purse.

Susan handed the purse to him. He investigated it. It was empty.

"Come here" Boris asked, waving his hand for Susan to come closer.

"Take me!" the young man exclaimed, following Susan.

"Sorry, brother, " Boris responded, pointing his gun at him. "You stay where you are right now. Who are you anyways?"

The young man stopped. "I am Kaleo Kahale, Susan's fiancé." Both Stella and Susan looked at Kaleo in surprise. Neither of them was aware of an engagement.

Boris laughed. "Well, I am sorry to interrupt your wedding plans, Kaleo. Susan and I have some other plans."

"Susan is not well, she needs supervision!" the young man exclaimed.

"Don't worry, I will take good care of her!" Boris chuckled. "In the meantime, you could do me a favor."

"What is that?" Kaleo looked at him with contempt.

"You will get the brain chips for me," Boris said. He tossed a burner phone towards Kaleo. "I will give you a call and let you know where you can trade the chips for her." He pointed the gun at Susan. "No word to anyone, or your fiancé is dead."

Boris looked at Stella. "You will also stay silent, babka," he said with a wry smile. "Make sure Kaleo brings the chips to me, and you will get your daughter back!"

Then he looked at Susan. "Let's leave, honey! We don't want to be late for dinner."

He pointed towards the door. Susan looked at him, the gun and back. *If I do not comply, he will shoot us,* she thought. She moved slowly towards the exit.

Suddenly, Boris turned around and gave the highchair with Stella a push. The chair and Stella flew backwards. Kaleo jumped towards Stella in order to catch her. Stella's left leg crashed into the second chair, which was lying on the ground. Kaleo managed to catch her with his good left arm before her head hit the floor. They both fell to the ground.

This maneuver had cleared the exit way. Boris quickly turned around, opened the apartment door and pushed Susan into the hallway. He grabbed Susan's left arm, pulled her closer towards him and pointed the gun under the cover of his jacket at her. Susan willingly followed his lead and they disappeared in the hallway.

Kaleo checked the cast around his arm and moved his fingers. The rescue jump had not caused any new injuries. He asked Stella if she was okay. She nodded.

Kaleo jumped up and ran to the door. But Susan and the man were already gone. Kaleo ran down the hallway and out of the building to the street. He looked in all directions. But there was no sign of Susan. Perhaps they had taken a different exit. Kaleo circled around the building three more times, then he ran up and down the street. But still, he could not find Susan anywhere. Finally, Kaleo returned to the apartment to check on Stella. She lay on the floor, tied to the chair. Kaleo went to the kitchenette, found a pair of scissors and cut the plastic ties around Stella's wrists and ankles. She moaned as he touched her left leg.

"Did you find her?" she cried, even though the answer was obvious.

"I am so sorry, Mrs. Pellegrini; it seems that they are gone."

Stella sobbed. "My leg hurts!"

Kaleo inspected her lower leg. It was clearly in disarray, likely broken. "You need to see a doctor. The General Hospital is just a few blocks away. I will call an Uber and get you there."

Stella was now sobbing uncontrollably. "We need to rescue Susan," she whispered. "This man will kill her!"

"I will not let that happen!" Kaleo said with a trembling voice. "I will get this guy what he wants. Let me bring you to the hospital first. That's what Susan would want if she were here now. Then I'll go, get the chips and bring them to this guy."

Stella's despair turned into anger. "This is all your fault! How could you get my daughter into this horrible situation?" she shouted at Kaleo.

Kaleo blushed. "Mrs. Pellegrini, stealing the chips was not my idea. This was Susan's project. I just went along to make sure she was safe."

Stella looked at him for a long time. She sensed that he was telling the truth. Kaleo was honest, considerate and *very* handsome. If they had met under different circumstances, she might have liked him.

They looked at each other for a while, both lost in their thoughts. Kaleo could not bear her gaze. He pulled his cell phone and typed something into it.

"I believe you," Stella finally said. "I just wished you had tried to talk her out of this!"

Kaleo looked up. "Believe me, I tried very, very hard. I am really sorry it turned out this way. Honestly, I was captivated by Susan's excitement. She can be very persuasive." A faint smile appeared on his face. "In addition, I thought that the university did not treat her well. They deserved to be punished."

Stella shook her head. "Well, who is being punished now?"

"I know, we messed up. Mrs. Pellegrini. I can assure you that I want to do everything to make this right. But first, we have to get you to the hospital. I just called an Uber and got a message that it will arrive in two minutes. Can we please go down to the street?"

Stella nodded in agreement. Kaleo helped Stella to get up on her feet. She moaned in pain as she tried to step on her left foot. Kaleo asked her to put her left arm around his shoulders. That was a little complicated as he also protected his casted arm. But they slowly made their way out of the apartment and down the stairs, where the Uber already waited for them. Stella had difficulty getting into the car. Her left lower leg had started to swell, and she couldn't bend her left knee. The Uber driver and Kaleo helped her into the backseat. Stella moved in sideways, with her legs extended. Kaleo took the passenger seat and they drove towards the hospital. While on their way, Stella noted Kaleo texting on his iPhone. She wondered who he was contacting now. She looked out of the window and saw the hospital coming closer. A minute later, they arrived at the driveway of the ER. The driver and Kaleo helped Stella out of the car. The Uber took off and Kaleo supported Stella again, as she slowly limped towards the entrance.

A young man with a familiar face crossed their way. Stella stopped to have a look at him. Then, she shouted, "Hello Amir!"

The young man looked at her in surprise. "Hello, Mrs. Pellegrini, it is good to see you!" He exchanged a quick look with Kaleo.

"What a coincidence!" Stella exclaimed. "Of all the days in my entire life, this would be the day when I would have wished to see you again!"

Amir looked at Stella and then at her leg. His face showed a worried expression. "Did you have an accident?" he asked.

"I'm afraid so," Stella answered. "That's why I came here." She pointed at Kaleo. "This young man was so kind to help me get here."

Amir looked at Kaleo with a blank face. "Thank you for helping Mrs. Pellegrini to get here. This is very kind of you!"

"Of course, no problem at all," Kaleo responded.

"In case you have some business to attend to," Amir said with a formal tone, "I know this lady and I can take care of her from here."

"That would be great," Kaleo said, looking at Amir with a blank face. He did not want anybody to notice that they knew each other. Kaleo turned to Stella. "I hope you're going to get better soon, Mrs. Pellegrini! I have your cell phone number and will keep in touch!"

Stella squeezed Kaleo's free hand. "Thank you for bringing me here, Kaleo. Please be careful and let me know as soon as you hear anything from Susan."

"I certainly will," Kaleo responded.

He nodded at Amir, turned around and walked away.

Amir offered Stella his arm and the two walked slowly to the ER reception. The receptionist had already seen them approaching and called a nurse practitioner, who waited for them with a wheelchair at the entrance. Stella sat down with a sigh. They checked in at the entrance and were brought to an examination room, where the nurse practitioner helped her to change into a hospital gown. Her left lower leg was markedly swollen and showed a large red-blue bruise. An x-ray technician came by to take a radiograph of her left leg. Amir waited outside and now came to join Stella, as they were waiting for the ER physician to come by. Stella was emotionally overwhelmed, moaning and sobbing uncontrollably. Amir held her hand and spoke to her in a calm, soothing voice. He had known Stella and Susan since he was a young child. They were like family to him. Amir wished he had seen them more often in recent years. Perhaps this whole tragedy could have been prevented if he had kept in touch. Sentence by sentence, he got a summary of the events in Susan's apartment. Stella slowly calmed down, looking into Amir's thoughtful, serene eyes. She somehow felt safe with him. She always had. After a while, a tall Black man in a white coat came in.

"Hello Mrs. Pellegrini, I'm Dr. Williams," he introduced himself. And he turned to Amir. "Good to see you, Amir! Do you know Mrs. Pellegrini?"

"Yes, we're old friends," Amir responded.

Dr. Williams nodded and turned to Stella. "Mrs. Pellegrini, I would like to discuss the findings of your left leg with you. Would you like Amir to stay in the room?"

"It is nice to meet you, Dr. Williams," Stella responded. "Yes of course, I would appreciate it if Amir would stay. He can explain the findings to me in more detail afterwards."

"Okay," Dr. Williams responded. "Let me show you what we found." He sat down in front of a desk and opened a computer file, which showed the radiograph of Stella's left leg."

"The x-ray shows a so-called Maisonneuve fracture," Dr. Williams explained.

What is that?" Stella asked.

"A Maisonneuve fracture is a combination of two injuries of the bones of the lower leg that happen at the same time," Dr. Williams explained. "The first is a fracture of the upper fibula, one of the two bones between your knee and ankle." He pointed to the fibula facture. "The second is an injury of the ligaments that hold the ankle joint together. This leads to a widened joint space between the distal tibia and calcaneus and results in an unstable ankle joint."

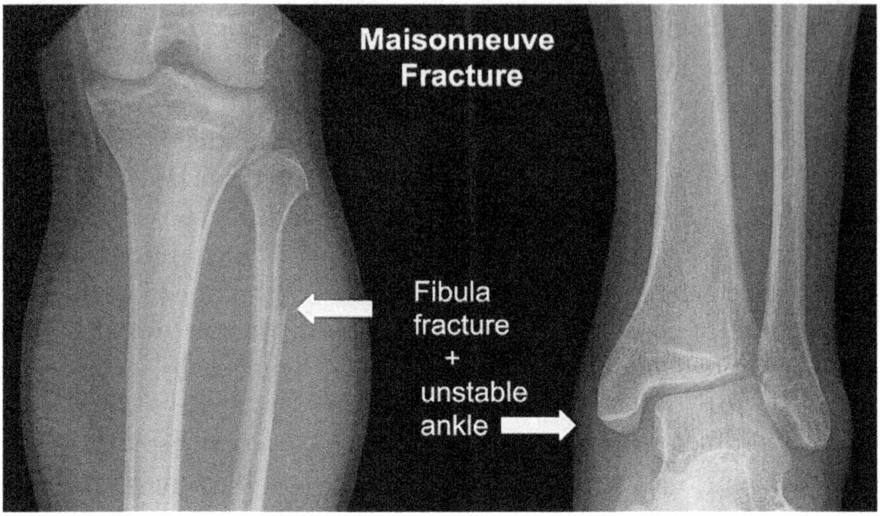

Dr. Williams turned to Amir. "You can see a widened medial ankle joint space here, which likely indicates a torn deltoid ligament. In this case here, there is also a small avulsion fracture of the medial malleolus, a tiny piece of bone that was ripped off during the injury." He pointed to a curvilinear density below the medial malleolus."

Amir nodded and asked, "Will this injury require an internal fixation?"

Dr. Williams responded, "Possibly. I suggest we obtain an MRI. I will also request a consultation with the orthopedic surgeons."

Stella said, "I am very sorry, but I cannot undergo a surgery right now. My daughter needs me."

Dr. Williams responded, "Mrs. Pellegrini, you cannot walk with this injury. I want to get you back on your feet. Our surgeons are very efficient. I am sure it won't take too long to stabilize your joint and get you home. Your daughter is most welcome to come visit or pick you up after the surgery."

Stella sent a pleading look to Amir.

"This is of course your decision," Amir said to Stella, "but it seems that we can only wait to hear from Susan or Kaleo at the moment. Why not fix your ankle joint in the meantime?"

Stella looked from Amir to Dr. Williams. She could not explain her agonizing fear to them. She was afraid that she would be in some surgery when Susan would reach out to her. What if her daughter needed her and she was under anesthesia? *What if I wake up and Susan is dead?*

Dr. Williams looked at her with a thoughtful expression. "You can give your cell phone to your nurse during the procedure if you like. The surgery should really not take very long, and it would be quite a co-incidence if your daughter would call you exactly during that time. But if she or anyone did call, your nurse can respond."

Stella thought about it for a moment, then she nodded in agreement. "I will keep my cell phone for now. But I would be grateful if a nurse can watch it while I am in the operating room tomorrow. I really hope the surgery won't take too long!"

Amir squeezed her hand. "I think you made the right decision, Mrs. Pellegrini. You need the surgery to get back up on your feet!"

Dr. Williams nodded and called the orthopedic surgery service for a consultation.

- 19 -
Lili
SCAPHOID FRACTURE

Tuesday, May 25, 2032, 5.15 pm.

On her commute to San Francisco, Lili called Stella, but she did not answer her phone. Lili arrived in the Mission Bay district shortly after 5 pm. She circled twice around the block until she finally found a spot. Lili parked the car and walked over to Susan's apartment. She rang the bell. Nobody answered. She tried again. No answer. Lili finally rang the bells of two other parties in the building. She heard the buzzer and the main door opened. She went up the stairs to the second floor. There, a long corridor led to multiple doors. Lili saw a head appearing from one of the doors and apologized that she had rung the wrong bell. The head disappeared and the door closed. Lili walked down the hallway and found Susan's name tag in front of one of the other doors. She rang the bell again. No answer. She took out a hairpin, inserted it into the lock and opened it. She had learned this little trick some time ago from her brother and it had served her very well on several occasions. The door flung open, and Lili walked into a sparsely furnished, single room apartment.

The room was a mess. Two highchairs were on the ground. Two pillows, a towel, some tape, an iPhone, lipstick, tissues, a pen, a few pennies and several plastic strips were spread over the floor. Lili looked at the plastic strips. Was there blood on them? She was not sure. *What had happened here?* She picked up the iPhone. It was dead. It had a girly, light-pink phone case around it, with numerous sparkles and a heart-shaped makeup mirror on the back. This was likely Susan's phone. Lili could not imagine that a teenager would voluntarily leave their cell phone behind. She could not quite put the pieces together. But something bad had happened here. Lili put the iPhone into the pocket of her jacket – perhaps it could provide useful information. She looked around some more. The bed looked like somebody had used it. Stella's jacket was lying on the nightstand. *Why was she not here?* Lili walked back to the living room area and found a business card in a corner under the table. She read. *Susan Pellegrini. Please call me when you get this. This is an emergency.* The other side of the card showed Terrel's name and phone number.

Lili sat down on one of the upholstered seats and tried to think. Susan, Stella and Terrel had all been here. The chaos in the room suggested some kind of fight. Susan and Stella were gone. They had left items behind which they would usually take with them. *Had Terrel Wright caused the chaos here?* Just as a precaution, Lili would be careful with him. If she wanted to find out what happened, she would have to talk to Susan or Stella. Lili called Stella again, and this time she did answer. "Hello?"

"Hello Stella, this is Lili."

"Lili, I am glad to hear your voice!"

"I just arrived at Susan's apartment and found a major mess here. What on earth happened?"

"Do you mean the stuff on the floor?"

"Yes, as a starter."

"I do not know how these things got tossed around. I slipped on a lipstick on the floor, fell and broke my leg!"

"Really? That is terrible! Where are you now?"

"I am in the ER at the San Francisco General Hospital."

"Is Susan with you?"

"No, I missed her. But she texted me that she is fine. So, perhaps I overreacted earlier today."

Lili was not sure what to make of Stella's story. It did not make sense to her. Earlier this morning, Stella could not wait to get to San Francisco to search for her daughter. Then, she arrived in Susan's apartment and slipped on a lipstick? Lili looked at the one and only lipstick on the floor. It showed no sign of damage whatsoever. She pulled the pink phone out of her pocket and looked at it again. It was locked. *Why was Stella suddenly not concerned about her daughter anymore?*

"Okay, I will come over there," Lili responded. "I just want to make sure you are alright."

"I will be glad to see you!" Stella said. "I hope they will let you in. There are several others here already. I will let the nurse practitioner know that you are on your way and ask for an exception to the visitor rules."

"Okay, see you soon!"

"See you soon!"

Lili hung up the phone, went back to her car and drove over to the General Hospital.

She was lucky. It was not too busy in the ER and the receptionist did let her in. She found Stella in one of the exam rooms, sitting sideways on a stretcher, with her legs elevated. As Lili walked in, Stella looked up. Her eyes were swollen, and tears were running down her face. "Lili!" she sobbed. "I couldn't protect her!" She looked exhausted. Lili walked over and gave her a big hug. Then, she pulled a chair next to her, sat down and put her arm around her to comfort her. "What happened?" she asked, gently. And Stella told her what she had missed in San Francisco that afternoon.

After Stella had brought her up to date, Lili asked, "Don't you think we should tell the whole story to the police? Or at least our friends from the FBI?"

"Nobody can know that Susan has been kidnapped!" Stella whispered. "Otherwise, we might endanger her life!"

"Perhaps you are right." Lili thought out loud. "Terrel asked you to wait in the apartment. But he did not join you there, right?"

"Yes, I did not think much of it at the time," Stella responded. "But now I am wondering why he did not come over to wait with me?"

The conversation was interrupted by two young men, who were entering the exam room. One was a tall Black man in a white coat. The ID on the front pocket declared him as an ER physician.

"Hello, my name is Dr. Williams," he introduced himself.

"Hello, I am Dr. Lili Pham, Stella's friend and a radiologist at SUEC," Lili responded. She did not usually introduce herself with her doctor title. But right now, it seemed helpful.

"Mrs. Pellegrini told us that you would be coming," Dr. Williams said. "I believe your support will be very helpful to her."

Lili noticed that Stella was exchanging some grimaces with the other man.

"Hello, I am Amir Nielsson, a nurse practitioner here at the

General hospital," he introduced himself. He had brought a ceramic cup with hot black tea, which he handed over to Stella. Since Lili was holding her right hand, Stella was reaching for it with her left hand. She gripped around the circumference of the cup, but then squealed and dropped it. The cup fell to the floor, splashing the tea in all directions.

"I'm so sorry!" she exclaimed. "I suddenly felt a sharp pain in my hand. I'm not sure what that was."

Lili fetched a few paper towels from the sink in the right corner of the room and wiped away the lake of tea.

"No problem," she said, "it is just hot water, easy to wipe away." Lili tossed a first set of wet paper towels into the trash can. She took a second set and moved it around with her foot to catch the splashes.

"No worries," Amir said. "I will call a cleaning service.

Lili looked at Stella's left hand. There was a dark blue bruise on the lower part of her hand, close to the wrist.

Amir also stepped closer and examined the hand. He pinched the area below the thumb and Stella responded with an "ouch."

"She has tenderness at the snuffbox," he said to Dr. Williams.

Dr. Williams stepped closer and had a look at Stella's hand as well.

"What is the snuffbox?" Stella asked.

"The snuffbox is a triangular depression found on the lateral aspect of the dorsum of the hand," Dr. Williams explained. "You can see it close to the thump when the thumb is extended. Historically, powdered tobacco was placed there for inhalation. Since nobody has found another use for this area, it kept the name. The powdered tobacco was also called dry snuff, hence the snuffbox. Pain in the snuffbox can indicate a fracture."

"Dr. Williams," Lili asked, "do you think it would be helpful to take a radiograph of Susan's hand?"

"Yes, absolutely," he responded. "We did have a look at this bruised area earlier. At the time, Mrs. Pellegrini localized the pain to the circumference of the wrist, which has some more superficial bruises. So, we assumed that this hematoma was secondary. But since she now indicates pain in this specific area, there could be an underlying fracture. We should definitely take an x-ray. I will submit a requisition for it."

Dr. Williams bowed slightly to us and walked out of the room.

This gave Stella some time to introduce Lili to the other man. "Lili, this is Amir Nielsson. His grandparents are my neighbors, and he grew up with them. I have known him since he was a baby. I was lucky to run into him today when I entered the ER. I also told him what happened to me and Susan today. He knows the whole story."

Lili looked at him. Amir was a tall and slender young man with a short, spiky haircut, a freckled, clean-shaven face and very expressive, intelligent green eyes. He looked concerned and a little tired.

"It is great to meet you, Lili. Mrs. Pellegrini spoke very highly of you, and I am so glad that she has a friend here in this difficult situation." He looked at Lili briefly, smiled politely, and then looked away. *He is avoiding eye contact,* she thought. *Is he hiding something?*

The x-ray technician came in and took a radiograph of Stella's left hand. A few minutes later, Dr. Williams came back in and showed the radiographs to Stella.

He pointed to a small bone of the lower hand, above the wrist. "Indeed, there is a fracture through the waist of the scaphoid bone," he explained.

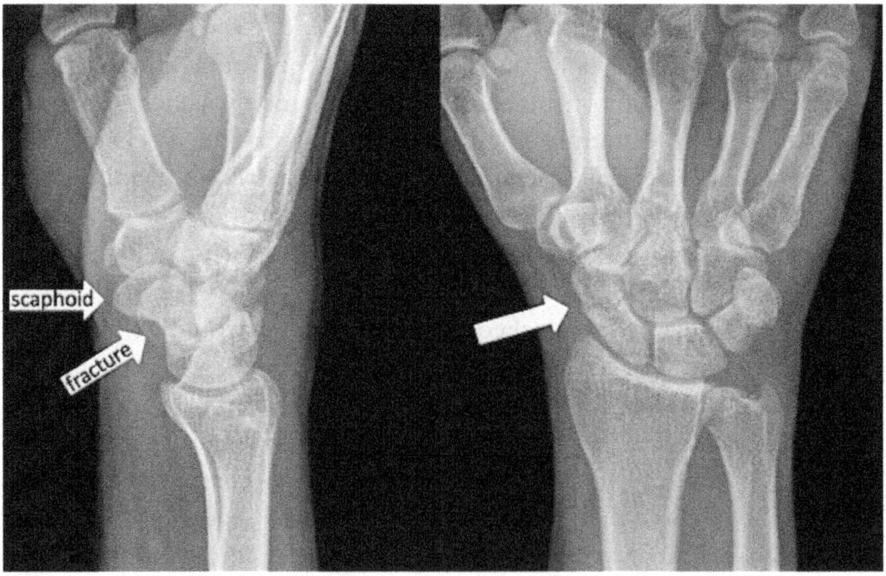

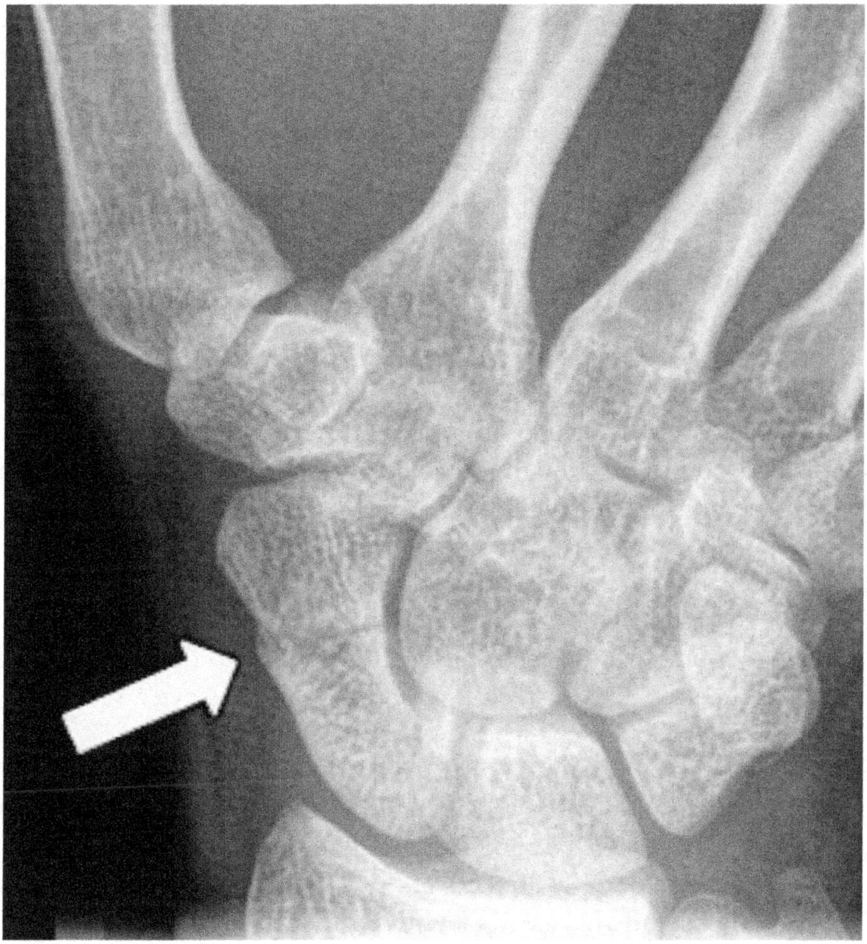

"Since the fracture is not displaced — I mean, the bone has not moved out of its usual place — we can try a treatment with a cast first. There is a risk that small vessels that supply this bone have been damaged as well. If that is the case, then the fracture might not heal, and further treatment might be needed. But at this point, we will try a cast first and hopefully the bone will heal."

"I certainly have enough trouble with one surgery!" Susan said. "If the hand injury can heal in a cast, I would very much prefer that."

"Of course, our team will do our best to make this as easy as possible for you Mrs. Pellegrini." Dr. Williams responded.

The door opened and Angus Weber and Terrel Wright walked in. Stella's eyes widened and she followed their moves closely. Their formal attire and serious demeanor conveyed authority and command.

Stella adjusted her blanket and greeted the two men politely. "Hello, Mr. Weber and Mr. Wright. What brings you here?"

Angus nodded at Stella, said hello and scanned everyone else in the room. His eyebrows frowned when he recognized Lili. "What are you doing here, Dr. Pham? I thought we had a very clear conversation earlier this afternoon. Which part of *do not get involved* did you not understand?"

"Hello Mr. Weber," Lili responded cheerfully. "It is great to see you too! I was just checking on my friend here, who had an accident. I am not aware of any law that forbids good citizens from visiting an injured friend in the hospital. Do you?" *She knew her rights.*

Angus Weber's face darkened. "I am watching you, Dr. Pham!" he said with an authoritative voice.

Terrel grinned, clearly enjoying the conversation.

"Of course, you need to do what you need to do." Lili flashed her most charming smile. "Would you like to have a seat?" She pointed to a free chair beside Stella's stretcher.

Lili prayed that Stella would not mention that she had been at Susan's apartment earlier today. But Stella had her own concerns, looking at Angus and Terrel with a weary gaze and tightened lips.

Angus only briefly looked at Dr. Williams and Amir. Their hospital gowns and IDs clearly identified them as hospital personnel. Lili made a mental note to not automatically dismiss hospital personnel as potentially related to a patient. Amir had stated earlier that he was working on a different ward. But he had turned his back to the new visitors and started to organize some paperwork on the small desk of the examination room, as if he were a nurse practitioner in the ER. *How strange!*

Dr. Williams sensed the tension in the room and apparently, was trying to change the subject. "Great to see you, Mr. Wright!" he said politely.

Angus looked from Dr. Williams to Terrel. "Do you know each other?"

"Dr. Williams treated me earlier today for a minor complaint," Terrel explained. "Remember, I asked you for authorization."

Angus nodded. "I remember that."

Terrel turned to Dr. Williams. "Thank you for taking care of me earlier today. I am feeling much better now!"

Angus Weber addressed Stella, "Mrs. Pellegrini, we were notified that you encountered an accident. We have been informed because this accident might be related to a matter of national security. Can you please tell us what happened? We also learned that your daughter went missing?"

Stella seemed overwhelmed. She looked from Lili to Angus. Perhaps his unfriendly behavior towards Lili made it easier for her to lie. "I went to my daughter Susan's apartment in the early afternoon today, to look for her. But I did not find her. There was quite a mess in her room. I tripped over something on the floor and broke my leg. That brought me here."

Terrel listened with a skeptical look on his face. He asked. "Mrs. Pellegrini, you called me in the early afternoon and told me that you wanted to wait for Susan in her apartment. Several hours later, you arrive in the ER with a broken leg. Are you telling us that this was just a simple accident in the apartment?"

Stella's face flushed. "Yes, exactly!" she responded with a defiant tone. "I tripped over a lipstick on the floor and broke my leg. Of course, I had to come here to get medical treatment."

Angus shook his head in disbelief. "Would you still like to find out where your daughter is?"

"Of course!" Stella shouted, getting clearly agitated by the interrogation. Tears reappeared in her eyes.

Terrel came closer. "Mrs. Pellegrini, I understand that you might be afraid. But we are here to help. We tracked Susan's cell phone and found that she stayed in a different apartment than her own in Mission Bay overnight. We could narrow the location of her cell phone down to four apartments in a building on the university campus at Mission Bay. We looked up the names of the residents in these apartments. Do you know any of them?" He handed Stella a piece of paper with four names on them. Terrel read them out loud. "Lucas Davis, Rebecca Green, Amir Nielsson, Sonya Meyer."

For a second, Lili saw a flash of surprise on Stella's face, which quickly turned into a blank expression. "I am sorry. I do not know any of them," she said, looking down on her bruised hand.

Lili tightened the grip around the pink cell phone in her pocket. She would have liked to hand it over. But how should she explain this to the FBI agents? She looked to the ground.

"Well, then I guess we have to check all of these people out," Angus responded. "Perhaps we will find your daughter in one of these apartments."

"That would be wonderful!" Stella said calmly, looking at the two FBI agents more annoyed than grateful.

Lili noticed that Dr. Williams and Amir had quietly stepped out of the room. She had seen Amir's ID. Amir Nielsson. And now the FBI was looking for the owner of an apartment where Susan had stayed last night, and one of them was Amir Nielsson. *Why was Stella covering up for him? He must know something!*

While Stella and the FBI agents were engaged in their conversation, Lili also retreated to the hallway and looked for Amir. *Where did he go?* As she stepped out, she saw him at the end of the ER corridor, turning around a corner. Lili rushed down the hallway and followed him from a distance. Amir walked through the foyer of the main hospital and up a flight of stairs to the second floor. Lili carefully followed him. He walked quite fast, and Lili had to almost run to not lose him. Fortunately, there were many people around, which made it easier for her to remain hidden. However, she almost ran into an elderly lady while trying to keep up with him. The lady yelled at Lili, Lili apologized and continued to rush up the stairs. On the second floor, she saw Amir turning around another corner. Lili arrived just in time to see him opening a glass door, that led to a roof garden. She arrived at the glass door a minute later. But her chase ended abruptly. She was not able to open the door, because it required her to swipe a hospital ID. Lili waited at the door for a minute. Then, a young man arrived, swiped his ID and opened the door. Lili stayed closely behind him, caught the door before it closed again and also stepped on the roof terrace. She looked around. She had entered a beautiful, serene garden terrace on the hospital roof, which was apparently reserved for hospital staff. The roof garden was flanked by the hospital building on three sides, which provided protection against the wind. Behind her was a cascade of potted palm trees, bushes, tall grasses and flowers of various colors. To her right was a living wall with blossoming lavender, which outlined several pretty benches. To her left was a living wall with succulent plants. The terrace was covered with white gravel and lime chippings. A water feature served as a focal point, flanked by an abundance of potted plants and several groupings of small rustic tables and wooden armchairs, where people in white coats were sitting. Some of them were engaged in discussions, others were reading, others were drinking coffee or eating an early dinner. The free edge of the terrace was lined by a transparent railing and provided a breath-taking view over the skyline of San Francisco. Lili saw Amir standing at the railing, looking towards the cityscape and talking on his cell phone in a low voice. Since he turned his back to her, it was easy for her to come closer and listen in on the conversation.

"…. two FBI agents are on their way to my apartment. You have to get out of there immediately."

He listened to the person on the other side of the phone.

"….no, I do not know how much time you might have left, probably not much. It takes about five minutes by car to get to my apartment."

Another pause

"…. yes, unfortunately she fractured her left lower leg and also her scaphoid bone."

"……That's a bone at the wrist."

"…… She is in good hands. Our team will take good care of her, and she will be safe here."

Lili came closer, trying to hear anything that the other person on the phone might say.

"….did the guy call you?"

Amir and Lili both listened. Unfortunately, Lili could not catch anything.

"… please be careful. This is very dangerous. And please text me the address of the trade when you get it."

"….of course. I do not want to interfere. But I want to help if you get in trouble."

Amir hung up the phone, turned around swiftly and crashed into Lili.

"I am so sorry!" he muttered. Then he recognized Lili. His eyes widened.

"What on earth are you doing here?" he exclaimed. "This lounge is for employees only!"

Lili tried to think of a plausible excuse but could not think of any. There was really no reason for her to be here at all. In times of crisis, honesty had always worked for her – as long as she was interacting with an honest person. Lili realized that Amir was somehow connected to the chip thieves. But based on her observations thus far, she got the impression that he was trustworthy. In addition, Stella trusted him with the life of her daughter.

"I saw Stella's look at you, when Terrel mentioned the apartment," Lili said, "and then you walked out of the room. I wanted to ask you about it and followed you. But you were on the phone. I am sorry, I overheard some of your conversation, and I believe I understand the connection now. Susan stayed at your apartment last night?"

Amir did not respond at first. He looked at Lili for a while, perhaps deciding what to do. Then, he nodded. "Please do not inform the FBI agents. They will learn it soon enough, I guess."

Lili lowered her voice. "Even if I wanted to inform them, that will not be possible. They are on their way to your apartment right now. Besides, I did not feel that Mr. Weber treated me in a way that I would be inclined to share any extra information with him."

"I noticed that," Amir responded with a sympathetic smile.

Lili was trying to make sense out of the fractions of the conversations that she had just overheard. "Is Susan's friend currently in your apartment?"

"He was there," Amir explained, "and hopefully, he will be gone before the FBI arrives there. He has the brain chips and will trade them to release Susan."

"He will bring the brain chips to the kidnapper in order to trade them for Susan?"

Amir nodded.

"When will that happen?"

"We do not know yet. The kidnapper will call Kaleo and tell him location and time of the exchange."

"I am not an expert on this," Lili said, "but every movie on this topic tells us that such trades usually do not work out. If Susan saw the face of her kidnapper, then he cannot let her go. Perhaps it would be good to get some help from the FBI after all."

"I agree that this is very dangerous," Amir responded. "But the kidnapper specifically said that we should not involve the police or FBI. I think we should be cooperative. I don't want to provoke him."

"Okay, let me at least help you," Lili said. "When you get the location of the meeting with the kidnapper, please let me know as well. I am no threat to anyone. I could just be in the area, a random passerby. In case Kaleo and you get caught in a fight or worse, I might be able to call for help."

"That would be the backup of the backup," Amir smiled. "Why would you risk your life helping us?"

"I understand that this might not be my smartest choice from a survival perspective," Lili responded. "But I am Stella's friend, and I don't want her daughter to die. And again, I would just be an observer in the background and call the appropriate service if I see a problem. I am a radiologist — that's what I do for a living."

Amir looked at Lili with a faint smile. *Was there some relief in his eyes?* "I will think about it," he finally said.

Lili searched in her pocket and found an old, crumpled business card. "Here you go." She handed it over to Amir. "Please send me the address and feel free to call me anytime."

Amir nodded. "It is possible that there will be a complication."

Lili did not understand. "What kind of complication?"

Amir looked at her again, his smart green eyes trying to connect. "Kaleo has only four brain chips, not five."

"I do not understand. He and Susan stole five brain chips, right? So, if he only has four brain chips now, what happened to the fifth chip?"

"I implanted one into Susan. I did not want to. But you know, she can sometimes be very persuasive." Amir looked to the ground.

"Are you out of your mind?" Lili exclaimed. "That could put both kids in grave danger!"

"I know. I am trying to fix it. If you do not hear from us by tomorrow around noon or so, please inform the FBI."

Lili shook her head. "I sure will! Amir, this sounds very dangerous! You have to tell Kaleo that he cannot meet this criminal without bringing him what he wants."

Amir looked at Lili. "I already did tell him that. But he thinks that he can convince the kidnapper that he stole only four brain chips."

"That does not sound like a winning strategy to me! This is a professional killer. He will know exactly what he wants."

Amir nodded. "I know. But there is nothing I can do about the four-chip problem. I have to leave now. Once the FBI agents realize that it was my apartment, they probably will start searching for me. I will wait for Kaleo's call in a secure location."

"Be careful!" Lili said.

"You too! Thank you for offering to help!" Amir turned around and left.

Lili went back to the ER, to check on Stella. But she was gone. Lili learned from a nurse that Stella had been transferred to the orthopedic surgery ward on the second floor. She went up to the ward. Stella was lying in her bed, sleeping. She looked exhausted. Lili did not want to disturb her and decided to come back early the next morning. She left the pink phone on the nightstand and left.

- 20 -
Susan
THE HOSTAGE

Tuesday, May 25, 2032, 5.15 pm.

Susan followed the boogie man down the stairs of her apartment building. She had difficulty processing the events that had just happened. She felt an endless love for everyone around her, including the man in the black jacket. Her sense of self had dissipated in a wonderful feeling of peace and joy. Yet a distant voice in her head told her that the man beside her had frightened Kaleo and her mother. As they walked down the stairs, Susan saw a ghostly afterimage of her mother, lying on the ground, tied to the chair, looking at her. The image invaded her happy space like a dark cloud, replacing sunlight with dreadful shadows. It seemed that visual perceptions of light or darkness affected her mood.

As the man rushed her down the dark hallway, it seemed to morph into a dark tunnel that opened its mouth to swallow her. Susan looked back and saw the man in the black jacket behind her. He was still holding her left arm and pushing her forwards. His grip was too tight – it hurt! The man pushed her further down into the gaping abyss. Susan wanted to stop, but the man continued to push her forwards. Susan saw the bright red emergency exit sign coming closer. Was there blood dripping down the red letters? The man extended his right leg beside her and kicked the exit door open. The door flung open, and beams of sunlight struck them, splintered into shards of multispectral rays. Susan gasped and stepped through the door, watching the amazing light show. She instantly felt better. A warm feeling of joy and gratitude embraced her. It seemed that everything around her was coming alive! The trees and the grass on the backyard were waving at her, whispering that everything was okay. She was part of a beautiful all-encompassing conscious universe. Susan felt so overwhelmed that she sat down on the stairs of the exit. The man almost toppled over her. He cursed. Susan looked at the man with pity. He looked so stressed and confused.

"What is your name?" she asked with a soothing tone.

"This is none of your business," the man shouted. He looked to the right and left, then at the watch at his wrist.

"Well, I won't go any further until you tell me your name!" Susan responded playfully.

The man rolled his eyes, anger building up in his face. He said slowly, "You will come with me right now or I will shoot your crazy head!"

Susan looked into his eyes with the same mesmeric gaze that he had encountered earlier. "My name is Susan," she said softly. "Your name?"

The man looked at her, clenching his teeth and fumbling with his right hand in his jacket. A pearl of sweat was running down his forehead.

"I am Boris!" he finally exclaimed between clenched teeth. "Let's go!"

"Thank you, Boris," Susan responded with a contented smile. She extended her non-casted left hand to Boris, like a princess who invited a hand kiss from her suitor. Boris was clearly irritated. He hesitated for a second. Then, he took Susan's hand and pulled her towards the street at the back of the building. Susan gave him a pleased smile and followed him down the street, away from the apartment and towards a small parking lot. After a few minutes, they arrived at a dark gray Mercedes coupé. Boris had exchanged it for the Tesla just in case anybody had seen him. The Mercedes featured black leather seats and tinted windows, perfect for the occasion. Boris opened the rear door. Susan looked at the dark rear seat, uncertain what to do. Boris gave her a push so that she flew into the car. Then he slammed the door shut and exhaled. *Mission accomplished. That had been the hardest part!* He got into the front seat, started the car and drove off.

***

It was dark inside the car. Susan emerged from her state of joyful delusion as if waking up from a beautiful dream. She found herself lying on the dark back seat of a car. Everything around her felt dark and tight, like a coffin. Things had happened too fast for her to process them. She was not sure if she had slipped or if Boris had pushed her. She sat up and looked around. There was a plastic partition between her seat and the front seat. She saw Boris in the driver's seat.

"Boris, where are we going?" she asked.

Boris did not answer. Perhaps he could not hear her through the partition. Susan brought her mouth closer to a small opening in the center of the plastic wall. "Boris, where are we going?" she asked again, louder.

Still no reaction. Susan only saw the back of Boris' head. He did not seem to move at all.

Anxiety crept up Susan's chest and encircled her throat. Her heart started pounding. *I hope he's not dead*, she thought. She looked at Boris again, trying to activate her stroboscopic vision to track his movements. She did not quite understand how her new ability worked. She sometimes saw the afterimages and sometimes not. But it seemed that she could activate the stroboscopic images when concentrating on a specific moving object. Susan focused on Boris arms and saw a trail of serial images revealing a right bend as the car turned around a corner. *Thank god, the driver is alive!* She thought. *Why does he not react?*

Susan tried the door handle on the right. It did not open. She moved over to the left, behind the driver's seat, and tried the door handle on the left. It did not open either. She pushed the button that would wind down the window. No response. She was trapped!

Is he kidnapping me? Her heart started racing and chills were creeping down her back. She remembered the newspaper article about Juan Perez's death. She looked at Boris and noticed the outline of a gun in the right pocket of his jacket. Susan's anxiety rose to panic. *He is going to kill me!* Susan started to tremble. The dark backseat seemed to become alive, engulfing her. She suppressed an urge to scream and tried to focus. Under normal circumstances, she was not easily intimidated. Boris probably still thought that she was lost in her delusion. Perhaps that's why he had not tied her hands or covered her eyes. She could use that to her advantage. Susan carefully patted her pockets for her cell phone. She could not find it. She remembered that she had tossed it in the apartment. Her mind started racing. She had to figure out where they were going. Susan looked through the tinted

window. Houses, trees and people appeared and vanished. They were driving through the city. Then, the car took a turn and drove up a ramp to a highway. They were leaving San Francisco. Susan focused her mind on the scenery outside.
They were not crossing the Bay Bridge or the Golden Gate Bridge. Susan noticed a change from cityscape to rolling greenery. Then, she saw a long, linear dark-blue lake to her right. A few minutes later, she saw a second, larger lake. Susan knew where she was. *This was San Andreas Lake and Crystal Springs Reservoir!* Her mother had explained to her that the longitudinal shape of these lakes was no coincidence. The main trace of the San Andreas Fault runs right under these lakes. They were driving down the I280 highway.

A few minutes later, the car changed from the fast lane to the right lane and took an exit. Susan saw a San Mateo sign. The car took several turns and Susan lost her orientation. They drove down a rural road, with patches of wood, scrub, wild greenery and the occasional herd of cattle passing by. After a while, the car took a turn onto a private road. They were bumping and bouncing over multiple cracks and potholes in the road. After about five minutes, they drove into a small patch of eucalyptus trees where a small log cabin was nestled under giant blue gums, with branches twisting, turning and reaching for the sky. The cabin was not much bigger than a shed and featured a small front porch, French doors, two adjacent windows and an A-shaped split roof with a row of small clerestory windows.

Boris stopped the car in front of the cabin. He opened the driver's door and stepped out of the car. Susan saw him walking to the entrance of the cabin, taking a key from his pocket, unlocking the French door and disappearing in darkness behind it. Susan frantically pulled and pushed on the rear doors of the car. But she could not find a way out. Boris re-appeared from the cabin and stepped towards the rear door on the left side of the car. Susan saw duct tape and the car key in his left hand. She heard her heart pounding in her head. Sweat was running down her temples. She hunched and prepared for perhaps her one and only chance to escape. As she heard the "blip" sound of the automatic door opener, Susan jerked towards the right rear door on the other side of the car, pushed it open, jumped out and ran towards the eucalyptus woods. Boris' jaw dropped wide open, completely caught by surprise. Then he took on the chase.

***

Susan was racing through the moist grounds of the eucalyptus woods, jumping over ferns, brushes and tree branches. Poison oak was striking her bare ankles, but she did not notice. The trees created a promenade for her, cheering her on and pointing towards the close by main road. She saw a car approaching in the far distance. *If I can reach the road in time, the driver can rescue me*, she thought, running faster. The mists of sunset were settling over the hills and the twilight was gently embracing her. She heard cracking tree branches and heavy breathing sounds behind her, coming closer. Then she heard a loud thump and crashing branches, followed by a flood of curses. *He fell! Do not look back!* she told herself. Susan continued to run away from her captor. She focused on reaching the road, making her way through the green alley between the trees, jumping over little hurdles in the underwood. She saw the approaching car in the distance. If she could make it out of the woods and into the meadow between the trees and the street, the driver might see her and come to her rescue. Susan sprinted towards the open field. But suddenly, her foot got caught under an exposed tree root. Susan crashed face forwards into the boscage. She stumbled to her feet and wanted to continue her race. But her fall had allowed Boris to catch up with her. Susan felt a sudden, brutal jerk on her ponytail. Boris had grabbed her braids and dragged her backwards with a triumphant laugh. She felt a blow to her head and lost consciousness.

- 21 -
Terrel
CALCANEUS FRACTURE

Tuesday, May 25, 2032, 7 pm.

Angus Weber and Terrel Wright drove to the apartment complex in the Mission Bay district of San Francisco, where Susan's cell phone had been last located. The apartment building was a modern, four-story house in a vibrant street with lots of shops, restaurants and bars. People were strolling by on the sidewalk or sitting under glowing heat lamps at dining tables with multicolored tablecloths and a variety of delicious looking food. As they walked by, Terrel smelled a mixture of turmeric-loaded curries, simmering seafood, freshly baked bread, sauteing onions and freshly grilled meat. He had almost forgotten how hungry he was. Dr. Williams had reminded him how important it was that he stayed hydrated, so Terrel stopped at a kiosk to buy a soda. Angus first protested in disapproval. They could not lose a minute. But then he joined Terrel. It had been a long day and a little caffeine would help them to stay alert. The two FBI agents gulped down their drinks as they continued to walk down the street.

The white facade of an apartment building emerged in front of them. The building had a sleek, contemporary design and large, floor-to-ceiling double exterior doors. Angus and Terrel entered the spacious entrance hall, where a concierge behind a beautiful walnut desk greeted them politely. The concierge was a man in his mid-30s with dark brown hair and a friendly smile. He wore a blue uniform with a name tag that identified him as "Jay." Angus showed Jay his FBI badge and explained that they were searching for a missing girl. Jay was thoroughly impressed. Angus asked him if he could lead them to the apartments of Lucas Davis, Rebecca Green, Amir Nielsson and Sonya Meyer. One of them had likely hosted the girl last night. Jay looked briefly at Angus with raised eyebrows, then he looked away. Terrel wondered. *Was the concierge holding something back?* Terrel made a mental note to follow up on that later. Jay led the two FBI agents up the stairs, to the third floor.

The three men first arrived at the apartment of Rebecca Green. They rang the door and a young woman in her early twenties opened it. She looked at them with agitated annoyance and groaned in irritation. She explained that she had been waiting for her boyfriend for more than an hour and they were late for a dinner party. No, she had not seen a teenage girl and certainly not hosted one. After some hesitation, she did allow Angus to enter her apartment, while the other two men waited outside. Angus walked through the main room, bedroom, office, kitchen and bathroom. Apart from a second toothbrush, which likely belonged to the boyfriend, Angus did not find any hint of a second person staying in this apartment. He certainly did not find any indication that Susan had been here.

The three men moved on to the next apartment, which belonged to Sonya Meyer. Angus rang the bell. Nobody answered. Angus rang the bell again, still no response. He asked Jay to open the door. The concierge brought up a bundle of keys, first tried two keys that did not match and then opened the door. Angus loudly announced his name and plan to enter the apartment. Still no answer. This time, both Angus and Terrel entered the apartment and searched the rooms. Again, there was no sign of Susan. Terrel started to wonder if this was worth their time. *What were they hoping to find?*

Next, Jay led them to the fourth floor, to two apartments which were located directly above those of Sonya Meyer and Rebecca Green. Jay first stopped at the apartment of Lucas Davis. Angus knocked at the door. No response. He knocked at the door again. "This is FBI agent Angus Weber, please open the door." They heard a smashing sound in the apartment, but nobody came to the door. Angus nodded at Jay, who produced his key chain again and opened the front door. Angus and Terrel entered and looked around. All the apartments were designed with a similar layout of living room, bedroom, study, kitchen and bathroom. The window of the study room was wide open. Terrel stepped into the study and went to the window. He saw a fire escape ladder below the window and a young man making his way down.

"Stop!" Terrel shouted at the man. "This is the FBI. We need to talk with you!"

The man briefly looked up at Terrel, then continued his way down the ladder.

Terrel cursed, then jumped through the window and followed the man down the ladder. The man had a good head start, but Terrel was in better shape and trained in the pursuit of fugitives. He quickly caught up. Meanwhile, Angus had seen the chase. He turned around, ran down the stairway inside the house, out of the front door and around the house, to meet the runaway on the ground. The man continued his way down the ladder as quickly as possible. Unfortunately, the ladder ended about three meters above the ground, to prevent intrusion of burglars. The man looked down, uncertain what to do next. Terrel caught up. The man briefly looked back at Terrel and then jumped from the ladder to the ground. He landed with a harsh crash and fell to the ground with a scream of pain, holding his left leg. Angus had reached him and pulled him up by his right arm.

"What on earth were you thinking?" he yelled at the man. "Do you really think you can outrun the FBI?"

"I am so sorry," the young man responded, clearly embarrassed. "I did not mean to cause any trouble!"

"Well, it seems that you did – mostly for yourself!" Angus responded with anger in his voice.

Terrel had also made his way down. He gripped the lowest part of the ladder, let himself slide down so that he was hanging on it with extended arms, then jumped to the ground. He walked over to the runaway and Angus.

"What is your name?" he asked.

"I am Lucas Davis," the young man responded. He was probably around twenty years old and looked at Angus and Terrel with wide open eyes. He reminded Terrel of a scared child.

"Why did you run away?" Terrel asked.

"Wouldn't you run if the FBI is after you?" The man responded.

Terrel shook his head. "If I had done nothing wrong, probably not," he said. "So, what were you afraid of?"

"I just got scared," the man said, looking towards the street, again avoiding eye contact. "Why would the FBI want anything from me?"

"We are investigating a double homicide and a missing girl," Terrel answered, "and your reaction looked pretty guilty to me."

"No, no, no!" the man exclaimed with wide open eyes. "I swear, I have nothing to do with this! And I did not kill anyone!"

"So, why were you running? Without an explanation, we can arrest you right now."

"I am so sorry, I just wanted to impress my girlfriend!" the man said, pearls of sweat running down his forehead.

"How did you want to impress your girlfriend?" Terrel asked, now seriously curious about the situation.

"I organized a sideshow," Lucas confessed, trembling. "I thought you found out and wanted to convict me."

"We are not interested in any shows! I don't even know what a sideshow is." Angus said, looking at Terrel for clarification.

"Sideshows have been a problem in the Bay Area for decades," Terrel explained. "Large groups of people gather to watch car drivers spinning doughnuts around each other. Sideshows can take place on parking lots, on public streets or on highway ramps. Sometimes, passengers are hanging out of the windows or sunroofs of the spinning cars. Sideshows are forbidden because they endanger others. Organizers and participants can be charged with a misdemeanor, fines of up to a thousand dollars and six months in jail."

"I see," Angus looked at Lucas Davis. "Should we release him to the police?"

"I will call our agency to check if somebody pressed charges. If not, I think we can work this out here," Terrel said. Then, looking at Lucas, he continued, "We might not press charges if you can help us out with some information."

Lucas looked from one FBI agent to the other. Then he sighed. "Of course, I can tell you everything you want. What do you want to know about the sideshows?"

Angus rolled his eyes.

"We are not interested in the sideshows," Terrel responded. "But we might be interested in your neighbor and his guests. Did you see this young man or this woman recently?" Terrel handed a photo of Susan and the phantom drawing of Kaleo to Lucas.

Lucas looked at the images carefully. "Yes, I saw both of them walking into Amir's apartment last night. I just came from work, and we walked up the stairs at the same time. I got out my key to open the door of my apartment. I saw them ringing the bell in front of Amir's apartment. The door opened and they entered. Amir rarely has visitors, so this was a bit unusual. They ordered some food later. I heard the doorbell again and Amir talked with somebody in the hallway. After that, there was noise until late at night, I believe they watched a movie. The walls are quite thin here, you know."

"Did you notice anything else, that seemed unusual?" Terrel asked.

"Tonight, this guy almost ran me over," Lucas pointed at the sketch that showed Kaleo. "He seemed to be in great distress. He came running down the hallway as I came back from the fitness studio on the second floor. He did not notice me at all. He had a key and entered Amir's apartment. I believe he just left about thirty minutes ago or so. I heard the entrance door opening and closing and I heard someone walking fast down the hallway."

"That is very helpful, thank you!" Terrel said.

Lucas nodded. He wanted to take a step back but moaned in pain when he stepped on his right foot. "I believe I might have hurt my foot when I jumped down the fire ladder," he said.

Terrel looked at Lucas' ankle, which was starting to swell and show different shades of blue bruises. "You need to go to a hospital!" he said.

"I am not sure I can walk," Lucas said.

"You can drive him there," Angus said to Terrel. "I will check out Amir Nielsson's apartment and then come to join you at the hospital."

"I don't think Lucas is going anywhere on his own," Terrel responded. "I can go back upstairs with you, and we can have a look at the last apartment together. That might be faster, and two pairs of eyes might see more than one."

"No worries, I can take care of it," Angus responded. "Lucas got injured as part of our investigation. Please make sure that he is taken care of. We have to document his injury and treatment in our report. In the meantime, I can have a look at the apartment. If the suspect has left as Lucas said, there is probably not much there anyways."

Terrel looked from Angus to Lucas, unsure what to do. He really wanted to have a look at Amir's apartment as well. Angus had missed several important clues earlier today. Terrel did not trust his colleagues' attention to detail. On the other hand, it was not his place to criticize a superior. That could have negative effects on his career. Angus had noticed Terrel's' hesitation and said, "Do not worry about me. The hospital is not too far from here. I don't mind a little evening walk and will meet you there."

Terrel sighed and nodded. "Okay, see you at the hospital."

Terrel turned to Lucas. "I parked my car about one block down the street. If you put your arm around me shoulder, do you think you can make it there?

"I am not sure if I can walk," Lucas responded, "my foot is really starting to hurt a lot."

Jay had come down from inside the building as well and quietly listened to the conversation. "I can stay with Lucas, while you are getting your car," he said.

Angus nodded. "That would be very helpful. However, I need a key to get into the apartment building."

"Here you go," Jay said, handing him a pair of keys. "Please leave the door open, I will come join you in a few minutes."

Angus took the keys and went back into the building. Terrel looked at Jay. This was his chance to follow up.

"Jay, I had the impression that you were holding something back when we asked about any unusual events today?"

"Well, there was a peculiar event this morning," Jay responded. "I saw the girl in your photo leaving the building. Then I heard a crash in front of the door. Amir came down the hallway shortly after her and when he opened the door, I saw that the girl apparently ran into a motorcycle. She reacted in a strange way, and I thought she was on drugs."

"In the morning?"

"Yeah, she looked up to the sky and held her arms out as if she wanted to embrace someone or something. Then, she crashed into a motorcyclist."

"Thank you, this is very helpful," Terrel responded. "Was there anything else out of the ordinary?"

"Well, when the other guy left this afternoon, a sticky note fell out of his pocket. I collected it and wanted to give it back to him or to Amir, when he would get home."

"Can you show me this note, please?" Terrel asked.

"Just a minute." Jay went back into the building and re-emerged after a short while with a small yellow sticky note in his hand. Terrel looked at it. It only contained a ten-digit number, perhaps a phone number. The number looked familiar. Terrel entered it into his phone and looked at Jay in surprise. This was Lili Pham's number! *How is Lili connected to all this?* he thought.

"Thank you, you helped our investigation tremendously," Terrel said to Jay, who shook his hand with a proud look.

"Always at your service, sir!" he responded.

Terrel turned to Lucas. "I will get the car. It should only take a few minutes."

"Thank you for taking me to the hospital," Lucas responded.

Terrel got the car from the parking lot. He understood the risk of leaving a suspect alone. But based on the information so far, it seemed that Lucas was not involved in the brain chip business. And if he did try to run, he would probably not get very far with his injured foot. When Terrel pulled into the driveway of the building, both Lucas and Jay were still waiting in the same place where he had left them, in front of the building. They helped Lucas into the car and Terrel drove back to the hospital, this time parking directly in front of the entrance door. By now, the security guard knew him and greeted him cheerfully.

"Hello, Agent Wright, looks like you have another customer for us!"

"Yes, indeed!" Terrel smiled. "It is good to see you again, Sam!

Terrel helped the limping Lucas to the entrance desk, where he was checked in and led to one of the examination rooms. Dr. Williams was still on duty and joined them shortly afterwards. Lucas asked Terrel to stay with him in the exam room. Terrel agreed. He had to include Lucas's diagnosis in his report anyways, so why not wait here? Dr. Williams examined the ankle carefully, which seemed to have doubled in size since Terry had seen it at the apartment building. Dr. Williams ordered an x-ray of the foot and ankle and left to see another patient. The x-ray technician came in and took the radiograph. Terrel and Lucas sat in the exam room, waiting for Dr. Williams to return.

"Would you like to call anybody to pick you up here later?" Terrel asked.

"I don't have anyone here that I could ask to come," Lucas responded. "My family is from the east coast and my girlfriend is visiting her family in Chicago this week."

"I see," Terrel responded. "Do you have another friend who could help you?"

"Well, I could ask Amir," Lucas responded. "He works here and could take me home with him after his shift."

"Amir works here?" Terrel asked, raising his eyebrows in surprise.

Lucas nodded.

The brain cells in Terrel's hippocampus connected. That was it! The name *Amir Nielsson* had sounded familiar the whole time. The nurse practitioner in Stella's room and the owner of the apartment were the same person! Terrel jumped to his feet.

"Can you call him?" he asked.

"Will you promise that you won't arrest him?" Lucas asked.

"Lucas, we are trying to find a missing girl whose life may be in danger. Amir may have important information that could help us find her."

Lucas hesitated for a moment, looking at Terrel.

"Remember we made a deal with regards to the sideshow."

Lucas' fingers flew over the keypad of his phone. *Hello Amir, FBI agents were searching your apartment for a girl.*

He showed the message to Terrel.

They waited.

No response.

Lucas wrote another message.

I believe I broke my leg. I am at SFGH. Can U take me home?

"Amir is the most caring person I know," he said to Terrel. "If he is alive, he will respond."

Ping. Lucas' phone announced an incoming text message.

WTF happened? Any other injury besides the leg?

Lucas showed the message to Terrel.

Terrel gasped. "Ask him to come back and pick you up," he said.

Lucas texted. *Long story. No other injury. Can you come pick me up?*

Ping. Another message.

Sorry. My shift already ended. Take an Uber? It is late. I'll check on U tmrw.

Lucas texted. *Of course, no worries. C U tmrw.*

Terrel stared at the phone. He had shown Stella the names of the apartment owners and one of them had been standing in her room. She must have known this! No wonder the suspect got away. *I need to talk with her!* Terrel thought. *What else was Stella hiding?*

They were interrupted by Dr. Williams who walked into the exam room and sat down at the small desk to the right of the exam chair. He opened the archiving system PACS (picture archiving computer system) on his computer and opened a file that showed the x-ray of Lucas' foot.

"Lucas, I am afraid, you broke the neck of your talus," he said, pointing at a bone below Lucas's ankle.

"What is my talus?" Lucas asked, looking at the picture of his foot.

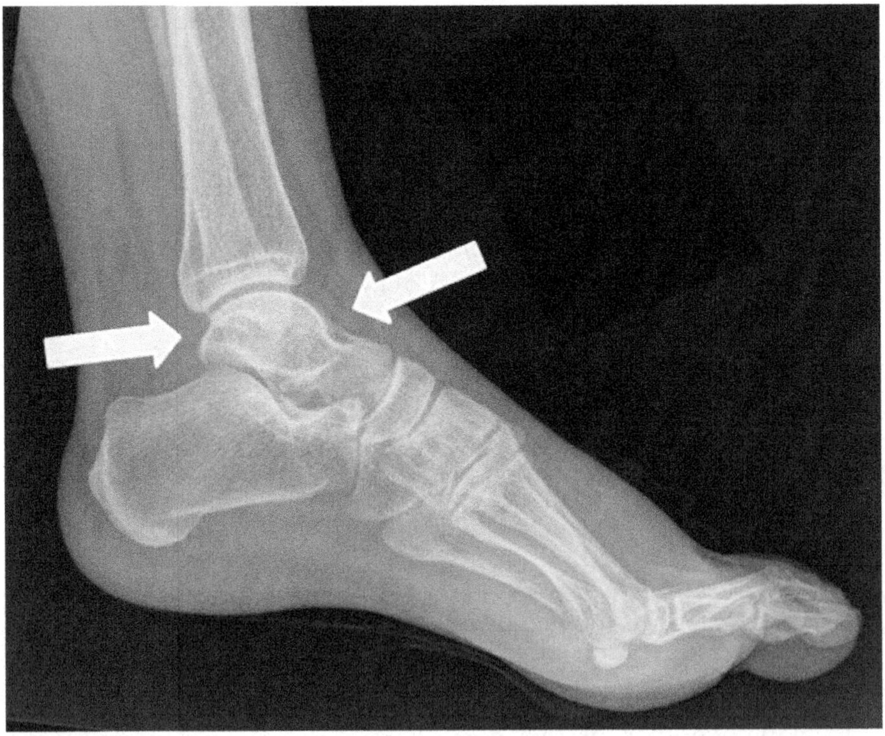

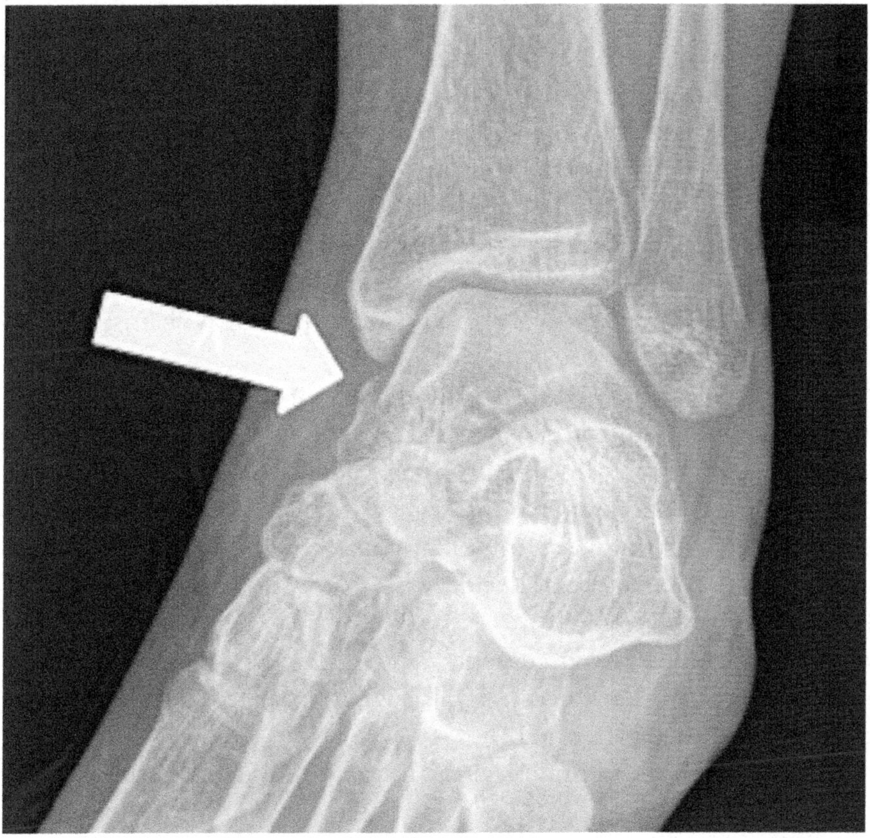

"Well, the talus is a small bone that sits between the heel bone (calcaneus) and the two bones of the lower leg (the tibia and fibula). It makes up the lower part of the ankle joint. The neck of the talus is the constricted portion of the bone between the body here and the oval head. This narrowed area can break when a major force hits the bone, such as your jump from the ladder." Dr. Williams pointed towards the neck of the talus.

"Do I need a cast?" Lucas asked.

"It is possible that our orthopedic surgeons would like to fix this with a screw." Dr. Williams responded. "I will ask them to come by for a consult."

"Oh no, I do not want any surgery!" Lucas exclaimed.

"We do not know yet, if a surgery is needed," Dr. Williams responded calmly. "Let's see what the surgeon suggests and decide from there."

Terrel smiled. By now, he had seen through the tactic of the emergency doctor. People were often afraid to take a big step forward. Dr. Williams guided them gently from one small step to another. And before the patient realized it, they had completed the necessary treatment.

"I assume this might take a little longer than you had initially anticipated," Terrel said to Lucas, "but I can assure you from my own experience that you are in very good hands with Dr. Williams. You do want to get better, do you?

Dr. Williams exchanged a brief look of gratitude with Terrel. They smiled in mutual understanding.

"Yes, of course, I do!" Lucas responded.

"The orthopedic surgeons will be here in a few minutes. No worries, they will only have a look at your foot and then discuss your options with you. You can decide what you want to do from there," Dr. Williams said.

Lucas nodded in agreement.

Terrel looked at Lucas. "I will have to leave now. I have to find the girl before she is harmed."

"Yes of course, I understand," Lucas responded. "Thank you for bringing me here."

Terrel nodded to Lucas and Dr. Williams and left towards the orthopedic surgery ward.

- 22 -
Susan
MONTEGGIA FRACTURE

Tuesday, May 25, 2032, 8 pm.

When Susan woke up, her head felt like it would blow up like a balloon. She was not sure how long she had been unconscious. It was dark around her. She tried to orient herself as her eyes got slowly accustomed to the dimness. She was inside the cabin, lying on a bed in a loft under the roof. Susan could see a full moon and dim twilight through the small skylights in the roof. Her feet were tied together, and her free left hand was tied to the cast of her right arm with duct tape. She felt a gag in her mouth and duct tape on her cheeks. She tried to remove it with her left hand but could not flex her arms enough due to the cast. Her right shoulder hurt like hell. Susan tried to suppress tears of pain and defeat. *This is not over yet. I will fight back!* she told herself. Susan sat up on the bed and looked around. She was in a small bedroom under the roof. There were two small nightstands, one on each side of the bed. She looked around to find anything that was sharp enough to cut the tape between her two wrists. But she could not find anything suitable. To her right was a ladder-like stairway that led to the single main room of the cabin. Susan let herself slide down to the hardwood floor in front of the bed. She used her tied feet to move her bottom towards the balustrade, careful to not make any noise. She peaked over the edge of the loft and saw Boris pacing back and forth in the main room, talking on his cell phone.

"Yes, I have her here and will exchange her for the brain chips," she heard him saying. Susan moved as close as possible to the balustrade without being seen, but she could not hear the response on the other side of the phone.

"I am sure they are eager to get her back," Boris said.

He needs me to get the brain chips! Susan thought, taking a deep breath. He cannot kill me now!

"No, nobody will make any connection."

What connection was he talking about? Susan wondered.

"Of course, I will make sure to steer the attention away from you. It will look like a suicide."

Susan felt her whole body tensing. *He will kill me later!*

"Nobody will track me down either. Once I have received my share, I will disappear for a while until the dust has settled."

"Yes, sir. This should be over tomorrow."

Boris hung up the phone. He looked towards the balustrade. Susan hobbled back towards the bed. She heard his footsteps coming closer, slowly coming up the narrow, squeaky stairway. Susan quickly let herself fall back on the bed, rolling on her left side so that her back was facing the stairway. She closed her eyes and pretended to be asleep. She heard Boris' footsteps coming closer. He stopped for a moment. Susan felt his eyes on her. Then, a bright light flashed through her closed eyes. Boris had switched on the light in the loft. Susan kept her eyes shut tightly and stayed as still as possible. *He cannot kill me now*, she told herself. *He needs me to get the brain chips!* Then, she felt a sudden jerk at her injured right shoulder, pulling her around. Susan screamed in pain, but her voice was muffled by the gag in her mouth. She looked at Boris with wide open eyes.

"There we go," Boris said, grinning. "You need to wake up, sleepy!"

Susan looked at Boris with anger. How could he be so rude and cruel. He still wore the same leather jacket and the same jeans as earlier today. She noticed dirt on his shoes. Not much time had gone by since he had caught her in the woods. Then, she noticed a baseball bat in his right hand. Boris noticed her gaze towards the bat. He leaned it against the bed and pulled his cell phone from his pocket.

"I wanted to show you some interesting pictures," Boris said as he opened the photo file in his phone. He scrolled through several photos, then turn the phone to Susan, so that she could see the picture.

"I was always fascinated by these fractures that were named after people," Boris said. "What an honor! See, for example this here is a Monteggia fracture, a fracture of the ulna (a bone of the forearm) with dislocation of the radial head. You can get this fracture with a blow to the lower arm.

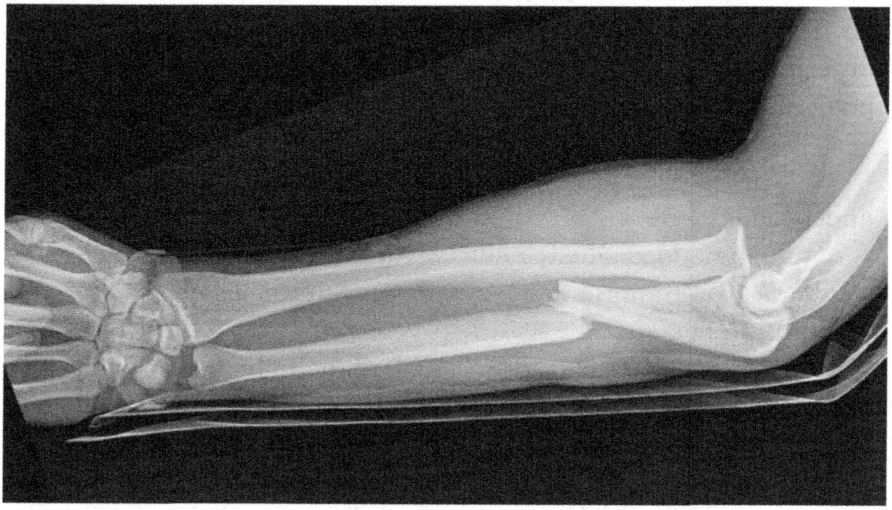

"And here is a Galeazzi fracture," Boris continued, "a fracture of the radius with dislocation of the ulna. I cannot quite decide which one I like better. What do you think, Susan?"

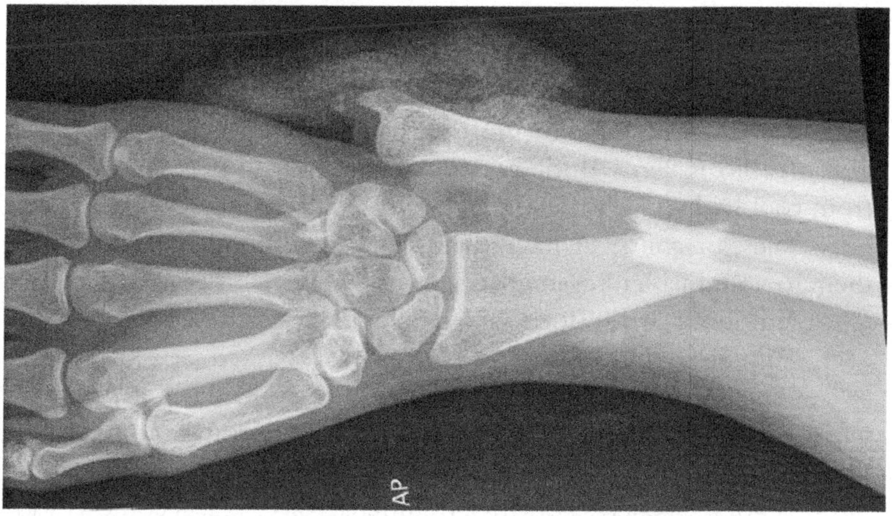

Susan looked at him with wide open eyes. *This man is mad*, she thought.

Boris looked back at her with a ruthless gaze. Susan swallowed and slowly shook her head.

"Well, I am also undecided," he said, "but I guess either one will do the job. You already have one broken arm. If the other arm is broken as well, you will not be able to get down this ladder." He pointed at the steep staircase that led to the main room downstairs.

Susan looked at him in horror.

"This is your place now"— he pointed to the bed—"do you understand?"

Susan nodded. She felt cold sweat running down her back.

"Do you promise that you will not scream again?" Boris asked. "Then I can remove the gag."

Susan nodded again. Boris grabbed the right corner of the tape over her mouth and removed it with one quick stroke. Susan flinched. She spit out the cloth in her mouth, moved her jaw to re-adjust and took a deep breath. Thank god, she could breathe freely again. Susan looked at Boris but did not say a word. Boris nodded with approval. "Good girl!" he said coldly. "One wrong move and you will get to know my bat here." He pointed to the baseball bat.

Susan stayed silent.

"We need to make a phone call." Boris moved closer to Susan so that their heads nearly touched. He took his cell phone and hit a number on the display. The phone self-dialed. The person on the other end picked up after the second ring tone. "This is Kaleo Kahale."

Susan's eyes swelled with tears.

"Hello Kaleo," Boris said in a calm voice. "It is great to hear from you! Did you get the brain chips?"

"Yes, of course, I have them," Kaleo responded. "I will bring them to you. Just let Susan go. She is not well."

"I noticed that!" Boris said, smiling at Susan.

"Where should I bring the chips?" Kaleo asked.

"I will text you the address," Boris responded. "Let me know when you get it." He sent a pre-typed message. Susan tried to read it, but it disappeared too fast.

"I got it," Kaleo said with a trembling voice. "I will come as soon as possible. I just ask you to confirm that Susan is with you and well."

Boris held the phone in front of Susan. Then, with a quick move, his left hand reached for the fingers of her right hand, which were sticking out of the cast. He squeezed them hard. Susan screamed, then pressing her lips together to regain her silence."

"Don't hurt her!" Kaleo shouted. "If I find her injured in any way, I will not tell you how to turn on the chips."

"*I* will tell you how to save your bitch," Boris said calmly. "If you do not bring me the brain chips, I will shoot her. If you do not come alone or if you tell anyone, I will shoot you both."

"I am on my way!" Kaleo responded.

Boris hung up the phone and turned to Susan, who sat on the bed next to him, watching him with wide open eyes. She was too afraid to say anything. Boris reached for the gag again, his left hand grabbed her jaw, so that her mouth opened and his right hand pushed the gag between her teeth. Boris produced a roll of duct tape from his pocket and secured the gag with another round of tape.

"I will be right back," he said to Susan. He went down the steep stairway to the main living room. Susan heard some rumbling downstairs. Then, Boris re-appeared with a wooden chair, which he carried upstairs and placed in front of Susan. He pointed to the chair. "Sit!"

Susan looked at him and lifted her feet, which were tied together. Boris brought the chair closer to her. Susan stood up and turned around to sit on the chair. Boris used the tape to tie her ankles to the front legs of the chair. Then, he wrapped the rest of the tape around her body and the back post of the chair. After he had used up the entire roll of tape, he turned the chair around, so that Susan was facing the railing of the loft. She could not move. Boris stepped a step back and looked at her. Then, he gave her a contented nod.

"This is perfect!" he said with a satisfied grin.

- 23 -
Lili
DELIBERATIONS

Tuesday, May 25, 2032, 8 pm.

After leaving the San Francisco General Hospital, Lili rushed to her car. She checked the time on her iPhone. It was 8 pm already – dinner time! Mark was likely waiting. He was the most reliable and trustworthy man she knew. He always kept his promises. And he expected others to live up to his standards as well – especially his wife! Lili sent him a quick text. *Am on my way, should be home in 20 minutes.* She jumped into her car and turned left towards Cesar Chavez street. There was not much traffic, and she made her way up the San Francisco hills quickly. As she drove up Fell street towards the Sunset district, Lili noticed a police car behind her with the alarm light on. *Had I been driving too fast?* she wondered. She sighed, turned on the blinker, stopped at the curbside and opened the window on the driver's side, hands on the wheel. The police car stopped, and a uniformed officer with a serious expression on his face got out. The tall man slowly walked towards her.

"Hello ma'am, driver's license and registration please!"

Lili handed the documents to the police officer.

He checked them. Then, he asked, "Do you know why I stopped you?"

Lili's brain raced. If she could make a personal connection, perhaps she could minimize the trouble. She smiled at the police officer. "Do I not get a ticket if I guess right?"

"You will still get a ticket."

"I guess I was driving a little fast."

"You were driving forty miles per hour in a thirty area. Do you have a really good explanation for that?"

Lili remembered a brilliant answer from an MIT student. She cleared her throat. "Well, when I got to my car tonight, I noticed that the tires were slightly underinflated, probably because it was very hot during the day, and it cooled down in the evening. I was driving just a little faster than usual to increase the heat and air pressure within the tires. By pressurizing the tires and increased the safety of the car."

The cop smiled back. "I haven't heard this excuse yet. But if this were true, then I could issue two tickets. One for speeding and one for knowingly driving an impaired vehicle. Besides, your tires look fine to me."

Lili decided to go with the truth. "I am so sorry, officer! I worked late today and am late for dinner with my husband. I was just trying to get home as quickly as possible. That plan clearly did not work out."

The cop looked at her and apparently, sensed that this was the truth this time. He said, "Well, today is your lucky day, Mrs. Pham! I give you one free pass. Don't let it happen again. If I see you again, you will be in trouble."

"I promise that won't happen!"

"Have a good evening, ma'am. Drive safely!"

***

Lili arrived at her home in the Sunset district at nine pm, an hour later than planned. When she entered the house, she saw Mark in the living room, sitting on the couch, working on his laptop. He looked up. "I started to get worried. What happened?"

"Mark, I am so sorry for being late. I really tried to get here as quickly as possible. I drove too fast and was stopped by a cop. But he was really nice and gave me a warning only."

"You did not get a ticket?"

Lili smiled. "No."

Mark grinned. "This seems to be your lucky day, indeed! You got away with speeding and your starving husband waited for you for dinner!"

"I really appreciate that!" Lili gave him a kiss.

Mark got up and they both retreated to the kitchen. Lili quickly fried two salmon fillets and Mark fixed a delicious summer salad. Lili prepared a table on the porch, under heating lamps. They both sat down, and Mark opened a bottle of Sauvignon blanc. Lili leaned back in the upholstered patio chair, taking a deep breath. *This here was her oasis!*

Mark first focused on his salmon. Lili had fried it in a pan with olive oil, herbs de Provence and a little bit of garlic. It smelled like rosemary and thyme and had a nice crunchy crust. Mark licked his lips as he looked at his wife. "You had quite a day today, hmm?"

Lili nodded and started to tell him all of her adventures. Mark listened carefully, sometimes asking questions for clarification. When she came to the part where she offered to help with Susan's rescue, Mark vehemently objected. "You will go nowhere near this kidnapper, Lili! You could be killed!"

"I want to help rescue Susan!"

"How do you plan to do that?" Mark asked. "Lili, you have many impressive strengths, but physical fights are not among them!"

"If the kidnapper is busy talking with Kaleo and Amir, perhaps I can release Susan in the meantime!" she said.

"Lili, you have watched too many movies! You are not an action hero. You cannot open a marmalade jar on your own!"

Lili looked into Marks intelligent, light-green eyes. *Perhaps he had a point.* When she had received her offer letter from SUEC, she wanted to tease him and told him that she could have a personal fitness trainer as part of her wellness program. He had just chuckled and responded, "Lili, I do not need to worry about that. You will never go there!"

So, physical fights were really not her strong suit.

Mark leaned over the patio table and gave Lili a kiss. "I love you anyways!" he said with a mischievous smile. "You are the smartest woman I know. With you, none of my days are ever boring!"

Lili started from a different angle. "Okay, let's wrap this up from the intellectual side then. It seems that somebody is leaking information. Only our small team knew that Juan Perez — or someone with his ID — had visited the ER after the theft of the brain chips. Yet, a few hours later, Juan Perez was killed. Who hired the killer?"

Mark took a sip from his wine. "It must be somebody at SUEC. Nothing else would make sense. I don't believe the domestic violence story."

"Agreed! Dr. Hill was very adamant that Juan and Juliana had a very loving marriage. It would be a really odd coincidence, if Juliana killed Juan out of jealousy on the day after he lent his ID to a criminal. And the teardrop fracture suggests that Juliana was severely injured when Juan was shot. She was not the shooter!"

Mark nodded. "The question here is. Who sent the killer to Juan Perez's home? I believe it must be a mole within your investigator team!"

"The FBI must have thought along the same lines. That's why they accused me!"

"Exactly! And there is another sign of the mole. A few hours after Stella identified her daughter on the FBI video, Susan was kidnapped in her apartment. Who informed the kidnapper that Susan was one of the thieves?"

"Besides Susan, Terrel and I, there were quite a number of other people who knew that Susan had stolen the brain chips."

"Perhaps. Let's play the situation through with each one of your team members," Mark suggested. "How about Annya?"

"Annya would never harm anyone!" Lili said.

"Emotions and judgements do not count," Mark countered. "Convince me with facts!"

"Annya knew that someone else had used Juan Perez's ID," Lili responded. "So, she would have no reason to hire a killer for Juan and his wife."

"Fair enough. How about Robert Hill?"

"He would not have to steal his own brain chips. He could just have built a few extra ones for personal use if he wanted to," Lili said.

"How about Terrel Wright?"

"You mentioned him before. I know personal judgements don't count. But I have the impression that Terrel has absolute integrity. In addition, he left his business card in Susan's apartment. What kidnapper would leave his business card behind?"

"I don't know. Perhaps a great tactic for disguise? I guess he's not off the list just yet. How about Ben Bennett?"

"The dean?" Lili chuckled. "You cannot be serious?"

"We cannot exclude anybody because of their status," Mark said.

"Well, I'm sure he would dread the negative publicity of technology thefts at SUEC. And he has a donor symposium coming up later this week, where he expects the largest donation in history. The news that critical technology got stolen from SUEC could jeopardize important business deals with major companies in Silicon Valley. But he is the dean!"

"No judgements! You never know what motivates people. Did he have the information to target Juan Perez and kidnap Susan Pellegrini?"

"I don't think he knew about Susan or her apartment."

"Okay. But Stella was his assistant, and she might have mentioned it?"

"I am not sure. Would you mention the address of your daughter's apartment in a conversation with your boss?"

"I don't know. It could come up. But you are right, it is probably a stretch. Finally, what about Agent Angus Weber?"

"He is directing the FBI investigation. He cannot be the kidnapper and investigator the same time," Lili said.

"Why not? Did he have the information to send the killer to Juan Perez and the kidnapper to Susan's apartment?"

"I guess he had the information. But he is the lead FBI investigator. He would not have a motive." Lili sighed.

"Didn't you say his partner was killed? Perhaps there is a connection we do not know about? Revenge is one of the most common motives for homicides?"

"I don't know. There could certainly be a connection we do not know about for any of the people we discussed."

"And, of course, there could be additional players."

Lili sighed. "We made a three-sixty and arrived where we had started. What did we miss?"

"We did not factor in that somebody broke into Dr. Hill's lab and tried to steal the concept paper about the chip," Mark added.

"This makes the least sense to me," Lili said. "Why did the thieves not steal the concept paper in the first place?"

"I think they must be different people," Mark concluded. "Susan and Kaleo stole the chips. The next day, somebody else tries to steal the concept paper. I think this is a copycat. Someone else must have learned about the theft and wanted to get the chips for themselves. The theft of the chips was kept highly confidential. This narrows down the list of people who could be the copycat."

"Yes and no," Lili said. "I realized this today. The kidnapper asked Stella to not tell anybody about the kidnapping. But she shared this information with at least two people, Amir and me. Amir told Kaleo and I told you. It seems that if somebody keeps a secret *confidential*, they will tell at least one other person. Humans are social animals. They have to share information, especially when they feel stressed or in danger. Just being listened to will create relief. If each of our core team members even shared their *secret* with two people, then the message spread exponentially."

"Apart from not remaining a secret for long, the other problem is that you feel connected when someone shares their secret with you. You want to guard them," Mark explained. "That was your reaction to Stella sharing her secret with you."

"Now, we truly arrived where we started," Lili said.

"I agree. And it is late. Did Amir contact you about a meeting with the kidnapper?" Mark asked.

Lili checked her phone. "No messages," she I said.

"Okay. I guess even a kidnapper will need some sleep at some point." Mark pulled her closer. "I cannot imagine he will contact Kaleo and Amir at midnight. Let's get some sleep. Tomorrow is another day."

- 24 -
Terrel
REVELATIONS

Tuesday, May 25, 2032, 9.00 pm.

As soon as he had completed all formalities with Lucas Davis, Terrel Wright left the emergency area of the San Francisco General Hospital and hurried up the hospital stairs towards the second floor, taking two steps at once. He had to talk with Stella Pellegrini about Amir Nielsson. She had known him, but not said anything. But it was already late in the evening. *I hope Stella is still awake*, he thought. *Why did she not tell us that she knew Amir Nielsson? What else had she held back?* As he reached the surgery ward, Terrel slowed down. He was not sure in which room he could find her. He went to the central nurse desk, showed his FBI badge and asked for Stella's room. A big, eagle-eyed nurse with a name tag "Tracy" inspected Terrel up and down. She grunted in disapproval. "It is late, sir! We have visitor restrictions in the evenings here. This is not a bar; this is a hospital! Our patients need rest to heal."

"I completely understand," Terrel said, flashing his most charming smile. "Tracy, I was hoping that you could grant me an exception. I am trying to rescue a missing girl and Mrs. Pellegrini might have important information about her whereabouts. Could you please check if she is still awake? I would not ask if it were not important. If she is sleeping already, I will come back tomorrow."

Tracy looked at Terrel for a moment, deciding what to do. Then, she got up from her seat and showed him to Stella's room. She knocked carefully on Stella's door. To Terrel's relieve, Stella responded.

She was still awake! He thought.

The nurse asked Terrel to wait at the door and went into the room.

Terrel heard her voice through the half-closed door. "Hello Mrs.

Pellegrini, there is an FBI agent in the hallway, asking to see you. Would you be willing to speak with him at this late hour? If you are not comfortable to see him how, that is completely fine. I can ask him to come back tomorrow morning."

Terrel heard Stella responding. "Yes, of course, I can see him. Please send him in."

Terrel heard footsteps approaching. Tracy opened the door and waved him in. "I would appreciate, if you could keep it brief, Mr. Wright."

Terrel nodded and entered the room as quietly as possible. "Hello Mrs. Pellegrini," he said. "Thank you for seeing me at this late time. I do not want to disrupt your sleep. But I have some really important questions for you, which could help me to find your daughter."

"No problem, Mr. Wright," Stella responded. "I am actually glad to see you. I already slept for a few hours. But then I woke up and could not fall asleep again. I am so worried about Susan!"

Terrel went straight to the point. "I just noticed that the nurse practitioner whom we met earlier in the ER, Mr. Amir Nielsson, is actually the owner of an apartment where Susan stayed overnight."

Stella sighed. "I wondered all evening if I should have told you. I was terrified that Susan might get hurt if I talk to you. But I have not heard from her or Kaleo until now. I am starting to think that they need help." She pointed to a chair next to her. "Please have a seat. I will tell you everything I know. But please promise that you will keep this absolutely confidential."

Terrel sat down and took Stella's hand. "Mrs. Pellegrini, I will do everything in my power to bring your daughter back. This is what I am trained to do. But you need to trust me. I need more information to find her."

Stella nodded, her eyes filling with tears. And she started to tell Terrel the whole story. How she got to Susan's apartment, how the man with the leather jacket had tied her to a chair and threatened her with a gun, how Susan and Kaleo had walked into his trap and how the man with the leather jacket had kidnapped her daughter and asked Kaleo to bring the brain chips as a ransom. Sharing her fears with the FBI agent emotionally overwhelmed Stella. Tears were running down her cheeks, as she explained, "Susan acted very strange, as if she was on drugs or something. She did not try to defend herself at all. She was not herself! And the man was ruthless and brutal! I am horrified what he could do to her!"

Terrel nodded, trying not to interrupt the flow of revelations. He held her hand when she shared her story, softly asking for details whenever he needed clarification.

Stella continued, "I know that the situation is grim. I have concluded that I cannot rely on Kaleo alone. I need all the help that I can get, and I am relieved that the FBI will take over. You surely are more experienced with kidnappers than Kaleo! But I am also afraid that breaking the silence could hurt my daughter! The kidnapper specifically told me not to talk with anyone. What if he finds out that I talked with you? I would never forgive myself if Susan got hurt because of my indiscretion!"

Terrel squeezed her hand. "Mrs. Pellegrini, I can assure you that you did the right thing! The FBI has much more experience and resources at their disposal than a graduate student. We will do everything to bring your daughter back!"

When he finally wished her a good night, Stella was exhausted. Terrel stopped at Tracy's desk and asked her to check on Stella, since the conversation might have upset her. Tracy looked at Terrel with a disapproving gaze. She grunted and walked over to Stella's room. From the distance, Terrel heard the two women chatting for a few moments. He heard Tracy offering Stella a sleeping pill. She had surgery tomorrow morning and needed to gain some strength. He sighed and left the ward. Stella would be in good hands here.

Stella took the sleeping pill that Tracy had offered to her. She tossed around in her bed for a few more minutes, then she fell into a deep sleep. She did not hear the soft buzzing sound of an incoming text message on her phone.

- 25 -
Susan
THE BAD TRIP

Tuesday, May 25, 2032, 9.00 pm.

Susan could not move at all. Boris had used an entire duct tape roll to tie her to the chair at the loft. In addition, she was afraid to move the chair at all. She anxiously looked at the bat that still leaned against the bed post. After a long time of waiting, Susan heard a car approaching. It stopped in front of the cabin. The car door opened and closed shut. Then, she heard steps on the front porch. Somebody knocked at the door. Susan raised her neck in order to peek over the front railing of the loft. She could see that Boris was sitting on a chair downstairs, facing the front door. The visitor knocked at the door again. Boris drew his gun from the inside pocket of his leather jacket and pointed it on the door.

"Come in, the door is open," Boris said in a cold, loud voice.

The door flung open and Kaleo stepped into the room. His eyes searched the room. He saw Boris and the gun, pointing at him. Kaleo stopped at the entrance and slowly extended his uninjured left hand, offering a small box on his open palm, as if offering food to a wild animal. His hand trembled.

Boris got up from his chair. He walked towards Kaleo and snatched the box from his hand. Kaleo sighed. He looked upwards and saw Susan, tied to her chair. Susan felt tears running down her cheeks.

"You promised to let her go," Kaleo said calmly to Boris.

"This is not quite what I said," Boris responded. "I said I would not shoot her. No worries, I am a man of my word." He opened the box and took out a small plastic bag. He opened it. Susan could see how he inspected the content. Then, he looked at Kaleo. "There are only four chips here, but there are supposed to be five. Where is the fifth chip?" He pointed the gun at Kaleo.

Kaleo looked at Boris. "We only got four chips, the fifth must have got lost when I fell in the lab."

"You are a liar," Boris said with a calm, icy voice. "I saw the video of your amateur departure from the lab. The box never opened, and nothing fell out of it."

Kaleo took a deep breath. "Man, we only had four chips. Why would I bring you four, if I had five?"

"I can think of many, many reasons," Boris responded.

"I swear, I have only these four chips!" Kaleo exclaimed, "Look, I would do anything for Susan. If I had another chip, I would bring it to you!"

Susan started screaming from the loft, but the gag in her mouth prevented her from forming any words. *Tell him I have it right here!* She screamed. *I have the fifth brain chip!* But the gag did not allow any words to form in her mouth. Nobody could understand her.

Kaleo looked at Susan. He waved a hand kiss in her direction. "I love you, Susan!" he said softly.

Boris looked at Kaleo, hate building up in his face. "Did I allow you to talk to her?" he asked. "Susan is with me now!"

"We made a deal," Kaleo insisted. "The brain chips against Susan! If you are a man of honor indeed, you'll have to let her go!"

Boris looked at him and said coldly. "The brain chips against Susan! That was the deal indeed. But you did not fulfill your part! You will bring me the fifth chip and you can have her back!"

"I don't have the fifth chip!" Kaleo exclaimed. "Let her go!"

Boris nodded. "I believe you, Kaleo," he said calmly. "Unfortunately, you do not make demands here. You failed." Boris pointed the gun at Kaleo's head.

Suddenly, Kaleo stormed at Boris, trying to push him to the ground. The gun flew across the cabin floor and landed in front of the fireplace. Both men fell to the ground and started to roll and flail across the floor. Kaleo was strong, but inexperienced in physical fights. He punched Boris' chest with little effect. Next, he aimed for Boris' chin, but missed. Boris had been surprised by Kaleo's offense, but he was an experienced fighter. With a quick grip, he throttled Kaleo's neck. Kaleo grabbed Boris's hair, trying to pull him backwards. The two men rolled around on the floor, towards the fireplace. Suddenly, Susan heard a sharp, brief, high-pitched sound. Kaleo was thrown backwards, and his head hit the tiles of the fireplace with a dull smash. A pool of red blood was quickly forming around him.

"Nooo!!" Susan cried through the gag. "Kaleo!" She tried to jump up from the chair but was unable to move. She started shaking uncontrollably. *Kaleo, I love you! Please don't die!* Susan sobbed uncontrollably, tears running down her cheeks.

Boris went to Kaleo's body on the floor and kneeled beside him. He put his right index and ring finger on Kaleo's neck for a few seconds. Then, he searched Kaleo's pockets. Boris took out the burner phone and an iPhone. He got up and threw the burner phone into the trash. He put Kaleo's iPhone into the outer pocket of his leather jacket. Then he gripped Kaleo's lifeless arms and pulled him in front of the kitchenette. He fetched a blanket from the sofa and covered Kaleo's body. Then he went to the dining table, sat down, pulled his own cell phone and dialed a number. Susan tried to control her pain and hold her breath, trying to hear as much as possible of the conversation.

"This is Boris." Boris said.

Susan could not hear the other side. *I wished I had implanted the chip over the hearing cortex of my brain*, she thought, tears running down her cheeks.

"I am sorry for contacting you, boss. I know this line is reserved for emergencies. But I need your input. We got a complication." Boris said.

"I got four chips back, not five."

What does he mean. He got the chips back? Susan wondered. *Did he have them previously?*

"Yes, I will come over tonight and put them in your mailbox." Boris said.

"No worries, I will wait until everyone is sleeping, probably around two or three am."

"I have no idea where the fifth chip is. Kaleo said that he lost one when he fell in the lab. But that was a lie. All chips were in one box. There is no way that one just fell out of the box. Perhaps he already sold one?"

"Yes, of course, I understand. We do not want to leave any loose ends anywhere. If you can find out a lead, I will be happy to pursue it."

"Yes, I will await your call tomorrow."

Boris hung up the phone. Then, he climbed up the stairs to the loft. Susan saw him emerging in front of her. Her heart started racing. *He will torture me to find out where the fifth chip is*, she thought. She looked at Boris's hands. He did not carry a weapon. Susan glared at Boris as he came closer. This time, he did not look into her eyes. *Perhaps he feels some remorse*, she thought. Boris walked around her. Susan realized that he was checking the tape around her feet, body, and face. *Perhaps he is too macho to think that I could know anything.* She prayed that this was the case.

"I have to leave for a little while," Boris said. "It won't be long. If I find you anywhere else than on this chair when I get back, you will get your favorite fracture. Is that understood?"

Susan nodded slowly.

"You will stay put," Boris said. "I might need you tomorrow.

Susan nodded again.

Boris turned around, climbed down the stairs, walked through the main cabin room, opened the entrance door and disappeared in the darkness of the night. Susan heard the cabin door's lock click shut. Then, a car engine started. The noise of the motor briefly got louder, then it slowly disappeared.

Susan looked around. She was alone. Boris had turned down all the lights in the cabin and the night had settled. She tried to look for Kaleo's body in the main cabin room below her, but Boris had dragged Kaleo somewhere under the balustrade of the loft, out of her sight. Susan felt completely overwhelmed by her emotions and started to weep uncontrollably. *What mess did I get us into? This is all my fault!* She knew how scared Kaleo must have been. Yet he came here to save her. *If Kaleo is dead, I do not want to live any more either,* she thought. The darkness seemed to embrace her. As Susan looked down, the shadows of the night seemed to become alive. The floor was breathing slowly, first moving up and down like a deadly lake, then moving sideways, opening a deep dark gorge below her. The chair legs seemed to mix with the floor and disappear in the darkness. Then, Susan saw her feet slowly merging with the roaring darkness as well. *This can't be real! It must be a hallucination!*

Susan tried to focus her mind and look in a different direction.

Light had always helped her to fight against nightmares. She looked for the brightest spot in the room, which was the balustrade of the loft in front of her. But it was hard to see anything clearly in the darkness. Susan realized that the sight of the black hole was streaking. It now appeared in front of her. It started as a small black cloud, the size of the palm of her hand. The black cloud expanded and started to spiral inwards, creating a horrifying abyss. Susan noticed a naked arm emerging from the hole, waving her in. She tried to look to the right in order to escape from this gruesome experience. But the abyss followed her. The arm duplicated into two, then four, eight, and many more. Within seconds, hundreds of arms appeared out of the hole, reaching for her, trying to drag her in. Susan wanted to scream, but her cry of horror was muffled by the gag in her mouth. *I am losing my mind!* she thought.

- 26 -
Boris
THE RESTAURANT

Wednesday, May 25, 2032, 10.30 pm.

Boris drove away from the cabin, his car bumping up and down the unpaved road. It was dark outside, and the narrow beam of the headlights did not outline the many potholes along the way. When he tried to avoid one, he bumped into another. Boris tried to contain his anger. The past hours had been a Deja vu of his most dreaded past. At first, the little bitch had manipulated his feelings. She had looked at him with her little puppy eyes and called his name with her sweet, melodic voice – like a little siren that lured him into the dark sea of betrayal. He had silenced her voice as a siren deserved. When she ran away from the cabin, her real nature had come out. She had reminded him of Inessa, his now-dead ex-girlfriend. Boris still did not understand how someone he loved and trusted could betray him with another guy. He felt pathetic for being fooled. He wanted *her* to feel his pain. After all, she had caused it. But then that wannabe movie star of a boyfriend showed up, like a little prince who came to her rescue. Boris was disgusted. The guy had not *listened*; what he was supposed to do? He delivered four chips instead of five. *What a fool!* Boris thought. *He thought he could change the rules! Now, everyone can see who is in charge here!* Boris tightened his grip around the steering wheel so that his knuckles turned pale. He had reached the ramp to the interstate 280 and drove towards Redwood City.

After a twenty-minute drive, Boris parked on the sidewalk in Redwood City, two blocks away from his favorite restaurant. He followed his security rule to separate his own location and the location of his car. That had saved his life many times. Boris got out of the car and walked to the restaurant. He loved this place for so many reasons. First, it was a hidden restaurant. It was located in a regular apartment complex, without any signs that there was a restaurant at all. Second, it was open until midnight, which suited his preference for late dinners. Third, it was run by only three people and had limited occupancy, which limited the number of people who could remember him and allowed him to keep an eye on everyone in the room at all times. And finally, the little restaurant had a backdoor, which would allow for a quick retreat in case of a security threat.

Boris had arrived at the entrance, a beautifully carved cedar double door. On the wall beside the door was a golden name plate, with the family name engraved in Japanese characters. Boris rang the doorbell and stepped back. He had learned that the doors opened outward in this building. A young woman opened the door and let him in.

"Hello, Boris!" she said softly, smiling at him.

"Hello, Ichika!" he smiled back. Boris had gotten to know the daughter of the restaurant owners. She was a slim young woman with a beautiful face and perfectly smooth, pale skin. Her movements were graceful, perhaps a little shy at times. Boris liked her – a lot. But this had to be his last dinner here. It was too risky if people remembered him. *Just one last dinner!* Boris got a little sentimental about the prospect of relocating.

He entered the dining room, which was not much larger than a standard living room — and that's probably what it was. The owner of the restaurant, Ichika's father, greeted Boris with a brief wave of his hand from the adjacent open kitchen where he prepared the meals. The dining room featured six dining tables, which were aligned in two rows with almost mathematical precision. The tables and chairs were simple, but decent, with a clear square teak design. On each table, there was a small white tablecloth and a vase with a single rose. Five tables were occupied, and one was vacant. It was late and most of the guests were finishing up their meals or paying their bills. The wife of the owner was busy attending to the customers. Nobody paid specific attention to Boris. Ichika led him to the vacant table, and he sat down.

"Would you like to order your usual dinner?" she asked.

"Yes, please! The dragon roll, teriyaki chicken and two Haku vodkas. Please bring two plates. I have a guest."

"Yes, sir!" Ichika bowed slightly and rushed to the open kitchen to give her father the order.

Boris checked the clock on his iPhone. He was five minutes early. He leaned back and looked around. Gentle koto music filled the room. He liked this restaurant. Life here was simple, attentive and respectful. The dining guests were seated with enough distance to enable private conversations. The windows were covered by sudare, traditional window coverings made from horizontal sticks of bamboo. The sudare let in a cool breeze and avoided unwanted spectators. Ichika brought two wet towels, two plates and the drinks. Boris wiped his hands and took a sip of Haku.

A mechanical two-tone chime announced a guest at the door. Ichika rushed to the door. She spoke briefly with the person at the entrance. Boris heard her polite, high-pitched voice. "Sorry, we are closed." A brief discussion followed. Her mother, who was collecting the payment from customers at one of the tables looked up to see if her daughter needed assistance. But Ischika had already turned around and closed the door softly. Boris grinned. Not everyone was welcome here. The owners reserved the right to refuse service to anyone they did not find suitable for their serene environment. But Boris was part of the family. He took another sip. A gentle wave of warmth filled his chest and stomach, slowly lulling his agitated mind.

The doorbell rang again. Ischika and her mother exchanged a quick look. The mother, an elderly lady with a resolute look on her face, went to answer the door. Apparently, it was a different guest this time. Ichika's mother spoke to the person outside briefly, then she invited him in with a gentle gesture. Bogdan stepped into the room with long strides and looked around. He saw Boris and walked towards him with open arms.

"Boris, it is so great to see you!"

"*Privyet*, Bogdan! It is great to see you, too!"

Boris stood up from his chair, he embraced Bogdan and kissed him on each cheek. They both sat down. Boris raised his glass and Bogdan raised his own. A few minutes later, Ischika arrived with the food. She placed a sushi plate and three bowls with teriyaki chicken, rice and salad between them. She had remembered to serve all the food at once, which prevented interruptions during dinner conversations.

"Thank you, Ischika! You are the most attentive woman on the whole planet!"

Ischika smiled politely, bowed slightly and walked away. Boris watched her as she retreated to the kitchen. He would have liked to cut open that pretty head to see what was really in there. From the corner of his eye, he also noticed the alert gaze of her mother on him. That woman was like a hawk! Boris focused his attention on Bogdan. He had started eating and Boris got right to the point.

"Did you get the construction plans of the brain chips?"

Bogdan carefully dipped a piece of sushi in the soy sauce, put it in his mouth, chewed and swallowed. "I am sorry, but our plan did not work out."

"What do you mean?"

"The scientist arrived in the lab earlier than usual. We got into a fight. I got away but could not retrieve the plans for the chip."

"Oh, man!"

"I know. It is a brilliant plan to return the stolen chips to SUEC for a hefty fee and sell the plans for the chips to the KGB. That's what I call baddie double dipping!" Bogdan chuckled.

"Well, I did my part. I have the brain chips here!" Boris pointed to the pocket of his jacket.

"Why don't you sell those to thc KGB?"

"First, the dean knows me. If I don't bring him the chips, he will send the FBI after me. Second, we can get twice as much money if we sell the chips and construction plans separately. That, of course, depends on you getting the documents!"

"I took a photo of the first page." Bogdan showed a photo of a document page to Boris. "But it was a twelve-page file. I will have to go back and take photos of the other pages – or just take the whole document."

Boris loaded rice and chicken on his plate. "Should I help with that?"

Bogdan shook his head. "Let me try again tomorrow. I work at SUEC and therefore, have a much higher chance of retrieving the plans without being noticed. You usually leave a trail of dead bodies. That will drop the price."

They both laughed. Boris looked at Bogdan. "Why don't you get the plans for the brain chips tonight?"

"They installed a new security system in the lab and placed an

FBI agent at the entrance for round-the-clock surveillance. I have to find a way around it. As you know, I am part of the security IT crew. I will figure out a way. But I will need some time to make a plan."

"Okay, you can try again tomorrow. If you are unsuccessful, then I will retrieve the documents on Thursday, during their big event."

The two-tone chime announced another guest at the door. Boris looked at the clock on his iPhone. It was almost midnight. Most of the guests had left. The restaurant owner had printed out their check and placed it on the kitchen bar, where Ischika's mother could pick it up. Ichika had retreated to the back of the house. Her mother went to answer the door. Boris automatically listened in. He heard her polite voice. "Sorry, we are closed!" From there, a lively conversation ensued at the entrance. But the voices were so low that Boris could not understand any details. Suddenly, the door flung wide open, and three men rushed into the room, pointing guns at Boris and Bogdan with extended arms.

"This is the FBI. Raise your hands and do not move! We are armed and will shoot if needed!"

Bogdan was sitting with his back to the three FBI agents. He looked at Boris in horror and slowly raised his arms.

Boris looked at the men at the entrance. They had pointed guns at them and were slowly coming closer. But they did not have a straight shot line at him. Bogdan was sitting between them. Boris quickly leaped towards the open kitchen and cowered behind the kitchen bar. He heard a gunshot hitting the oven behind him. Ichika's mother cried out and the old man dug in behind the kitchen counter. Boris looked backwards, planning a run for the back door. But to his left, he saw Ichika in a door frame behind the large refrigerator. He had never seen this door; it was hidden from restaurant customers by the large appliance. Ichika waved at him. Boris made a decision in a split-second. He was not sure where Ichika wanted him to go. But it was very likely that FBI agents had already secured the back door. Ichika was smart and she lived here. She was his best bet to get out!

Boris jumped towards Ichika, and they both ran down a staircase into the basement of the building. It was dark here. Ischika did not turn on any lights. She took Boris's hand and led him swiftly down a hallway.

Boris heard the FBI men running after them. But they had difficulties finding their way in the darkness. Ischika ran around a corner and stopped abruptly. The hallway ended blindly in a small storage room. There were two more refrigerators, a freezer, and three large shelves, which were overflowing with various food items. Boris cursed. This was a dead end! But Ischika gently pushed one of the shelves at the end of the room. The shelf moved to the left and revealed another hallway. It was a hidden door. Ischika pointed towards the dark hallway behind the shelf and Boris ran through. He briefly looked back. Ischika did not follow him. She waved him goodbye and gently closed the shelf door behind him.

Boris sighed. This little girl had just saved his life. He would reward her handsomely. Boris carefully walked down the dark hallway, more feeling the way with extended arms than seeing it. He heard loud voices in the room behind him, but no more footsteps followed him. The hallway connected to another apartment next door. The voices slowly faded in the distance. Boris walked up the stairs to the living room. All the lights were out here. A faint glow from streetlights came in through the windows, outlining shadows of furniture. The room was calm and empty. Perhaps the restaurant owners lived here.

Boris tried to orient himself. The restaurant was on the left side of the apartment building. Boris went as far as possible to the right side. He found a bathroom on the right-hand side of the building. Boris opened the bathroom window and looked outside. There was a small empty street, which was faintly illuminated by streetlamps. A car drove by. There were no pedestrians around. A racoon watched him with great interest from the other side of the road. Boris grabbed the window frame and jumped feet first through the window. He landed like a cat on the sidewalk. He got up, straightened his leather jacket and took a deep breath. Then, he walked slowly to his car, got in and drove away.

- 27 -
Angus
THE ARREST

Wednesday, May 25, 2032, 11.55 pm.

Angus had investigated Dr. Hill's lab earlier today and found several hairs in the area of the fight with the intruder. He had submitted those to the forensics lab. An hour ago, he had received a match. Bogdan Smirnoff, a member of the SUEC security team. To his dismay, he also received FBI intel that the last name was a fake name. Bogdan's real last name was Sokolov, and Bogdan Sokolov had a long history of felonies, including grand theft, arson and sale of illegal drugs. Dean Bennett had missed this when he conducted Bogdan's background check before hiring him to the security team at SUEC. The security team! Angus asked his team to locate Bogdan immediately. They found him – or rather his cell phone – in a local restaurant at Redwood city. Angus had ordered an immediate response team from the FBI and stormed the restaurant.

When the FBI team got into the small restaurant, Bogdan was sitting with his back to the door. This was really a beginner mistake. Angus concluded that Bogdan was not a professional criminal, but probably just a casual thief. Nevertheless, the stolen items were a matter of national security. The FBI team had arrested him. But the other man at Bogdan's table got away. Angus' decades of experience told him that this man was important. A regular dinner guest would not just disappear into thin air. Angus asked the owners of the restaurant, an elderly Asian man and his wife, if they knew the other man or remembered how he looked like. But they only shrugged and shook their heads. Angus also asked the daughter. She looked at him with an unrevealing gaze, shaking her head as well. Angus was not sure, if the family did not understand him if they did not know anything or if they did not want to say anything. In any case, they were clearly not interested in sharing any information.

Angus turned his attention to Bogdan. His colleagues had handcuffed him and placed him on the back seat of the FBI van. Bogdan looked at Angus with an uneasy smile.

"Hello Mr. Sokolov, I am FBI agent Angus Weber, and I am investigating an attempted theft of classified materials in a research lab at SUEC University."

Bogdan raised his tied hands. "Hello, Agent Weber, I remember you! I saw you at SUEC. This must be a misunderstanding. I am a security guard at SUEC. I do not steal classified materials, I protect them! Why would you interrupt my dinner and arrest me? I am an innocent citizen!"

"Well, for a starter, you applied for a job as a security guard with a fake name. In addition, we found your DNA in a SUEC lab, where a researcher was attacked. You are under arrest for attempted grand theft, Mr. Sokolov!"

Bogdan scoffed. "I am innocent! Perhaps I slightly misspelled my name when I signed up for the job. My mother's name is Sokolow. This was just an honest error!"

"We found your DNA at a crime scene!"

"Of course, I had to check the security of the lab. I am a security guard, not a thief. You do not have any proof for your insulting accusation."

Angus Weber looked at him. "Mr. Sokolov, I am from the FBI. I can arrest you based on reasonable evidence that you threated the national security of the United States of America. You had no authority to be in this lab and yet we found your DNA at a crime scene of attempted grand theft. I suggest you consider carefully if you would like to make a voluntary statement. That might have a positive effect on your charge."

Bogdan insisted, "I do not know how my DNA got there. Perhaps I ran into the researcher in the cafeteria, and he had it on his clothes."

This conversation was clearly not getting anywhere. Angus changed the subject. "Who was the man who was dining with you in this restaurant?"

Bogdan shrugged. "I do not know him. I only joined him at his table for dinner because there was no other free table available in the restaurant when I arrived. A very nice man. He did not tell me his name."

Angus gave up and cited the Miranda warning. "You have the right to remain silent. Anything you say can be used against you in court. You have the right to talk to a lawyer for advice before we ask you any questions. You have the right to have a lawyer with you during questioning. If you cannot afford a lawyer, one will be appointed for you before any questioning if you wish. If you decide to answer questions now without a lawyer present, you have the right to stop answering at any time."

Bogdan exhaled noisily. "I didn't do anything wrong."

Angus looked at him. Then he talked briefly with his colleagues. They nodded, got into the van, closed the doors and drove off. They would take Bogdan Sokolov into custody, photograph and fingerprint him. But Angus was not sure if the evidence would allow him to bring Bogdan to justice. He sighed. Life was definitely not fair.

- 28 -
Annya
PTSD

Wednesday, May 26, 2032, 2.00 am.

Annya was tossing around in her bed, trying to sleep. The news about Juan and Juliana Perez's death had taken a bigger toll on her than she would admit to herself. She stared at the ceiling of her featureless, small bedroom for a long time, trying to calm her nerves. Finally, she dozed off into a hollow, superficial sleep. She dreamed of a man in a dark leather jacket, pointing a gun at her. The barrel was wide enough that she could see the bullet in the chamber. She froze in horror. Then, she heard the gunshot in her head and the dull sound of a body falling to the ground. *Was it Juan or Juliana? Or her own body?* She felt a dull pain behind her forehead and blood running down her temples. *Was she injured?*

Annya jerked up from her bed, soaked in sweat. She reached for her forehead, trying to hold back the blood that was gushing out of the gunshot wound. But there was no injury. She only felt her old scar. *It was just a dream!* Annya's heart raced. She switched on the little rococo lamp on her nightstand, catching her beath. *Stay focused! These are just memories from the past! You are safe now!* she told herself over and over again until the attack slowly vanished. Annya checked the time on her iPhone. Two-fifteen am. The whole night was still in front of her. But she was too stressed out to lie down again. As a physician, she knew that she had just experienced a panic attack from her posttraumatic stress disorder. It was by far not the first time, and she did get better handling these attacks.

Annya got up and sat on the side of the bed for a moment, adjusting her eyes to the gentle light of the nightstand lamp. She had to get the horrific picture of the man with the gun out of her head. She focused her attention away from her forehead and towards her feet.

She had learned this as a coping mechanism in meditation class. The plush carpet under her naked feet felt nice and soft. Annya stood up and walked around the bed to the bathroom.

She opened the bathroom door and stepped onto the cold tiles. She looked around. The dim-blue phosphorescent night light dipped the appliances into a soft-velvety haze. Annya went to the faucet and turned it on. She collected water with both hands and threw it into her face. Again. And again. The cool liquid prickled on her skin and refreshed her senses.

Annya looked into the mirror. The water had soaked her long bangs. She stroked her hair backwards with the extended fingers of her hands. She looked at the large scar on her forehead. It had been more difficult to conceal when it was still dark and red. Meanwhile, the color of the scar had turned to a faint white. She applied makeup to her forehead every morning to cover it. The bangs did the rest, covering the tragedy of her story like the front curtain in an old theater. Annya was pretty sure that nobody at SUEC had ever seen her scar. That was good. She did not want to talk about her past. She did not want to think about it. She wanted to erase all the miserable and gruesome memories in her brain and overwrite them with experiences of joy and fulfillment. She was living in a different world now.

Annya took a deep breath, savoring the moment. When the hospital leadership had invited her to join the physician team at SUEC hospital, she had been intrigued by the ability to provide high quality medical care at the most famous university in the world. At SUEC hospital, everyone was under constant surveillance, and she was in control. She was not the victim. She was the savior. But as much as work at the hospital had intrigued her intellectually, the SUEC campus had *enchanted* her at a deep emotional level. The sight of the octagonal university building and the small village underneath, embraced by towering redwood and sequoia trees, had hit her like a scene from a fairytale. This was the first place in a long time where she had instantly felt at home. The remote location of the university campus, the gated entrance and the abundance of security guards who patrolled the campus around the clock added to a feeling of protection and serenity. In her contract, she had agreed to a rather modest salary but negotiated accommodation in one of the few faculty apartments on the SUEC campus. She was aware that she was the only physician who lived on campus. All the other faculty tenants were researchers. The university leadership had agreed to her request to live on campus because they considered it convenient to have an emergency physician on site. On multiple occasions, Annya had been called at night to check on minor accidents or other health problems of the campus residents. She did not mind. On the contrary, every time she helped someone out, she felt a gratifying sense of belonging to this community.

Before the Perez killing, Annya had thought that everyone would be fascinated by the important work at SUEC. Surely, nobody would want to harm people who were working on the most important innovations of our time! But she now realized that not everybody thought this way. SUEC workers were not superhuman and they were not invulnerable. Her belief system had been shuttered and the deaths of Juan and Juliana Perez had disrupted her sense of safety.

Annya took a deep breath. She hadn't felt so shaken for quite some time. She needed to clear her mind. She went back to the bedroom and got dressed in her jogging outfit. She had learned in her coping classes that walking or running could break her out of a PTSD episode by interrupting her body's stress response and grounding her in the present moment. That was exactly what she needed right now. Annya put on her dark gray sports hoodie, her black running leggings, her sneakers and a pair of red headphones. As usual when she was going out at night, she also took her Glock out of the drawer of her nightstand and put it into the pocket of her hoodie. Becoming a legal concealed carrier had significantly accelerated her mental recovery. At 2.30 am, Annya stepped out of her apartment and made her way to the visitors' promenade on the left, that led up to the main university building. The path was lined by redwood trees and multiple solar-powered torches, which sent a fairylike flickering light over the pavement of the walkway. Annya briskly walked up the softly illuminated path, taking in the emerging view over the valley. The university buildings in the valley to her right looked calm and serene. They were outlined by little streetlights, like a fleet of starships on a starry night sky. There was no other human in sight. Even the chipmunks were sleeping in their underground dwellings. The air was fresh and cool, with a light scent of pine trees.

Annya continued her walk up the promenade. After about fifteen minutes, she arrived at the stairs to the visitors' terrace on the left-hand side of the main university building. She walked up the stairs, crossed the visitors terrace, stepped towards a gate at the back end of the terrace and activated the door opener by pressing the fingers of her right hand on an ID pad. The door flung open and Annya walked to the terrace in front of the octagonal university building. Even at night, the view was breathtaking from here. A full moon gently illuminated miles of redwood hills around her, like a sea of shimmering dark green emeralds which embraced the SUEC valley. Annya took a moment to enjoy the beautiful view. As always, this walk had calmed her mind and created a feeling of peacefulness and gratitude. *She was a different person now than she had been a decade ago! She was not an easy target anymore! She was strong and powerful!* Annya sighed with content and continued her way down the promenade on the right side of the building.

The two promenades created a nice loop. The pathway on the right was similarly outlined by redwood trees and illuminated with solar torches, mirroring its complement on the left. As Annya walked down the hill, she noticed the outline of a dark shadow in the far distance. This was most unusual at about three in the morning. Nobody was supposed to be here, except for the security guards. This person did not stroll up the promenade as if they had endless time. They almost ran towards the main SUEC building.

Annya's senses immediately switched back to alarm mode. She quickly stepped into the darkness of the adjacent redwood trees, away from the torch light, and observed the approaching shadow from a safe distance.

The shadow came up the promenade. It was probably a man, and he clearly did not wear the uniform of the security guards. Was he limping? Annya's physician eye sensed a slight asymmetry in the gait, barely visible.

As the shadow came closer, Annya felt a baffling sense of familiarity. His silhouette and his movements reminded her of her past. *She knew this man!* Annya froze. *No, this was impossible! This must be another panic attack!* Annya tried to calm herself down and get a better view of the person's face. But the man was looking down onto the walkway, apparently trying to spot and avoid any obstacles along the faintly lit pathway. Then, as he came closer and passed one of the torches, he looked up to the octagon building and Annya got a good view of his profile.

She had to conceal a cry of surprise and horror. *This could not be true! This person looked like Boris Sokolov!* Perhaps she was still in the middle of her nightmare! Annya pinched her arm to make sure she was awake. Even though she was already concealed by the darkness of the redwood trees, she cowered lower to hide herself. She watched the man as he passed her and walked up the promenade. He stepped up to the terrace on the right of the main building and approached the entrance area. The main entrance of the building was illuminated all night with spotlights. Annya could see the man approaching the entrance area, pulling something from his pocket and reaching for the door. Annya held her breath. Was he trying to break into the building? He could not be serious. This was one of the best secured buildings in the country. But the man had already turned around and walked away from the building, down the promenade and towards her. Annya held her breath. Hopefully, he had not seen her. The man came closer again, passed her and walked down the hill.

Annya was torn about what to do. If this was Boris indeed, then he was here to hurt someone. Should she walk up the hill, trying to find what he had done at the entrance? No! She decided against it. Boris was an expert. Whatever he was up to, he would not leave any traces. Annya carefully stepped out of the trees and followed the man from a distance. Perhaps she could find out where he was going. For her own sanity, she had to make sure he had left the campus.

Boris walked with long strides down the hill, albeit putting more weight on his left rather than his right foot. He was limping for sure. Boris passed the SUEC village and walked towards the parking lot. Annya continued to follow him, trying to stay under the shadow of the trees, away from the torches. Boris approached a parked car on the left-hand side of the parking lot. It was a BMW. Annya saw a security guard at the far-right end of the parking lot. That encouraged Annya to come a little closer. Perhaps she could see the license plate of the car. Boris walked towards the right side of the car and opened the passenger door. Then he walked around the car, opened the driver's door, got in and closed the door.

Still under the protection of the trees, Annya came closer. She could see parts of the license plate. AMC3... Suddenly, she heard the man calling her. Annya froze instantly. A shiver went down her back. It was Boris' voice! But he apparently had not recognized her in the darkness. He called over to her. "Hello, can you please close my passenger door? I am handicapped and have a hard time walking around." Annya took a gentle turn around, as if on a stroll, and walked away from the parking lot as calmly as possible. Boris continued calling her while Annya continued to ignore him. She slowly walked up the promenade, her heart racing. Boris started cursing at her. Annya knew that he had a gun. He always had. But he would not have a straight line towards her, as she walked up the promenade under the protection of the trees. The more distance she could gain, the more the darkness would embrace her. From the corner of her eyes, Annya saw the security guard walking over to the parked car. Then, she heard the passenger door slammed shut and the car speed away.

Annya's heart was racing. She was sure she had just escaped an assault. Whatever Boris was up to meant pain and destruction for her and her fairytale world. She would not let that happen again. Annya briskly walked all the way back, up the promenade and towards the entrance of the SUEC building. At the entrance, she looked around carefully. As expected, she found nothing unusual. *What did Boris want here?* She thought. She looked around once more. Nothing.

Annya finally decided to go back to the village. It was approaching four am now, and she had to get ready for her morning shift in the ER. Annya walked back to her apartment, took a shower and brewed herself a strong coffee. With this little sleep, work in the ER would get extra stressful today. But this was not her first sleepless night. She would manage.

- 29 -
Amir
THE ADDRESS

Wednesday, May 26, 2032, 5.30 am.

Amir had asked Jimmy, one of his friends, if he could crash at his place. He had told Jimmy that painters had painted his apartment and that it stank too much to sleep there tonight. Jimmy worked as a nurse practitioner on the intensive care unit at the California Pacific Medical Center (CPMC). Amir thought that it was highly unlikely that the FBI agents would reach out to Jimmy, at least not tonight. It turned out that Jimmy was on night shift. Amir considered this a great coincidence as he would not have to explain his situation any further. Amir was unfailingly sincere. After a beer or two, he would probably come out with the truth. So, he was glad that he could just pick up the key to the apartment at CPMC and spend the night at Jimmy's apartment on his own. He had been exhausted, had gone to bed early and had fallen into a deep sleep.

Amir woke up in the early morning, physically refreshed, but worried. He checked his phone every few minutes, but there was no message from Kaleo. He went to the kitchen and made a coffee in the "one cup only" espresso machine. *Who wants only one cup of coffee in the morning?* he thought. Fortunately, there were plenty of capsules. Amir made himself a second coffee. He looked around the kitchen and found some bread to toast and some marmalade. That would do. He would stop at the grocery store later today and replace it. Amir ate his breakfast and waited for a message from Kaleo. The time seemed to stretch endlessly, and Amir's mind spiraled into great anxiety. He was worried about Susan.

Susan and Amir had known each other since they were small children. They had gone to kindergarten and school together, they had celebrated their birthdays together, they had routinely slept over at each other's house, and they had gone to the same summer camps. Amir had held Susan's hand on her first day at primary school, he had wiped away her tears in times of pain and disappointment, he had punched that guy at the bus stop who wanted to intimidate her and he had brewed his famous pomegranate tea for her whenever she was sick. They had argued and fought with each other, they had laughed about each other's jokes, complained about their parents' rules – or grandparents, in Amir's case – and celebrated each other's accomplishments. Amir had been Susan's date for the proms. He had felt uncomfortable, but she had insisted.

Amir sighed. He was not sure when his friendship for Susan had changed to romantic feelings. Susan was the most beautiful girl he had ever met. She was smart, strong, passionate and overwhelmingly positive. Amir was constantly amazed by her ability to beat the odds of her underprivileged upbringing. He and Susan connected on a deep metaphysical level. They could exchange thoughts by just looking in each other's eyes. They were soulmates.

But Amir had told himself that it was pointless to express his feelings to Susan. She was still just a teenager. He was six years older, and it would have been inappropriate to delve any further into his emotions. So, he went to the city to train as a nurse practitioner. This surely got him occupied and Amir lost sight of Susan in the process. It was the most painful experience of his life, when his doorbell rang in San Francisco, and he found Susan on his doorstep — with Kaleo. Which cruel fate in the world had placed the woman of his dreams in his doorstep with superman on her side? *Yeah, it did help that he had learned to keep his emotions in check.* Susan had looked so happy. But what a stupid plan to steal brain chips from the most famous university in the world! Amir wished he had stayed in touch with her. Perhaps he could have prevented the recent events. He took a sip from his second morning coffee and sighed again. It did not help to dwell in the past. He had to look forward. All that mattered now was to get Susan back safely. Amir paced back-and-forth in Jimmy's apartment, staring at his phone. Nothing.

After waiting for what seemed an eternity, Amir finally decided to call Kaleo. But Kaleo did not pick up his phone.

Amir called Stella next. She picked up the phone right away. "Hello Amir, it is great to hear from you! Have you heard anything from Susan?"

"No, sorry, I haven't. That's why I am calling you, Mrs. Pellegrini. I was wondering if you heard from Kaleo? He wanted to contact me, but he did not."

"No, he did not contact me. I am so worried, Amir!"

"Are you sure he hasn't sent you any text messages?"

"Well, I did not hear any text message coming in. But let me double check."

Amir heard a rustling noise in the background.

"Hello Amir, you were right! I did get a text message from Kaleo! I am not sure how I could have missed it! He has told me that he is on his way to Susan and sent me the address!"

Amir's heart started to race. "Mrs. Pellegrini, can you please forward it to me?"

"Of course, just a second…. I sent it to you. You should receive it shortly!"

A "ping" tone on Amir's phone signaled the incoming message. He opened it and looked up the location on google maps.

"Did you get it?" Stella asked with a trembling voice.

"Yes, thank you, Mrs. Pellegrini. I looked it up. It is not far away from San Francisco, an address in San Mateo, perhaps a twenty-minute drive."

"Amir, last night, the FBI agent visited me here to ask me a few more questions. I was so anxious about Susan that I told him about her. Now, I am very worried if this was the right thing or if that put her in danger."

"I think you did the right thing, Mrs. Pellegrini. We are dealing with an experienced criminal. We can use any help we can get."

"Should I call him now?"

"Perhaps give me some time to check out what is going on. This guy has never seen me, so he cannot assume that I am a threat."

He heard Stella chuckle. "Nobody would think that you are a threat, Amir!"

"I know. We can use that to our advantage. I will drive to the address and check it out. If you do not hear back from me in an hour or so, please call the FBI agent for help."

"Okay. But please be careful, Amir! The man has a gun!"

"I will do everything I can to bring Susan back safely!"

"Thank you, Amir! I am so glad that we ran into each other yesterday! If we get out of this alive, I never want us to lose contact again!

"I missed both of you as well, Mrs. Pellegrini! You will hear back from me shortly!"

Amir hung up the phone, fetched his jacket, left Jimmy's apartment, jumped into his car and drove to the address in San Mateo.

- 30 -
Imani
THE CABIN

Wednesday, May 26, 2032, 5.30 am.

Imani Wright, Terrel's wife, loved to start the day with an early morning run between five-thirty and six am. The weather was cool in the morning, making it comfortable to run before the summer heat set in. In addition, watching the sun rise felt enchanting. The solitude of the early morning hours gave her a quiet, uninterrupted block of time to boost her energy and collect her thoughts before the day got underway.

Meanwhile, Terrel used the first hour of the morning to spend some quality time with his son, Niles. When he heard the alarm clock, their three-year-old son came to join Terrel in the primary bedroom. Curled under the warm blanket, they read Niles's favorite books together, such as Llama and the Gruffalo, while Imani got an energy boost from her morning workout. After Imani was back and had a shower, the whole family had breakfast together and everyone would leave for work – or Kindergarten – around seven-thirty am. Both Imani and Terrel cherished this morning ritual.

Imani had filled out a tentative adoption form for Oscar, the goldendoodle, through the pet clinic where she worked three times a week. The dog did have an implanted chip. The colleagues at the pet clinic had confirmed his identity, called animal control and allowed Imani to foster the dog while giving relatives of the Perez family a chance to come forwards if they wanted to adopt him as well. So far, nobody had cxpressed interest. If this continued, then the Wright family would have priority for an adoption later in the process. Imani had found the name of the dog engraved on his collar. Both she and Niles had instantly fallen in love with him. On the first day at their home, Oscar had been deeply disturbed, hiding behind the sofa in the family room and shaking whenever he heard some noise on the street. Yesterday, Imani and Niles had spent almost the entire day trying to comfort the dog and connecting with him. Oscar's personality slowly emerged. By the time Terrel got home at night, the goldendoodle greeted him playfully at the door.

Imani had created a dog bed in the family room by retrieving an old dresser from the attic and placing a pillow in it. However, when she and Terrel went to bed yesterday, they had heard the dog whining outside. He was lonely and clearly still processing the loss of his previous owners. So, they decided to move the dog bed into the main bedroom, just for the time being, to allow Oscar to adjust. The dog clearly appreciated the gesture. When Imani got up in the morning, she almost had the impression that he was smiling at her, happily wagging his tail.

She decided to take Oscar along for her morning run in order to bond with him further. Imani liked to explore new routes for her morning run and considering the anxiety of the dog, she wanted to find a route that might not be congested with people or traffic. She checked out her trail app and found a suitable wooded area between Montara and the city of Pacifica. Imani put the dog on the leash, went outside and walked towards her dark blue Honda Odyssey. Oscar followed her with a little hesitation at first but did get excited when he saw her opening the side door of the minivan. He was clearly used to excursions that involved a car ride. Oscar jumped on the back seat and settled there without any issues. Imani closed the side door, got into the driver's seat and drove to the selected area, which was only a few minutes' drive from her home.

Imani parked her car on a small parking lot and let the dog out of the car. She looked around, did not see anybody and decided to take Oscar off the leash. The dog constantly looked at her and therefore, she was optimistic that he would follow her. Running without holding the leash would make the exercise much easier. Imani started to run down a small unpaved path into the woods and the dog happily followed her. *This is great!* Imani thought, *I feel much safer running with Oscar than running on my own.* The path led deeper into the woods and Imani inhaled the fresh scent of eucalyptus trees and pine trees. Golden rays of early morning sunlight entranced her track. Imani felt the blood running through her veins, clearing the mental fog of the night's sleep. Running in the morning felt as though her brain clicked on. She ran faster, the dog following her.

All of a sudden, Oscar stopped to sniff at something on the ground. Imani stopped as well about twenty meters down the path. She called the dog, but Oscar did not respond. She called again. No reaction. Oscar was busy checking out whatever he had found. *Perhaps it was premature to let him run on his own*, Imani thought, taking out the leash from the pocket of her jacket and walking back to the dog. Was there a piece of garment caught in the cracks of a tree stump? Perhaps a piece of a sock? Oscar looked up at her. Then he looked at the leash in her hand, understanding Imani's plan. The dog quickly turned around and ran into the woods.

"Oscar, come here!" Imani shouted in frustration. She was on a tight time schedule in the morning. But the dog continued running away from her. Imani let out a curse and followed him as fast as she could, trying to avoid snaping branches, leafy poison oak and moisty moss on the uneven forest floor. She tried to catch up with the dog. Oscar had his nose on the ground and was racing towards a clearing in the forest. Imani followed him closely, crisp leaves and twigs crunching under her sneakers. She noticed a cabin emerging in the middle of the woods. Oscar raced towards the front door and started barking frantically.

"Oscar, what are you doing? This is private property!" Imani shouted in part for the dog and in part for the owner of the cabin. *Hopefully, nobody will file a complaint*, she thought. She ran towards the dog, finally managed to grab him by the collar, clicked on the leash and pulled him away from the door. As she turned around, she noticed an odd noise from inside the cabin. It sounded like a muffled voice. Or was she imagining something? Oscar barked frantically, which made it difficult to listen to anything else. Imani turned around and looked for a doorbell. There was none. She knocked at the door. There was the same noise again. It seemed to come from a distance, but definitely from inside the house. However, nobody answered the door.

Imani waited a few more minutes but nothing happened – except for Oscar not calming down. Perhaps the owner had just left on the radio? A gut instinct told Imani that something was not right here. But she could not figure out what it was. She finally decided that she would tell Terrel about it. Perhaps he could check it out further. Imani turned around again, dragging the barking, distressed dog with her. She clearly had to get Oscar away from here. Something completely freaked him out. As she walked down the steps in front of the house, Imani noticed something in the dirt in front of the porch. She got closer and saw that it was an iPhone. With her free hand, she grabbed for her own iPhone and took a picture. She had learned from Terrel that this was the first step to retrieve evidence. She also took a picture of the cabin, the adjacent forest and the street in the distance. Then, she took one of the plastic bags out her pocket, that she used to retrieve dog poop. She picked up the iPhone with the plastic bag and sealed it, carefully avoiding any touch. She then ran back to the car with Oscar and drove home.

- 31 -
Annya
JONES FRACTURE

Wednesday, May 26, 2032, 6.00 am.

At six am, Annya walked into the ER of SUEC hospital, dressed in her usual scrubs-plus-white-coat outfit. She was surprised to find a new receptionist at the entrance. He introduced himself as Samuel Grey. He explained that Aiko had been transferred to the reception desk of the main SUEC building, to fill in for Stella, who was being treated for a fracture in a hospital in San Francisco. Annya made a mental note of this information. Perhaps Aiko could help her find out what Boris had been up to last night.

Annya went to the main conference room to attend the morning huddle, where the night shift personnel oriented the morning shift team about the occurrences of the night and the status of patients who were currently in the ER. Several patients were in the process of being examined or treated. Annya's internal alert system was activated again when Laura Chin, the chief nurse, mentioned a patient with a foot injury who had forgotten his ID. He had checked in as Boris Romanov. The patient had reported that he fell while jogging in the woods and injured his right foot. An x-ray had already been obtained and he was waiting in one of the exam rooms for an ER physician. After the orientation, Annya went to the main nurse station, which provided views of all exam rooms through cameras in each exam room. Indeed, she saw Boris sitting on a stretcher in room 6.

This nightmare of a man seemed to show up wherever she went. *Does he know that I am working here?* Annya wondered. But she decided against this. She had changed her name and if he had been looking for her, there would have been better opportunities to catch her than here in the ER. But she had to make sure that Boris would not see her. That would be devastating. Fortunately, her most experienced fellow, Santiago, was with her on the morning shift. Annya asked Santiago to go and see the patient while she would check the result of the radiograph. Annya walked over to the radiology reading room, where the radiology resident Lucia was reading out radiographs.

Annya greeted her. "Hello Lucia, could you provide me with a preliminary review of the radiographs of patient Boris Romanov."

Lucia continued dictating the report for another radiograph. Once she was finished, she put down the microphone and smiled at Annya. "Hello Dr. Segond, thanks for letting me finish this case. And of course, let me have a look at your patient."

Lucia searched through the patient list on her computer. After a few seconds, she clicked on one of the icons on her display and brought up a radiograph of the foot, labeled with Boris' fake name.

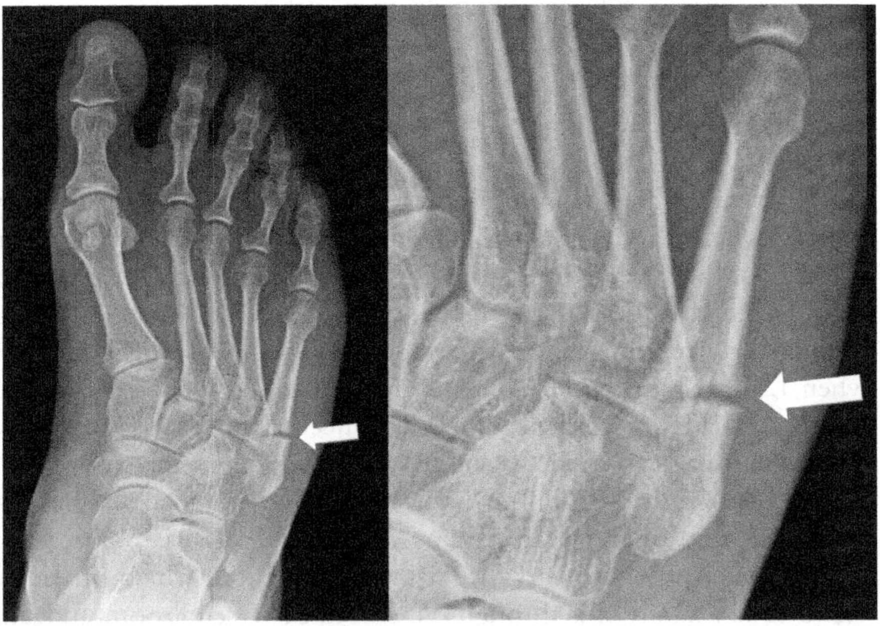

"Oh, it looks like your patient has a fracture of the fifth metatarsal bone," Lucia said.

Annya looked over her shoulder. "Yes, indeed, he has a Jones fracture!"

"What is a Jones fracture?" the resident asked.

"Well, a Jones fracture is a transverse fracture at the base of the fifth metatarsal bone, the long bone in the foot that connects the ankle with the little toe. A Jones fracture is located at the metadiaphyseal junction, approximately two centimeters from the tip of the fifth metatarsal bone. This is different to an avulsion fracture, which is located at the tip of the fifth metatarsal bone, or a stress fracture, which traverses the shaft of the bone. See this figure here…." Annya pulled up a drawing from a teaching file on her iPhone and showed it to Lucia.

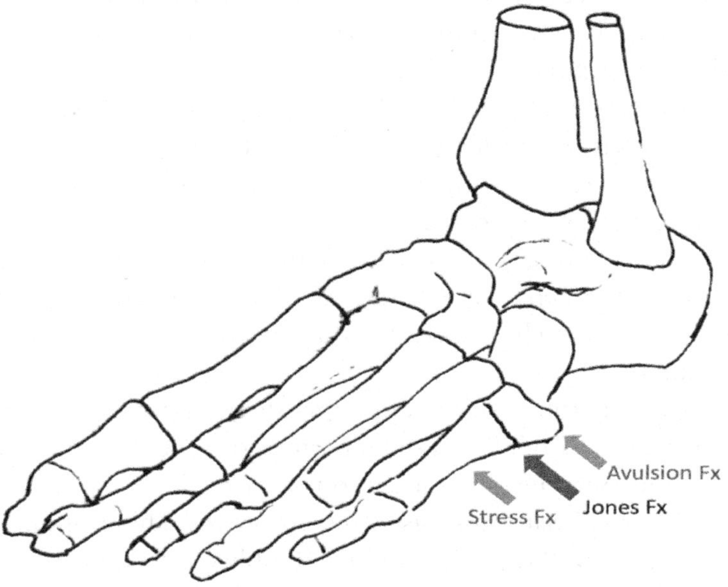

Lucia inspected the drawing carefully. "Thanks for explaining that to me, Annya!" she said. "I love working with you! I always learn something new when we discuss cases together."

"No problem, I enjoy working with you, too. If you are on service, none of my patients have to wait too long for their radiology report."

"Thank you, Annya! Can I ask, how do you treat a Jones fracture?"

"A Jones fracture has a high risk of non-union and prolonged pain. Therefore, the usual approach is a surgery with fusion of the broken bone with a small screw," Annya explained.

"That is a great teaching case," Lucia said, marking the radiograph for her own file. "I will keep that in mind and watch out for the post-surgical radiograph! Thanks again!"

"Of course!" Annya responded. She waved goodbye and left towards the central nurse station, where she found Santiago waiting for her. Santiago described the findings of Boris' physical exam, which were also consistent with a fracture.

"The patient had been walking on the injured foot for some time. The foot is severely swollen," Santiago reported, "I told him that a surgery might be needed, but the patient vehemently opposes this plan. He said that he had to complete a very important work assignment within the next few days."

Annya shrugged. "Well, in that case, it might be good to give it a few days so that the swelling can improve. Then, we can re-assess, if a conservative treatment might be possible or if we can offer an outpatient surgery. Can you relay that to him?"

"I believe that would work for him," Santiago responded. He hesitated for a moment. Then he asked. "Dr Segond, don't you want to have a look yourself and see if you can convince him towards a surgical repair?"

"No, I don't think we need to duplicate our efforts," Annya said, shaking her head. "I think you did a perfect job! We have many more patients waiting who need our attention as well."

"Of course." Santiago raised his eyebrows. This response was out of character for Annya. She usually double checked every patient. But he trusted her and did not want to press the issue.

Annya noticed his hesitation. "To be honest, the patient looks like someone who matches one of the suspect photos, that Terrel Wright showed me yesterday," she lied.

"And that explains why *you* don't want to see him?" Santiago asked. He looked at her with his head tilted, trying to understand.

"Well, if he was one of the chip thieves and then reappeared on campus, I could possibly spot him without his recognizing me," Annya explained.

"But you haven't seen him yet?" Santiago responded.

"I did see him on the camera at the nurse station," Annya explained. "That's when I recognized him and asked you to see him."

"I understand," Santiago responded. It was clear that he still did not fully buy her story. But he trusted her enough to not ask further questions.

"So, I will prescribe a non-weight bearing cast and two crutches." He summarized the treatment plan. "I will also make an appointment for a follow up visit in about a week from now, to re-assess alignment of the bones."

"That sounds like a good plan." Annya responded. She focused on a spot on the ground, trying to figure out how to best approach the subject. "I have to ask you one more thing." *Now came the hard part. Please let him cooperate!* she prayed. Annya reached for a pen in the front pocket of her white coat. She twisted the end cap and retracted a tiny little chip. Until now, only her sister knew about this chip. She carried it around at all times. If she ever got missing, her sister could locate it via a GPS tracking function.

"I got this from the FBI agents," she lied again and handed the chip over to Santiago, whose jaw dropped almost to the ground. "Can you please put this chip in his cast. This will allow the FBI agents to track him."

"Wow, I feel like James Bond!" Santiago exclaimed. He carefully took the chip between his thumb and index finger and inspected it.

"Please keep this quiet, will you?" Annya responded. "The success of this mission depends on your ability to plant this chip without anyone noticing. I will inform the FBI in the meantime."

"Why can they not just come here and arrest the man?" Santiago asked.

"I don't think they have enough evidence yet to make an arrest," Annya responded. "If we can track him, he might lead us to the evidence."

"Are we allowed to track someone without his consent?" Santiago asked. "Or could I get in any trouble for planting the tracker?"

"I take full responsibility," Annya said, "and I will inform the FBI right away."

Santiago looked at her for a minute. Then, he nodded in agreement. "Okay, I will get the chip into the cast. Undercover operation in progress." He smiled at Annya; his cheeks flushed. He slipped the chip into his pocket and left towards the patient exam rooms. Annya sighed. She took out her cell phone and activated the tracking system for the chip. *That went better than she could have imagined. She was in control now! She would face her demon and put an end to her nightmares once and for all!*

- 32 -
Terrel
SEGOND FRACTURE

Wednesday, May 26, 2032, 6.00 am.

When Imani shared the story of the frantic dog with Terrel, it all sounded much less logical.

"Oscar invaded a private property, and you stole an iPhone from it?" he asked, shaking his head in disbelief.

"Something was off there," Imani insisted. "Both Oscar and I felt it. You should have seen him, he completely freaked out!"

Terrel looked at Oscar, who was lying in front of him on the kitchen floor, completely calm, glancing back at him with his big, round eyes. Niles was kneeling besides the dog, offering him the rest of his morning sandwich, which the dog happily accepted.

Terrel's phone rang. Angus Weber was on the phone. "Hi Terrel, we have some news here. I just received a call from Dr. Ben Bennett. He informed me that four of the brain chips have been returned."

"Returned?" Terrel echoed in disbelief. "What do you mean? The thieves returned the brain chips?"

"We do not know who returned them," Angus said. "Dr. Bennett found them in his mailbox this morning and called me right away. They were in an anonymous padded envelope, addressed to him. There was no other note or explanation inside the envelope."

"How bizarre," Terrel exclaimed. "I just learned last night that a middle-aged white male in a leather jacket kidnapped Susan Pellegrini. Susan is one of the chip thieves and Stella Pellegrini's daughter. The man demanded the chips in exchange for Susan. The other thief was Susan's friend Kaleo Kahale, and he was apparently determined to respond to the demand in order to get Susan back. I do not understand who returned the brain chips to you. It cannot be one of the thieves. One has been kidnapped and the other wanted to buy her free."

"It gets even more bizarre," Angus said. "We ran DNA analyses on the envelope and the returned chips. Of course, whoever returned the chips made every effort to not leave any fingerprints anywhere. However, we found touch DNA on the envelope and the chips. We ran tiny amounts of shedded skin cells in the envelope against our database and got a match with a murder suspect for an unsolved crime a couple of years ago. His name was Boris Smirnoff. We know that this is a fake ID. But the interesting part is that an iPhone has been bought recently under the same name. Surely, this could just be a coincidence, and this could be an entirely different person. However, we tracked that iPhone's location and to our surprise, it seems to be in your home."

"In my home?" Terrel responded. It took him a few seconds to put all the pieces together.

"Imani went for a run in a nearby forest this morning and found an iPhone close to a cabin that looked suspicious to her," he explained. "We were just discussing what to do about it."

"Perhaps the thieves staged the kidnapping to cast themselves as victims," Angus speculated. "Then, they made a deal with the dean to return the chips against a hefty reward."

"But then Susan should be back, and the dean should have received five chips back, not four," Terrel countered. "This whole story does not make sense! Let me see if I can find any useful information on the iPhone that Imani found. It is locked, but I have unlock software in my home office. Give me a few minutes. I will see if I can access the phone and check it out."

"Okay," Angus responded. "I am at the SUEC campus now and will question both Dr. Bennett and Dr. Hill. If the chips were returned by a criminal, there must have been some incentive for him. Therefore, I suspect that either the dean or Dr. Hill must be involved, at the very least providing a reward for returning the chips and possibly hiring this person to kill the Perez family and abduct Susan Pellegrini."

"Let me see if I can find any related evidence on the iPhone. I will get back to you shortly," Terrel responded. He hung up the phone and gave Imani a long, passionate kiss. "You are amazing," he said to her. "You brought us key evidence for a homicide!"

"So, now you believe me!" Imani stated with deep satisfaction. "Why does it always need another man to verify what a woman says?"

"My apologies!" Terrel exclaimed. "Angus provided crucial additional information that explains your bad feeling about the cabin and the iPhone. Let me check out what is on the phone." Terrel took the iPhone and walked to his office, which was located next to the kitchen. He could activate the unlocking software through a wireless connection, without opening the plastic bag. That could help later when they checked for fingerprints. Or perhaps there was more touch DNA on the phone.

A ring tone signaled that the phone had been unlocked. That was faster than expected. Terrel opened the phone, first checking the email boxes. Interestingly, all mailboxes were empty. Same for text messages and recent phone conversations. No current messages, no saved messages, no histories, no trace of previous conversations. That was odd, but also consistent with the suspicion that this was the phone of a crime suspect. Terrel opened the health app. Interestingly, the guy was monitoring the number of steps he took every day. Or perhaps he was not aware that he measured his movements. Terrel opened the photo app. There was a folder named "fractures" that contained numerous photos of x-rays of broken bones. There was another folder named "clients," which contained photos of stunningly beautiful women. After each photo, there was an x-ray with a fracture. Terrel flipped through the contents of this album. Photo, x-ray, photo, x-ray...

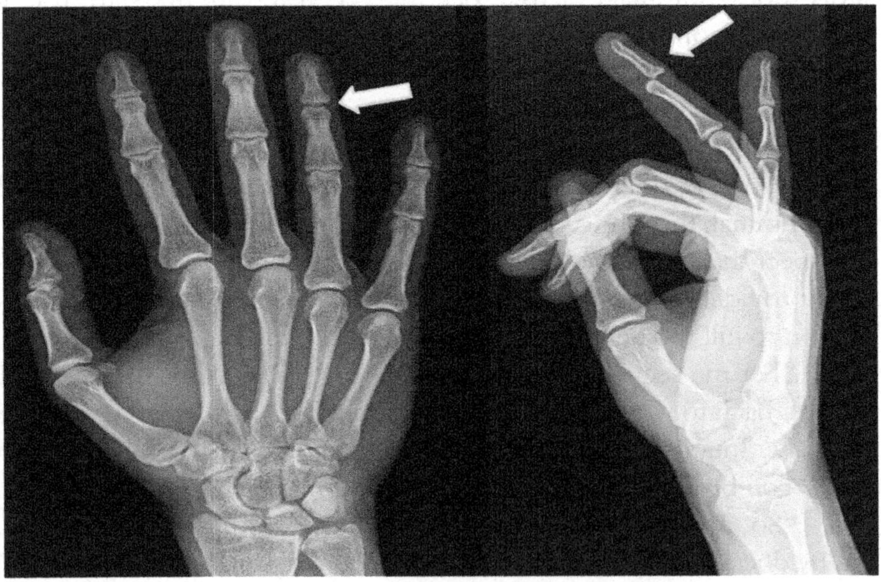

Terrel saw a radiograph with a label that indicated a dislocation of the distal phalanx of the ring finger. It was interesting to him that the frontal view showed only a slight widening of the distal interphalangeal joint, while the lateral view showed a dislocation of the distal end of the fourth finger.

The radiographs of the next woman in this file showed dislocated fractures of the spinous processes of the C7 and T1 vertebral bodies. The fracture lines were labeled with arrows. On the lateral view radiograph, the fracture lines could be clearly delineated and were marked by arrows. On the frontal view, the fractures could be identified by the downward displacement and double shadow of the spinous process.

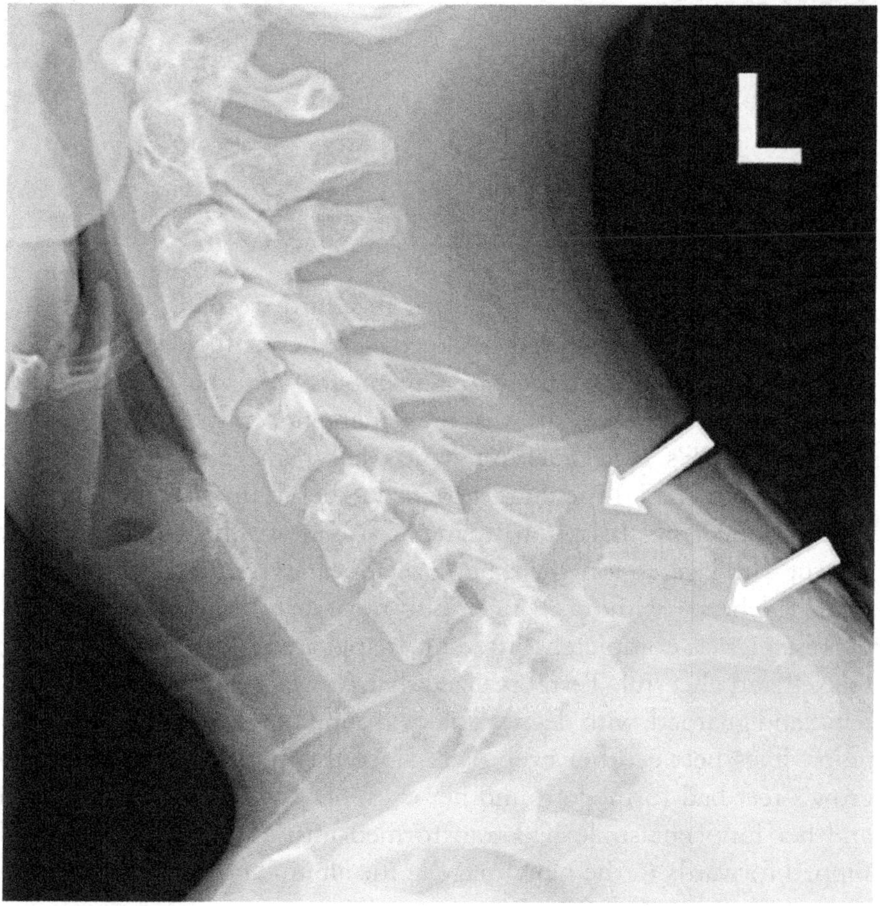

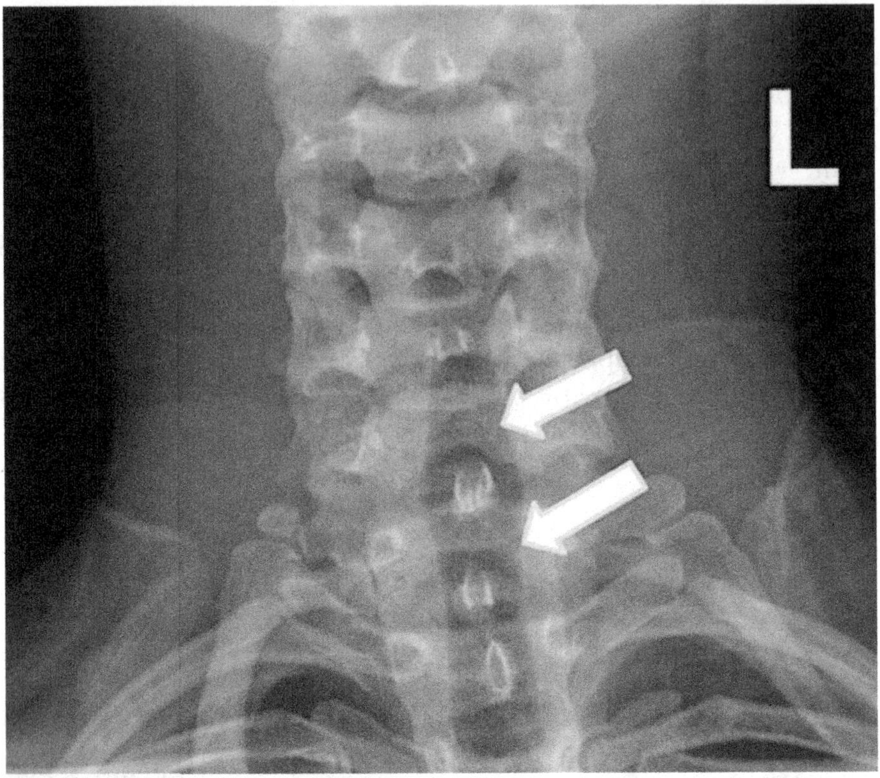

Terrel stopped at the photo of the third woman. He was sure that he knew her, but he did not recognize her at first. He looked at the photo carefully and tried to remember where he had seen her. Then, he remembered. It was the emergency physician at SUEC University, Lili's colleague! What was her name again? Dr. Annya Segond. Terrel had difficulties recognizing her at first because she was much younger on this photo than she was now. She had a different haircut with layered long hair, her face appeared thinner and she had a clear forehead, without bangs. But most astonishingly, her facial expression was completely different. It appeared much more juvenile, relaxed and cheerful. Terrel realized that Annya's expression now was tense and guarded, with deep wrinkles around her eyes and mouth, and worry lines between her eyebrows. Since this photo was taken, deep crow's feet had formed around her eyes, her full lips had turned thin and her innocent smile had transformed into a tough mime. Terrel flipped forwards to the next image in the album and saw a radiograph of a leg. He was not sure what it showed. He airdropped both the photo and the radiographs to his own photo gallery. Then he sent a text with Annya's radiograph from his phone to Lili Pham. *Hello Lili, can you provide a diagnosis for this x-ray ASAP? Thank you! Terrel*

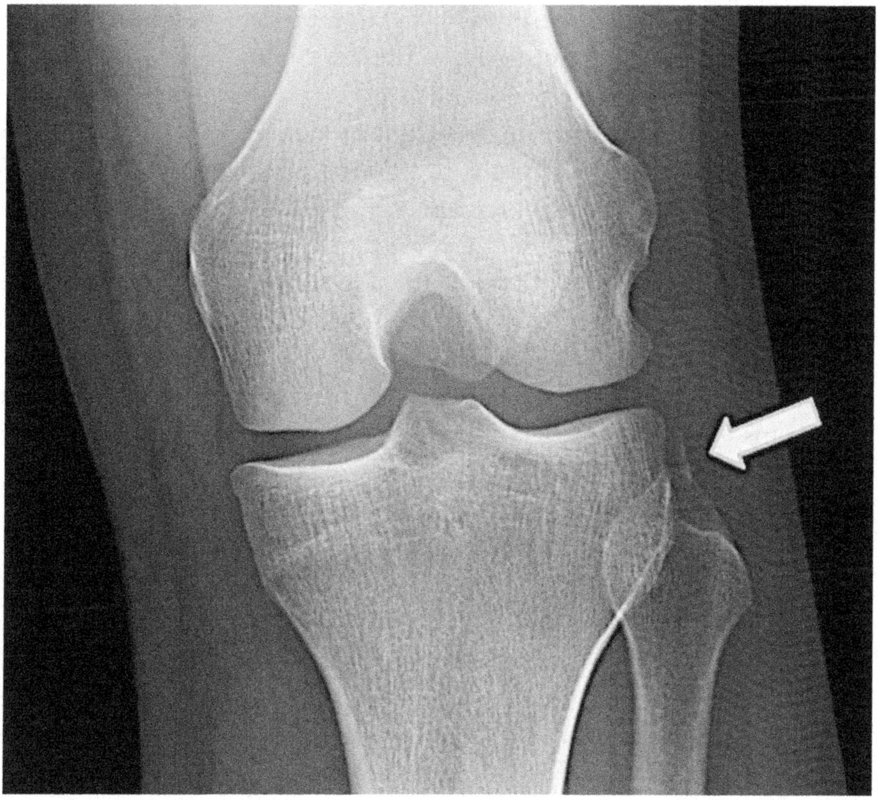

His phone buzzed just a few seconds later. *Hi Terrel, this is a Segond fracture = an avulsion fracture at the anterolateral tibia (lower leg bone). You can see an elliptical bone fragment parallel to the lateral tibial plateau. I placed an arrow on the abnormality. This is often associated with a rupture of the anterior cruciate ligament. Therefore, if we see the curvilinear bone fragment that I outlined with the arrow, we suggest an MRI to look for additional injuries of the knee joint. Best, Lili.*

Thank you! Terrel texted back. He really wished Lili were on the FBI team. She was smart, knowledgeable, quick and efficient! He had to report his findings. He dialed Angus Weber's number.

Angus answered right away. "Hi Terrel, what did you find?"

"Unfortunately, not much more information about this guy," Terrel reported. "But surprise! I found a list of women on the phone, each of them associated with a photo of a bone fracture. They might have been victims of abuse or harassment. Among these was a photo of Annya Segond. I assume she was another victim of this guy. In addition to her photo, there was a radiograph of a Segond fracture, that is a fracture of the lower part of the knee joint."

"Isn't her last name Segond?"

"Yeah, I assume that might be a fake name."

"I will look into it," Angus responded. "How many women are on that list? Anyone else you recognize?"

Terrel flipped through the photo collection. All these women were stunningly beautiful. Towards the end of the photo collection, he recognized Juliana Perez.

"There are twelve women here. I see Juliana Perez and a radiograph of her cervical spine fracture," he reported to Angus. "This guy seems to be some pervert who enjoys looking at images that document suffering of beautiful women. And I wonder how he got access to Mrs. Perez's radiograph!"

"Perhaps he inflicted the injuries, and he keeps the x-rays as trophies," Angus suggested. "These will be helpful evidence when we lock him up!"

"Yes indeed, he seems to specifically target women, and exceptionally beautiful women!" Terrel responded. "You should see the photos! Perhaps he was rejected by one of them and this is some kind of revenge. If this guy kidnapped Susan Pellegrini, she might be in great danger."

"Let's find that bastard!" Angus said. "I just got a list of previous locations of the phone. Looks like he was in San Francisco yesterday and he was at Susan Pellegrini's apartment. That makes him a prime suspect as her kidnapper and will be sufficient to arrest him. He apparently left towards San Mateo. But we could not track the exact location of the phone from there. It was somewhere in the forest, about 5 miles from your home. After that, we located it at your home."

"My wife can explain where she found the phone," Terrel responded. "In addition, she took photos of the cabin and its surroundings. The photos have coordinates on them and can be linked to their exact location. Perhaps Susan has been held hostage in this cabin. I can be there in a few minutes and check it out."

"I agree that this is urgent," Angus said, "but do not go there alone. If this guy is responsible for Juan and Juliana Perez's death, he is likely a professional killer. Ask for backup first. That's an order. I lost one partner and I do not want to lose another one. I will come there as well as soon as possible!"

"Of course, I will ask for backup first and then go back to the cabin," Terrel responded softly. "I am glad we have a solid lead now! Let's get this rolling! "

- 33 -
Lili
THE PHONE

Wednesday, May 26, 2032, 6.00 am.

Lili slept only lightly, as if she were on call, checking her phone for a text message every few hours. She was tired and wanted to sleep. But her brain insisted on staying awake, perseverating on the recent events, talking to her agitated self and waiting for a message from Amir. Her mind went into an endless cycle of dozing off and waking up. When the sun finally rose, Lili had the feeling that she had not slept at all. When she got up at six am, there was still no message. Mark was already up. Lili heard the roaring noise of the coffee machine and clattering porcelain in the kitchen. The smell of freshly brewed coffee filled the air in their home. Lili got up, dressed and went to the kitchen, where Mark had prepared three sandwiches, two for himself and one for her. Her hubby sat at the kitchen table in front of a half-eaten sandwich and a steaming coffee mug, chewing and checking his phone. Lili gave him a soft, loving kiss on his cheek. Mark looked up at her. "Good morning, detective! Any messages about your crime case?" he asked with a smirk.

"Nothing," Lili responded.

"So, what's the plan today?"

"I thought I'd stop by the General Hospital to see Stella before I drive to SUEC. Perhaps she has new information."

Mark looked at his watch. "Will you have time for that? You might be late for clinical rounds."

"I got this week off from clinical assignments, so that I can help the FBI agents with their case. Although at our meeting yesterday afternoon, Dean Bennett and Angus Weber told me that they did not want me involved any more. So, I guess I have some extra time. I will first check on Stella, then drive to SUEC and help in the reading room.

My colleagues there will be happy to see me coming in unexpectedly. I am quite sure they did not get a replacement for me and have to put in extra hours to manage the work."

"The usual drill," Mark responded. "I wonder when someone will change this abusive system. It is not healthy for healthcare workers or our patients if we work extra hours on a daily basis. Numerous studies and lawsuits have shown that tired clinic personnel can miss important diagnoses."

"Who knows?" Lili considered. "Perhaps they did hire a replacement for me."

"First, they will have to hire two people to replace you," Mark said, smiling at his wife with pride. "You work really hard, and you are very experienced. Second, the Accreditation Council for Graduate Medical Education implemented rules for limited work hours of resident physicians in training. But there is no rule or lobby for appropriate work hours of attending physicians. That is the reason for the burnout crisis!"

"I know. I believe that the system will change eventually. But it will take time. In the meantime, I will check out if my colleagues in the reading room are overwhelmed and need some help."

"If you have a different assignment, then the administration really should place someone else in the reading room," Mark responded. "It is not okay to continuously count on our sense of duty to help out on our days off, after hours and on weekends, when we are not officially on service. The next generation surely will not continue this madness."

"You are absolutely right, as always!" Lili smiled at Mark. "In addition, I really want to help Stella. Remember, she already lost her husband. She cannot also lose her one and only child."

Mark got up from his seat, hugged her and gave her a long kiss.

"I know you will do the right thing. Just be careful," he whispered. "I don't want you to get hurt!"

"Mark, what is on *your* schedule today?"

"I have three biopsies scheduled, in addition to our usual work in the reading room. And I have to interview two candidates for next year's clinical fellow positions. As you know, there is never dedicated time for that either, we'll just have to squeeze it in somehow. It will be a very busy day!"

"Make sure you get a break! I love you!"

"A break? What is that?" He smiled as he fetched his computer bag and hurried to the door. His clinical service started thirty minutes earlier than Lili's and he always left even earlier in order to read his emails in his office before his clinical duty started. Despite his complaints about the system, he was the most duty-bound and responsible man she knew.

"Dinner at eight!" he shouted from the door.

"I will do my best to be on time tonight!" Lili called after him. "I'll keep you updated in case I face any delays!" She heard the main door of the house being opened and shut. Then, there was silence. Lili finished her breakfast, put on her jacket, got into the car and drove to the General Hospital in San Francisco.

She arrived at the hospital around six-thirty am. The hospital building appeared quiet and calm, almost sleeping. Golden rays of the rising sun were burning their way through the morning fog. A few people, presumably healthcare workers, were rushing into the entrance. Lili parked the car in the visitors parking lot, walked to the main entrance and checked in as a visitor. An elderly man in a green uniform with an ID that identified him as Gentry, Volunteer, led her to the orthopedic surgery ward and handed her over to a nurse practitioner with the ID tag Gloria, who informed her that Stella was being prepped for her surgery later this morning. Gloria went to ask Stella if she wanted to see a visitor. Fortunately, Stella agreed and a few minutes later, Lili sat at her bedside.

"Good morning, Lili!" she greeted her. "It's great to see you!"

Her face looked pale, her eyes were puffy, and it seemed as if multiple wrinkles had appeared around her mouth overnight.

"You look very tired," Lili said, taking her hand.

"Well, I was really exhausted last night and slept until about three am. But then, I could not sleep any more. I was so worried about Susan! Do you know the saying that if you cannot sleep, it is because you are awake in someone else's dream? I hope that would be Susan's. That would mean that she is still alive!"

"What a lovely thought!" Lili responded. "I hope that Susan will be found soon! Have you heard anything from Kaleo or Amir?"

"At first, I did not hear anything," Stella responded, "and I got so worried last night that I also told the FBI agent, Terrel Wright, the whole story. Now, I am worried that that might have put her in danger!"

Stella looked at Lili for a while, as if holding back a thought.

"I think it was a good decision to inform the FBI," Lili responded. "I feel much better knowing that they are involved. They are experienced in dealing with criminals and kidnappers. We are not."

"You are probably right," Stella responded. "I just feel so guilty. Perhaps I could have done something to avoid this whole disaster in the first place."

"Unfortunately, crimes happen to the best people. I don't think you could've done anything. Susan is an adult now and she is making her own choices."

"Well, for a starter, I think I was a bad role model," Stella said. Tears were again welling up in her eyes. "You know I am a single mother, and our budget was always short. I made a deal with Dr. Bennett that I could take leftover food home from the SUEC buffets. You know, when he meets with VIPs from the industry, they are getting fantastic lunch plates or dinner buffets and they eat less than half of it. So, when I cleaned up after the meeting, I took home whatever was untouched. That helped me out quite a bit with my small budget and provided Susan with high-quality food on an almost daily basis. I also took the flower bouquets on the table, if nobody else wanted them."

"I cannot see anything wrong with that, if the dean approved it," I said.

"Well, then there were the SUEC conferences where beautiful notebooks, pens, pencils and flash drives were distributed to attendants. There was always at least one extra packet, and I took that home as well."

"Looks like SUEC is supporting their administrative assistants in ways I had not imagined," Lili chuckled.

"Yea, and then there was the toilet paper."

"The toilet paper?" Lili asked, now really surprised.

"Well, a pack of toilet paper these days costs five to seven dollars," Stella responded. "There was always a pile in our restroom at SUEC and I just took one or two home every week. I rarely had to buy one. Over a year, that can save you a lot of money."

"Now I understand why toilet paper dispensers in public restrooms are locked!" It had never occurred to me that anyone would take them. "Well, Stella, that would likely be considered a theft. I will just pretend I haven't heard about it and would strongly suggest that you stop that habit immediately."

"Yes, of course," Stella responded. "I understand that now. But what I'm saying is that almost every day, I brought something home from SUEC. Susan might have gotten the impression that it is okay to take things from the university. So, in the end, I might be responsible for the idea forming in her head that she could just take these brain chips home."

That was an interesting thought. Tears were now running down Stella's cheeks. Lili felt sorry for her. As a single mother, her intention had clearly been to take care of her daughter as best as she could within the constraints of a very limited budget and living in the expensive Bay Area.

"You never know what motivates people," Lili responded. "Perhaps Susan wanted to impress her boyfriend with superpowers. Who knows? It does not help either of you if you torment yourself with these thoughts. Let's look forwards, not backwards. Can you think of anything I can do to help ?"

"Well, I'm terrified that I will go into surgery and miss something important while I am anesthetized," Stella responded. "What if anyone contacts me and I do not respond? Then I wake up and Susan is dead!"

"Should I take your cell phone for the day?" Lili asked. "I can call the ward as soon as I hear anything. You will likely want to sleep after the surgery, and I can bring your cell phone back in the evening."

Stella looked at her and thought about it for a while. Then she nodded. "That might be a good idea. Actually, I am awaiting for an urgent message from Amir. If he sends a text, will you promise to act right away?"

"Of course, I will!"

"Thank you for being such a wonderful friend, Lili."

Someone knocked at the door. The door opened and Gloria, the nurse practitioner, stepped in. "Mrs. Pellegrini," she said to Stella while ignoring Lili, "it is time to leave for the operating room."

Stella pressed her cell phone in Lili's hand. "The password is Susan," she whispered. Lili shook her head in disbelief. *Had she ever heard of a secure password?* But of course, this one would be easy to remember.

"No worries," she said, trying to hide her heavy heart with a light voice. "I hope I will have good news for you when you wake up from your surgery. It is most important now that you get back on your feet!"

"Thank you for everything, Lili!" Stella exclaimed and squeezed her hands. Meanwhile, Gloria had released the brakes from the wheels of the hospital bed and started to pull it out of the room. Lili waved Stella goodbye, put her phone into her pocket, walked down the hallway, down the stairs and out of the hospital to the parking lot. She had a feeling that Stella had withheld some information when she talked with her. It was just a feeling about how she hesitated when she talked about the FBI agent. But she could not quite put her finger on what it was. She would ask Stella about it after the surgery. Lili got into her car again and drove to SUEC.

- 34 -
Amir
THE PUNCH

Wednesday, May 26, 2032, 6.30 am.

Amir arrived at the cabin at seven-thirty am. He parked in the forest, on the side of the unpaved road, and walked the rest of the way by foot. He did not want to alert a kidnapper with the noise of a car. If he ran into him, he could just pretend to be a local hiker. Amir carefully approached the cabin from the back. There was no sign that anyone was there. Amir noted tire tracks in front of the cabin. There was no car. His heart sank. *Perhaps they have left already*, he thought. He slowly walked around the cabin and peeked through the window.

The morning sun reflected on the glass of the windows, and he could not see much of the interior. As he walked around to the entrance, he thought he heard some muffled noise from the inside. He stopped and held his left ear against the wooden exterior wall. But he could not hear much. One moment, the noise was there. Then, it had disappeared. It was difficult to make out what it was exactly. Amir walked to the front door of the cabin and tried to open it. Of course, it was locked. His growing concern and anxiety had reached a peak. He kicked the door hard. The lock gave in, and the door flung open.

Amir walked in. His concern for Susan had overwritten his concern for his own life. He could only think of rescuing Susan. Amir stepped into the cabin and looked around. The large living room on the ground floor was a combination of wood, glass and steel, which created a rustic and industrial feeling. The cabin windows allowed views of the forest, which he might have called beautiful under different circumstances. A steel ladder led to a loft. Amir looked up. There, she was! Susan was tied to a chair at the edge of the loft. She was alive! Amir rushed to the kitchenette in the back of the cabin, grabbed a knife and jumped up the ladder as fast as he could. He cut the rope and duct tape that tied Susan's arms and feet to the chair. Then, he removed the tape and cloth that covered her mouth.

Susan screamed in horror. She looked through Amir with blank eyes that were devoid of any recognition.

Amir felt tears of despair running down his cheeks. He tried to stay calm. "Susan, it is me, Amir!"

Susan did not react, she continued to look through him, screaming.

Amir talked to her in a soft, composed voice. "Susan, you are safe now! I am here to bring you home!"

At the word *home*, Susan seemed to hesitate for a moment. *Was there some reaction?* Susan looked towards Amir, but her eyes remained empty. After a few seconds of silence, she continued screaming with renewed energy.

Amir tried to stroke her hair and embrace her gently. But she continued to scream with a horrified, high-pitched sound. *If the kidnapper is anywhere close, he will come here now,* Amir thought. Sweat started running down his back.

Meanwhile, Susan had noticed that Amir had released the rope and tape that tied her to the chair. She jerked up from the chair and started jumping around, waving around her casted arm. Amir was afraid that she might hurt herself. Her mind was *gone.* Susan looked in horror at the floor and walls. Apparently, she saw something there that scared her. She jumped from one spot to another, apparently trying to avoid some imaginary threat that only she could see. Amir was worried that she might fall down the loft.

Suddenly, he realized. *The chip does this to her! I have to remove the chip!* Amir walked towards her, the knife still in his right hand, trying to pull her towards him with his left hand. Susan flung around, crashing her cast against his chest. Amir caught his breath and let go. He put the knife down on one of the nightstands. Then, he gently took her free left hand, pulled her towards him and embraced her. Susan tried to kick with both arms and legs. But this time, he got her. He grabbed some of the rope which he had cut earlier and tied it around Susan's arms and body. Then, he gently lifted her up and moved her to the bed. Susan continued screaming. Amir rolled her on her left side, secured her with his left arm and reached for the knife.

He continued talking to her. "Susan, you are safe now! I am here to bring you home!" It was almost like a chant. Amir waited. After a few minutes, Susan stopped screaming. *I have to be fast,* he thought. Amir let go of her body, felt for the chip under the skin of her lower head, pushed her long hair to the side, made a quick cut with the knife and squeezed out the chip. Susan screamed in pain and jumped up from the bed. The rope was still around her. Amir put the blood smeared chip into his pocket, ran after Susan, grabbed her and threw her over his left shoulder. Susan screamed and kicked, trying to free herself.

Now comes the hard part, Amir thought, *I have to get her down the ladder.* He walked towards the ladder and tried to make his way down the first steps of the ladder. But Susan continued to kick and scream. Amir tried to talk to her and calm her down. But she did not react. Amir let out a curse. It was not possible to get her down this way. They risked falling from the loft and at this height, that could lead to serious injury. He was sweating profusely by now, horrified and exhausted by Susan's pain and the prospect of the kidnapper coming back any minute. He put Susan down on the floor and sat down beside her, gently holding her uninjured left arm.

Think. He tried to calm himself down. *We got this far, and we will also get down there safely*. Suddenly, the solution popped up in his mind. He ran to the bed, pulled out the mattress and threw it over the railing of the loft. The mattress landed on the floor, at the base of the ladder. Then, he steadied himself at the upper end of the ladder, grabbed Susan and shoved her headfirst down the ladder. To his relief, Susan calmed down a bit, perhaps surprised by this new action. Amir finally grabbed her feet, leading her down as far as possible, with her head dangling over the mattress. When he could not let her down any further, there was only about half a meter left between her head and the ground. Blood from the wound in her scalp was dripping on the mattress. The injured arm in the cast nearly touched the floor. Amir prayed that she would not fall at any weird angle that would cause another fracture. He let go of her feet. Susan let out a surprised cry as she fell down. She landed on the mattress and immediately jumped up.

Thank God! That went well! Amir felt overwhelmed by a wave of joy and relief. He fetched the knife, jumped down the ladder, ran after Susan and untied the rope.

"Susan, we have to run now!" he shouted at her.

Susan looked at him. Amir saw a flash of recognition in her eyes.

"Amir!" she cried.

"Yes, it is me!" Amir hugged her gently, "I am so glad you recognize me now!"

Susan looked at him. "Thank you for coming to rescue me, Amir! I had a horrific nightmare!"

"I know! You have been kidnapped, Susan. The kidnapper could come back any minute. We have to leave!"

Susan nodded. She walked towards the door. But suddenly, she stopped in the middle of the cabin and stared at the kitchenette. She started sobbing uncontrollably.

"Susan, we have to run!" Amir shouted at her again.

Susan pointed at the dead man on the floor. "He killed Kaleo!" she cried.

This was the first time that Amir saw the body on the floor of the kitchenette. It was incompletely covered by a blanket; two shoes were sticking out underneath. Amir rushed to the body and removed the blanket. It was Kaleo indeed. His chest did not move. Amir kneeled beside him and put his ear and cheek over Kaleo's mouth and nose to check if he was breathing. He was not. Amir felt the vessels on Kaleo's neck. There was no pulse either. In addition, Kaleo's body already showed signs of the rigor mortis, a stiffening of the joints and muscles which sets in a few hours after death. Kaleo was dead.

"I am so sorry, Susan!" Amir looked at her with great compassion and took her in his arms. This time, she did not fight him off. She leaned against his shoulder and sobbed uncontrollably.

"He shot him because Kaleo brought him four chips and not five!" she sobbed. "I wanted to tell him that I have the fifth chip, but my mouth was gagged. It is my fault that Kaleo died!"

"Don't say that," Amir said softly. "Kaleo saw the man's face. The guy would have killed him either way."

"I love him!" she moaned.

"I know." Amir stroked her hair. He wondered, if the shock had catapulted her mind back into reality or if the influence of the chip was weaning off. Perhaps it was a little bit of both.

Suddenly, Amir heard a purring engine outside of the cabin. He peeked through the window and saw a dark gray Mercedes approaching. He felt a hot flash running through his body and anxiety encircled his throat. Amir turned to Susan. *Perhaps we can run to my car and get away*, he thought. But when Amir looked at Susan, he dismissed this plan. She was still completely lost in her grief. Amir doubted if she would have the focus and determination to recognize and reach his car. Likely not. If this man captured her again, then Amir's entire mission was for nothing. Or worse, he might shoot her. He clearly had no scruples. Amir grabbed Susan's shoulders, so that he could look straight into her eyes. She shrieked as he touched the shoulder with the clavicle injury.

"Susan, listen to me," Amir said as calmly as possible. "Your kidnapper has just arrived."

They locked eyes for the first time since Amir had arrived at the cabin. Amir captured a snapshot of the tantalizing pattern of her amber eyes. It was one of those moments where their minds united without saying anything. Amir felt the gravity of her sadness, her pain and despair. All he could think of was how to keep her safe.

"He does not know that I am here and that you are free," he whispered to Susan. "We can surprise him. I will open the door and you'll run into the woods. Run as fast as you can and don't look back. If you make it to the road behind the forest, I'm sure you will find help there. Stop the first car that comes by and ask them to bring you to the police station."

Susan nodded. She did not want to tell him that she had tried that tactic before. "What about you?" she asked.

"I will run in a different direction. He cannot come after two people at the same time. If he runs after you, I will stop him."

"I cannot lose you too!" Susan exclaimed.

"Do not worry," Amir said, trying to sound convincing. "I have a plan." He didn't. But they also didn't have more time.

"Okay, if you want it this way," Susan gently stroked his cheek. Then she gave him a long kiss on the lips.

"I'm sorry, I did not tell you that I love you, too. I always have!"

Amir felt his heart exploding. He had dreamed about this moment a million times. But his deepest desire came true in his darkest hour. There was no time for emotions now. Amir gently took Susan's left hand and they walked to the door. The car had stopped in front of the cabin.

"I will count to three," Amir explained, "and then I will open the door and we will run. Don't look back, just run to the forest as fast as you can."

Susan nodded. Amir counted. "One – two – three!" He opened the door and Susan raced down the porch and towards the forest. By now, she knew the fastest path to the woods, and she remembered the obstacles along the way. She didn't have time to notice how scared she was, and her competitive mind cheered her on. She had lost the last race against Boris and she would not lose this one. Susan ran across the clearing in front of the cabin, where she was an easy target in the glaring sunlight. She heard her own heavy breaths and the hushed noise of her running feet. She felt some relief as the shadows of the towering redwood trees embraced her. She ran as fast as she could, jumping over fallen trees and tree stumps, avoiding squirrel holes, finding her way through dense underbrush and sliding down muddy inclines. She ran and ran. After a while, she started to feel a side stitch. But she did not slow down. She did not look back. She ran away as quickly as possible, trying to escape the greatest horror of her short life. *God, please let Amir get away as well!* she prayed.

Boris had just opened the door of his car when he saw Susan sprinting towards the forest. He left out a curse and – just as Amir had predicted – reached for his gun. Amir raced towards the car and punched Boris with his bare fist into the face. Amir felt a sharp pain in his hand and a warm feeling of deep satisfaction. Boris's head did not move an inch. But he was completely puzzled. He looked at the pale, thin man in front of him, not sure if this guy was real or if he was dreaming.

"Man, you have courage!" he exclaimed. "I heard your hand break!"

Amir quickly turned around. He wanted to run to his car. But Boris leaped towards him, grabbed his shirt and pulled him back. Then, he grabbed Amir's neck with both hands and choked him. Amir realized that he was dealing with a predator who was willing to kill. He frantically tried to think of the man's weakness. *Was that a cast on his right leg?* he thought. He saw the white outline of a leg cast to his right and his inner voice responded. *The toes are always sticking out!* Amir stepped back as far as he could while hunched. He lifted his right leg and took all of his strength to stump on the man's exposed toes. Boris cried in pain. He stumbled backwards, losing his balance. They both fell to the ground and Boris released his grip around Amir's neck. Amir rolled around and jumped to his feet, ready to run. But Boris was faster. Still on the ground, Boris kicked Amir into the back of his right knee joint. Amir's leg gave out, and he fell back to the ground. Boris leaped towards him, and his grip encircled Amir's neck again. Amir grasped for air and tried to get away from the man, while the grip around his neck tightened. Amir's vision started to blur. He felt that he was losing his consciousness. But when he looked at the forest and saw no sign of Susan behind the fog in his eyes, Amir knew that Boris had lost, and he had won.

- 35 -
Lili
HANGMAN'S FRACTURE

Wednesday, May 26, 2032, 8.00 am.

Lili arrived at SUEC hospital around eight am. She went straight to the radiology reading room, to check out if she could help. Her colleague Dr. Matthew Holmes was on service, together with a first-year resident, Dr. Saira Clark, and the chief resident, Dr. Felipe Diaz. As she walked in, Saira and Felipe were completely absorbed discussing newly incoming imaging studies. Was this a professional discussion only or did she see a spark in their eyes as they looked at each other? The two reminded her of Mark and her, when they first met in the reading room. Mark had shown her a Tillaux fracture on a teenager. He explained to her that a Tillaux fracture is a Salter 3 fracture where only the anterolateral tibia epiphysis breaks off.

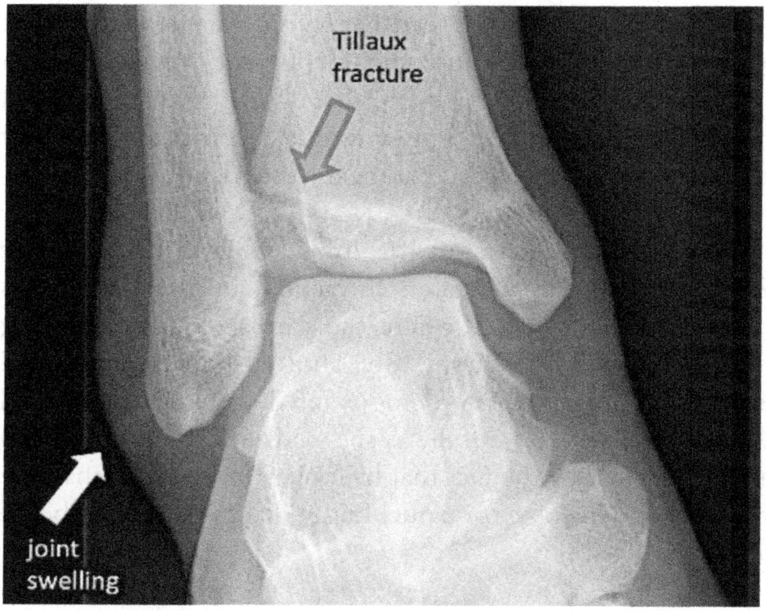

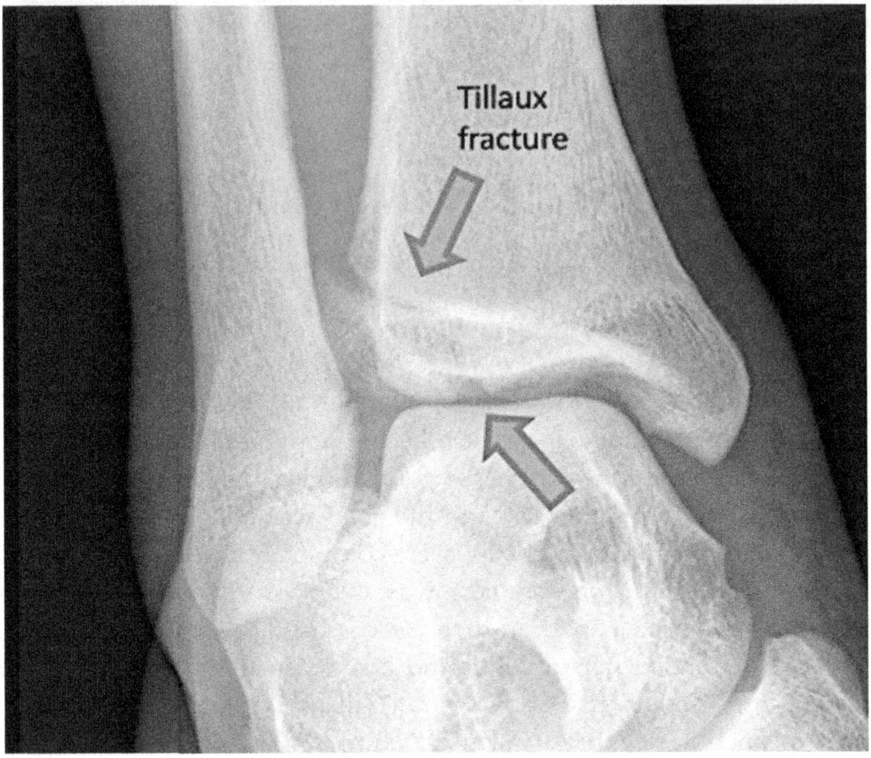

This happens when the growth plate is partially closed. The growth plate closes first medially. When a teenager with such a partially closed growth plate sustains an ankle injury, the fracture line extends through the still open lateral part of the growth plate. When it hits the closed part of the growth plate, it extends downwards, towards the joint. Lili remembered the radiograph as if it had been yesterday.

Lili had been fascinated and wanted to impress Mark with a similar cool case. She showed him a Freiberg infraction, an osteochondrosis of the second metatarsal head, where the cartilage of the growing skeleton fails to convert into bone. She showed him the abnormal second metatarsal head, which demonstrated an impression and sclerosis. Mark had listened carefully as she explained the findings. Lili had been quite irritated by the fact that he looked more at her than the radiograph. That had been so romantic! Lili smiled as she remembered the encounter.

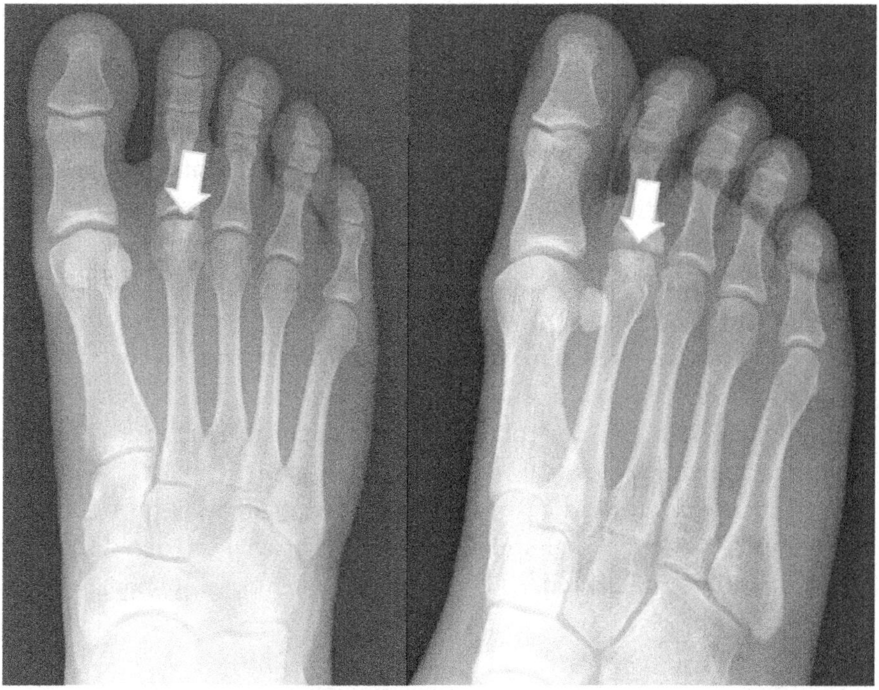

Matthew looked up, interrupting her rosy memories. "Hello Lili, I did not expect you today. I thought you were not on service?"

"Hello Matthew, that is true indeed. I just had some extra time and wanted to check if you are okay with the workload?"

"Thanks for checking. It is not too bad, especially considering the immense help I got here from Saira and Felipe!"

Lili smiled. Saira and Felipe were very smart and hard-working indeed, not shy of helping with a pile of work. Although currently, they were completely absorbed by each other. Matthew saw her look and smiled as well.

"Actually, I came in at six-thirty am today to present imaging studies at the surgery conference. After that, I started dictating urgent ER cases right away and did not get a chance to fetch a coffee yet. If you don't mind watching the reading room for a while, I would love to get some breakfast."

"Of course, go ahead!" Lili responded. "I would be happy to dictate a few cases while you take a break."

Matthew left with a grateful nod. Lili settled down at the

workstation and logged into the PACS system. She looked around. She had hoped to meet Annya here as well. Lili still felt uneasy after the incident with the dean and Agent Weber last night and would have loved to discuss it with her friend. Annya had encountered her share of disrespect and microaggression and would probably have some great advice for her about what to do when she met them again. Hopefully, it would not take too long until Annya stopped by the reading room to review a case with them. Meanwhile, Lili looked through the worklist and started dictating. After a few minutes, Saira and Felipe noticed her. They greeted each other and reviewed a few cases together. Lili loved the process of reviewing interesting cases with the trainees. They brought so much enthusiasm and positive energy to the workplace.

"Here is a very sad case from this morning." Saira brought up a radiograph of the cervical spine. "This woman was involved in a car accident and got paralyzed."

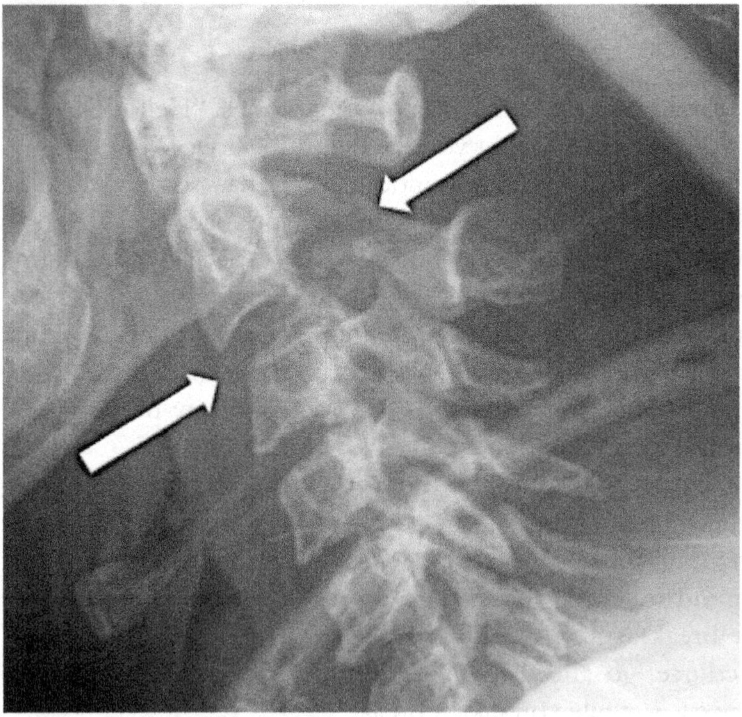

"Looks like a Hangman's fracture," Felipe countered.

"What is a Hangman's fracture?" Saira asked.

"A Hangman's fracture is a fracture through the pars interarticularis of the C2 vertebral body," Felipe explained. "The pars interarticularis is the bony connection between the front and back of the vertebral body. A fracture through the pedicles separates the neural arch of C2 from the C2 vertebral body."

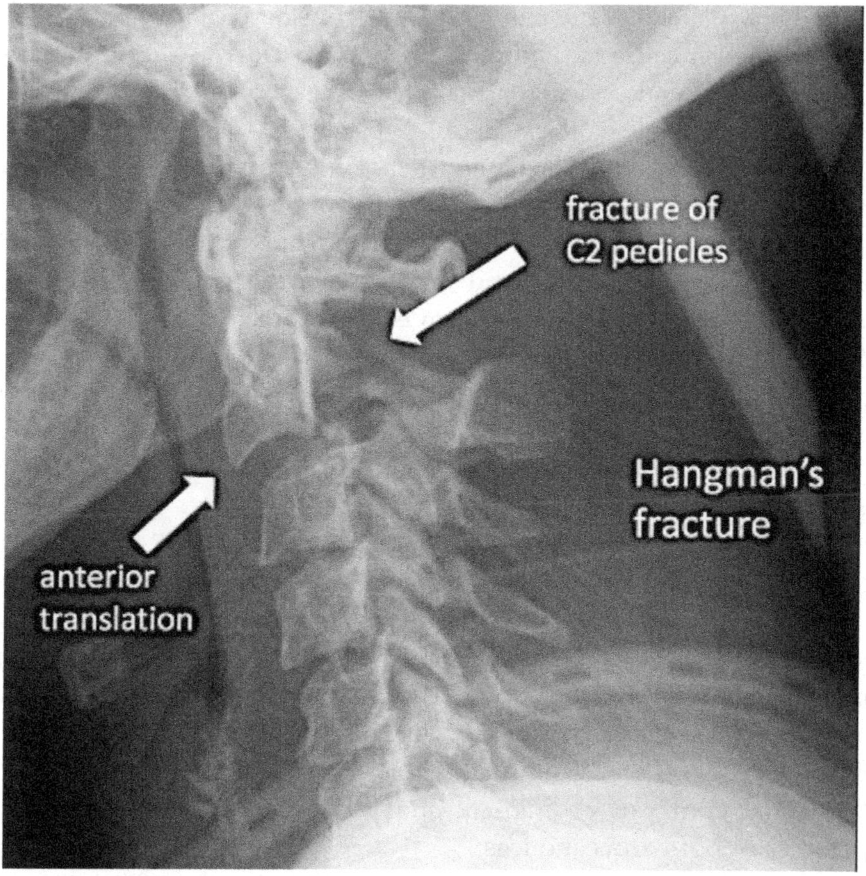

Lili added, "There are different types of Hangman's fractures. The injury can cause the C2 vertebral body to move out of alignment with the bone right below it, the C3 vertebral body. This is the case here as well. In addition, it is important to check if the C2 vertebral body is angulated anteriorly. That can lead to injury of the spinal cord. The fractures were initially classified according to Effendi and later according to Levine and Edwards. A type 1 fracture is a hairline fracture without displacement. A type 2 fracture demonstrates significant translation (> 3 mm), which is the case here. A type 2A fracture demonstrates severe angulation (> 11 degrees) and a type 3 fracture demonstrates severe angulation with facet joint dislocation."

Saira asked. "Why is it called Hangman's fracture? Does it usually happen when somebody commits suicide by hanging themselves?"

Lili explained, "The name could be considered a misnomer. The most common cause is a motorcycle or car accident. The fracture is almost never seen in suicidal hanging, and it is very rare in people who were judicially hanged. These people typically die due to asphyxiation, that is suffocation due to lack of oxygen. Let's see what the mechanism was here."

Lili looked at the file of this patient. To her surprise, she noticed that the patient had indicated "Cybersecurity/Technology special agent, FBI" as her profession. Even more surprisingly, under primary contact, she found. "Angus Weber, special agent, FBI." Lili did not mention anything to the trainees, as this was clearly unrelated information. She concluded that it was probably not appropriate to look at the exact description of the injury. On the summary page, she saw a note. *Car accident, paralysis.*

"There are no further details here about the injury," Lili told the trainees. "The most common mechanism of injury is the head of an unrestrained driver striking the dashboard or a passenger's neck being thrown backwards into extreme hyperextension during a collision. In many instances, a fracture of the lateral aspect of the vertebral body increases the space of the spinal canal and does not cause spinal cord injury. However, especially for instable type 2A and type 3 fractures, the spinal cord can be injured, and this can result in a complete paralysis of both arms and legs."

"I am so sorry for this poor woman," Saira said.

"Take home point for a radiologist is to always carefully check the vertebral bodies of the upper cervical spine when a patient presents after an accident," Lili said. "You as radiologists can prevent complications by informing the clinicians about such a fracture, so that they can treat it."

Saira and Felipe studied the radiographs carefully. Felipe wrote some notes in his notebook.

"Lili, can you please explain the difference between a Hangman's fracture and an odontoid fracture?" he asked.

"This is a very good question and very timely, as we have another patient here with this injury," Lili responded, while bringing up the radiographs of another patient.

"Hangman's fractures are vertical fractures through the second vertebral bone, while Odontoid fractures are horizontal fractures through its tooth-like anterior process. There are three types of Odontoid fractures. What you see here is a type 2 fracture. It is a horizontal fracture through the base of the odontoid process. Since the vertebra is located high up in the spine, we often add an 'open mouth' radiograph to look for this fracture if there is a clinical concern about it. In this case here, we proceeded directly towards a CT scan. You can see the fracture line here in the bone."

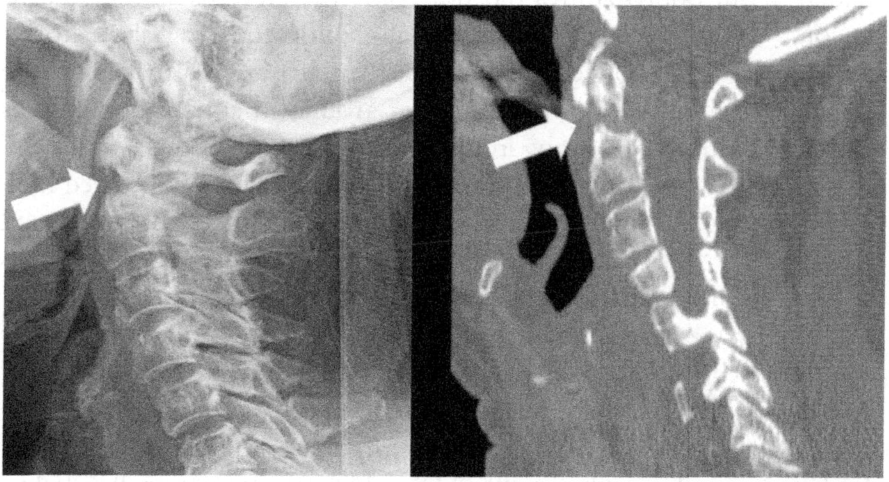

"Lili pointed to the fracture line on the radiograph and CT scan. "It is very important to recognize this fracture because it is unstable and can lead to neurological complications. A type 1 fracture is higher, it extends through the tip of the odontoid and is usually stable. A type 3 fracture is lower, extending through the body of the C2 vertebral body and is also stable most of the time. Type 1 and 3 fractures may be treated conservatively, while a type 2 fracture might require surgery."

"Thank you for explaining this to us!" Felipe said.

"I really like how you explained this in general terms!" Saira added. "I understood it, even though I only started a few months ago!"

"My pleasure!" Lili responded. She thoroughly enjoyed teaching the trainees. They were so interested and engaged, filling the room with youthful enthusiasm. They continued to review a series of other images. Then, they all started dictating reports for the images that they had reviewed together. It was gratifying solving new cases and providing patients with a diagnosis, so that they could be referred to appropriate treatment. The radiology team served as the eyes of medicine.

While dictating her cases, Lili continued to peek towards the door. *I would really like to talk with Annya,* she thought. They had reviewed at least thirty radiographs. Surely, a few of those must have been her patients. But oddly, Annya did not come by. Her absence started to become unusual. *Perhaps she is sick?* Lili wondered. After about forty-five minutes, she noticed from the corner of her eyes that someone was approaching the door. Lili turned around in anticipation. It was Matthew, with a coffee mug in his hand.

"Thank you for covering for me," he said with a contented look on his face. "A little break was all I needed. I feel refreshed and refueled!"

"No problem at all," she responded. "I had great help here!"

"Yes, we have a fantastic team here today," Matthew said. "I was so happy when I saw Saira and Felipe walking into the reading room! I thought with their help, I will be fine. Even if I am the only attending today." Saira and Felipe had overheard the conversation and were looking proudly at them. "We like this rotation as well," Felipe responded. "There are always great cases here and the attendings take time to teach us!"

"Have you seen Annya this morning?" Lili asked all three of them, changing the subject.

"Lucia told me that she discussed cases with Annya this morning," Saira responded, "but I believe she left. Santiago is here. Perhaps he knows where she is."

"Yes, let me check with him," Lili responded. Looking at Matthew, she continued, "Are you okay here now?"

"No worries, we have the business under control," he said.

"Thank you for helping out!"

"No problem! See you later!"

Lili left the reading room and walked towards the ER, where she met Santiago in the hallway.

"Hello, Santiago," she greeted him. "I was hoping to find Annya.

"Good to see you, Lili," he responded.

Lili noticed an unusual, almost haunted look in his eyes.

"Hmm, can I perhaps talk with you for a second? The exam room here is free. We could talk there a little more privately?"

"Of course!" Lili responded, hiding her surprise. *What did he want?* Perhaps part of being a good detective was just to be around and talk with people. They stepped into the exam room and Santiago closed the door.

"I think Annya left," he whispered. "We had a very unusual morning together. I feel really uncomfortable and have to share what happened. Will you please keep our conversation confidential?"

"I will do the best I can, Santiago," Lili responded, "but in case it is needed for anyone's safety, it is possible that I will have to pass on information."

"Well, I don't think it's a safety issue," he responded, "but we had a very unusual incident here this morning."

"What happened?" Lili asked, getting curious.

"We had a patient with a Jones fracture here. Annya said that she recognized him as the man the FBI team is looking for. She refused to see him in person and asked me to plant a GPS tracking chip in his cast."

Lili's jaw dropped to the ground. The last twenty-four hours had been extremely eventful, but this was the most amazing story she had ever heard.

"You dropped a GPS chip in a patient's cast?" she asked, not believing her own words. "Where did you get that GPS chip from?"

"Annya had it in a hollow pen in her front pocket," he responded.

"What? And she got that chip-pen from the FBI?"

"I am not sure about that," Santiago said. "I believe I've seen the same pen in her front pocket many times in the past. But of course, it could have been a different pen. But anyways, Mr. Weber, the FBI agent, was also here this morning and he did not seem to know about the suspect or the chip."

"Did you tell him?"

"No. Firstly, he wanted to know everything about a patient with a spine fracture, who apparently was his previous partner. Then, he asked if I had seen Annya. I looked for her and realized that she had left. She had not told anyone that she was leaving or when she would be back. This was very much out of character for her. Usually, she is very diligent and responsible. Agent Weber did not ask anything about the man with the cast and I did not tell him anything either. I was too afraid that I might have done something wrong. If I endangered the patient somehow, perhaps I could lose my license or go to jail!"

"You acted at the order of your superior," Lili said. "I don't think anybody can lock you up for that. But planting a GPS chip in a patient's cast, that is quite a stunt and clearly an invasion into his privacy. That could have some disciplinary consequences. But I cannot imagine that it would harm the patient in any way. Perhaps you could get away by stating that it's a new SUEC invention. If a patient ever gets lost, we will find them right away!" Lili grinned.

"Please do not make jokes about it. I feel terrible!" Santiago looked at her, his lower lip trembling. It had clearly taken him some courage to talk with Lili and she admired his trust in her.

"I am sorry," she said. "I don't mean to trivialize the situation. I do respect Annya, and I believe she had her reasons to ask you to plant this chip. However, I agree with you that placing a GPS chip in a patient's cast would require their consent. But this was a crime suspect."

"Well, Annya disappeared this morning before her shift ended. The FBI agent was looking for her and she was gone. It sounded more like Agent Weber considered her a suspect."

This reminded Lili of her encounter with Angus Weber and the dean last night. *They must be desperate to find somebody, whom they can blame,* she thought.

"I will see what I can find out," she said, "and most importantly, I will see if I can find Annya. I am sure there's a good explanation for her actions."

"I really hope so!" Santiago responded.

"No worries, we will get this straightened out." Lili clapped him on his shoulder. "We have managed many difficult situations together. You, I and Annya are a team! We will manage this situation as well."

Santiago gave her a faint smile. "Thank you, Dr. Pham. I am really glad I talked with you. I feel much better now."

"Take care!"

Lili left the exam room and walked out of the ER towards her car. Her mind was spinning. *What a day of mind-blowing revelations!* She arrived at the parking lot, got into the car, sat back in the driver's seat and took a deep breath. She was grateful for the normalcy of her surroundings. If she didn't have the dull simplicity of the car rides today, her brain might as well explode! *Was Annya a spy? Why was the FBI looking for her? Why did she run away?* Lili was determined to find out. She dialed Annya's phone number, but only reached an answering machine. Lili texted. *Hello Annya, I was hoping to talk with you. Could you please call me back when you get this*? She waited a couple of minutes. No answer. Perhaps Annya was at home. Lili had never been at her apartment, but it should not be too difficult to find it. Lili started the car and drove up to the SUEC University campus.

- 36 -
Amir
TWO DEAD BODIES

Wednesday, May 26, 2032, 8.30 am.

Amir was not sure how long he had been unconscious. When he woke up, he felt a dull pain in his head and a sharp, excruciating pain in his right hand. He tried to orient himself. He had freed Susan. He had a fight with the kidnapper, who had knocked him unconscious. Now he was back in the cabin. He was lying on his belly on the floor of the loft. He remembered the hardwood floor, where he had held Susan's hand. He looked around. Susan was not here. *Hopefully, she had escaped!*

Amir's hands were tied together behind his back. He tried to move. His feet were tied as well. Amir slowly rolled around onto his left side. He saw the bed not too far from him, with pillows and blankets scattered around it on the floor — the result of his struggle with Susan. The mattress was still missing. Rays of sunshine fell through the skylights. Amir saw the sun high in the sky to his left, which should be the east side of the cabin. So, it was likely still morning.

Amir listened. He heard clattering dishes in the cabin downstairs, and he smelled the wafting aroma of freshly baked pancakes and the smoky scent of freshly brewed black tea. Apparently, Boris had a late breakfast in the cabin downstairs. Amir rolled to his right side, carefully avoiding making any noise. He saw parts of the cabin down the stairs, but he could not see Boris. Amir looked around the loft once more, but he could not see anything that could be used as a tool to untie his hands. And even if there were one, it was unlikely that he would make it past Boris and out of the cabin.

Amir rolled back on his belly, keeping his head facing to the right, towards the railing of the loft. This would allow him to observe the situation while trying to come up with an escape plan. He could also pretend to still be unconscious if Boris checked on him. Amir was not sure what he would do if Boris would start interrogating him about the fifth brain chip. He could pretend not to know anything, but he was a terrible liar. He could just hand the chip over. But he did not want to be responsible for more accidents or mental horror trips if the chip were implanted into another human being. At the same time, he wanted to survive.... Amir let his tongue outline his lips, remembering Susan's sweet kiss. Was there still a faint taste of her strawberry lip balm? Amir sincerely hoped that she had made it to the road by now. Since Boris was here, he apparently had not tried to follow her. Or he had followed her and did not capture her. Otherwise, she would probably be here in the cabin again. Unless Boris had shot her dead. Amir tried to erase that thought, which creeped into his mind like a dark shadow. All his energy and determination right now was based on the assumption that Susan had escaped. *I saw that she got away! She is safe now!* he told himself over and over again.

Amir heard steps on the ladder to the loft and quickly closed his eyes. Boris came up and walked towards him. Amir heard the uneven sound of a shoe and a cast on the hardwood floor. He could not suppress the thought. *This is not a walking cast!* After a pause, Amir felt the warmth of Boris body in front of him. Then, he felt Boris fingers on the right side of his neck. Amir had to control his reflex to flinch. He held his breath. *Do not choke me again!* He thought. But Boris did not grab the circumference of his neck, he felt his pulse. Amir tried to calm himself down as much as possible. His heart was racing, but he managed to produce a shallow, rhythmic breathing pattern. He now wished he had turned the head away from the railing. Boris was likely also inspecting his face carefully. Amir tried to not move his eyes, eyelids or any part of his face. After what seemed to be an eternity, Boris got up and Amir heard his footsteps disappearing across the loft and down the ladder. Amir carefully opened his left eye, which was closest to the floor. It was still possible that Boris was watching him. With a beating heart, Amir opened his right eye as well, just a tiny little bit, then more. When he saw that Boris was gone, he sighed. *So far so good!* Amir knew that he had only delayed another confrontation with Boris. But if everything went well, Susan was safe by now and she would send someone to his rescue. Hopefully, he would manage to survive until then.

Amir heard Boris talking downstairs. Amir slowly shuffled a little closer to the railing in order to hear him better, carefully staying out of Boris's sight. His voice came from the direction of the dining table. Presumably he sat there. He probably could not walk around much with his leg cast. Amir inched forwards so that he could see the outer edge of the dining table. Two crutches were leaning against it. Amir heard Boris's voice more clearly now.

"....I am using a new burner phone and will discard it right after I have received my payment. Nobody will find the phone or me."

There was a pause, where the other party apparently responded.

Then, Boris continued, "No, I do not know where the fifth chip might be. Perhaps it did get lost. I checked the usual contacts on the black market in San Francisco. Nothing. There was no trace on the dark net either."

"Yes, she escaped. She seemed pretty wasted on drugs or something. But as soon as she gets sober, she will be able to describe me. I have to disappear, or I will endanger the entire operation."

He is talking about Susan! Amir thought. *She did make it!* Amir's heart jumped in excitement. He felt overwhelmed by emotions. Ecstatic happiness, gratitude, relief, satisfaction and pride that he had rescued her.

Another pause. Then, Boris spoke again. "The operation *has* been completed successfully! The chips are back and only a handful of people know about their journey. The FBI has a self-interest to keep the chip theft confidential. The public does not know about the brain chip research and the FBI probably wants to keep it this way. You need to deal with your staff. I can always come back and shut them up if needed."

Another pause

"I have two dead bodies here. Two friends on a weekend trip. They will burn down with the cabin. It will look like a terrible accident."

Two dead bodies? It took Amir a moment to comprehend who else Boris was referring to, in addition to Kaleo. *He is referring to me as a dead man! He will kill me!* Amir's senses heightened.

Another pause.

"Four chips were all there was. I already told you, I do not know where the fifth chip is! The operation needs to be terminated now. I have to disappear, or the entire project could be uncovered."

"If the fifth chip emerges, you will just state that you have nothing to do with it."

"I do expect the full payment. I eliminated multiple unexpected threats to the operation. I will offset this extra work against the fifth chip, which disappeared. Four chips were successfully retrieved and returned."

Boris's voice became toneless, threatening. He said slowly. "Dr. Bennett, I will say this one last time. I will find my payment on my account tonight. If I find one cent less than agreed upon, I will inform your sponsor that any amateur can just walk into your research labs, grab classified materials and walk away."

Dr. Bennett? Amir tried to remember where he had heard the name before. Then he realized. The dean of SUEC had a name like that. *Had Boris just talked with Dean Bennett? Had the dean hired a killer to retrieve the chips? Considering the high stakes, it was surprising that nobody had thought about this possibility before.*

Amir heard a slamming sound. Perhaps Boris had slammed the phone on the wooden table. Whatever it was, the phone call had ended. Boris stormed to the middle of the room, fists clenched, then kicked the chair beside the dining table.

Amir slowly rolled back to his previous position on the loft and held his breath. *I hope he won't come up the ladder now!* he thought, closing his eyes and repeating his wish as if he could alter reality with a chant to his mind.

Amir's wish was fulfilled. Boris did not come back up to the loft. But he did get busy in the room downstairs. Amir could not see him directly, but he heard fluid smashing on the ground floor. Then, he heard a sizzling sound. Flickering lights illuminated the lower floor. Amir heard the squeaking front door being opened and shut. A key turned in the door. *Boris had left the cabin!* Amir rolled on his back. He lifted his upper body, getting into a seated position. He shuffled on his butt towards the balustrade, pushing himself forwards with his tied feet and hands. He felt that his right hand was severely swollen. It hurt when he tried to push himself forwards on the floor. So, he used mostly his tied feet to move his body forwards on the floor like a caterpillar. He felt an increasing heat in the cabin. A smoky odor came from the living room below him. Amir carefully peeked over the balustrade. What he saw made him turn pale. Menacing flames were rushing over the ground floor to his left, in front of the kitchenette and cabin door. Through the window, Amir saw Boris standing in front of the cabin. He was leaning against the Mercedes with arms folded in front of his chest, watching the fire taking over the cabin.

- 37 -
Lili
A REASON TO KILL

Wednesday, May 26, 2032, 9.00 am.

Lili parked in the employee parking lot and checked her phone. There was no message from Annya, Amir or anyone else. Lili got out, locked the car and went to the gate, where she showed her ID to the security guard. She then walked up the beautiful tree-lined promenade, which led to the main octagon university building. The towering redwood trees were providing much-needed shade as the late morning sun started to send intense summer heat into the valley. Along her path up the hill, Lili heard birds chirping in the trees and she saw hummingbirds fluttering around flowerpots with multicolored columbines. A few busy students were passing by, walking up or down the promenade. Some looked at her briefly, but most of them were busy with themselves, chatting with each other or talking on the phone. Lili arrived at the hilltop, passed by the café to the right of the octagon building and entered through the main entrance, where she met Aiko Tanaka at the entrance desk. She had remembered that Aiko was filling in for Stella and was hoping that she would help her find Annya's apartment, even though she knew that Aiko did not like her.

Aiko was the daughter of immigrants from Osaka, Japan. She had grown up in San Francisco's Japantown, between the Western Addition and Pacific Heights districts. Her parents had come to San Francisco in the post-internment era. They had overcome financial constraints, anti-Asian racism and local gang activities. They identified as Nikkei, which was used to refer to Japanese people who emigrated from Japan and their descendants. Aiko's father had worked at the Benkyo-do confectionary. Her mother had taken care of her and her brother. Aiko knew what immense sacrifices her parents had made to attain the status of a middle-class American family. She was grateful for the opportunities afforded to her. She was independent, she had married the manager of the SUEC cafeteria and they had two healthy children. Aiko's parents were immensely proud of their daughter, being the mother of two beautiful, smart children and working as a senior administrator at the most famous university in the world. Aiko was sharp, focused, conscientious and an excellent communicator. She would have loved to become a physician. But when she was young, she did not have access to dedicated training and preparation for entrance exams to medical school. She knew that she had made it far beyond the constraints of her first-generation upbringing. She also knew that with a little more mentoring and a little more cash, she would be walking in Lili's shoes now. And whenever Aiko saw Lili, she saw her lost opportunities in her. It did not help for Lili to point out that she had made sacrifices as well. As a physician-scientist, she had completed twelve years of training, she worked ninety-hour weeks and she had faced microaggressions, bullying and discrimination on a regular basis. Lili was so absorbed with her work that she did not have the bandwidth to care for a child. She admired Aiko's ability to combine a rich family life and a fulfilling job. But Aiko did not see this. She hated Lili for everything that she had achieved and Aiko had not.

"Hello Lili," Aiko greeted her with an authoritative voice as Lili walked into the lobby of the octagon building. "It is really good to see you! I was just looking up your phone number. Dean Bennett would like to talk with you."

"Is that so?" Lili said, hiding her surprise. "What would he like to talk about?"

"He will discuss that with you," Aiko responded. Lili concluded that she might not know or if she knew, she did not plan on telling her.

"Of course, I would be happy to talk with him!" she responded, smiling at Aiko.

"Well, I did not expect to find you so quickly. He's currently in another meeting. Could you please wait outside and come back in about thirty minutes?" Aiko pointed at the door. She could have easily invited Lili into the lobby, which featured private waiting areas and free coffee. But it did not look like she was in the mood of discussing Lili's waiting arrangements.

"Sure, no problem!" Lili said with a cheery voice. This was probably not the best time to ask for Annya's address. In fact, she probably had to rethink her plan to find Annya's apartment. Lili turned around, walked out of the building and towards the coffee shop on the hilltop terrace. She was annoyed. She despised Aiko's condescending tone, the disregard for her own time and the prospect of meeting the dean again.

Lili got a café latte at the Starbucks counter and added a sugar-coated biscotti to recharge her positive energy. She looked around. Most of the tables were occupied by chatting students, some of them apparently discussing contents of their electronic textbooks, others munching a late breakfast and yet others leaning back in their chairs, enjoying a break. Lili spotted a small unoccupied bistro table at the edge of the terrace, walked over there, sat down and drank her coffee. Her cell phone buzzed to indicate an incoming text message. It was one of our ER residents. *Hello Lili, can you have a quick at this case. Dr. Holmes is busy presenting cases in the surgery conference. Is this a radial head fracture?* Lili opened her laptop and brought up the image in question via the Web-PACS. There was a clear radial head fracture with a cortical step off and fracture line. She placed arrows at the abnormalities, took a screenshot of the radiograph without the patient's name on it and texted the image back.

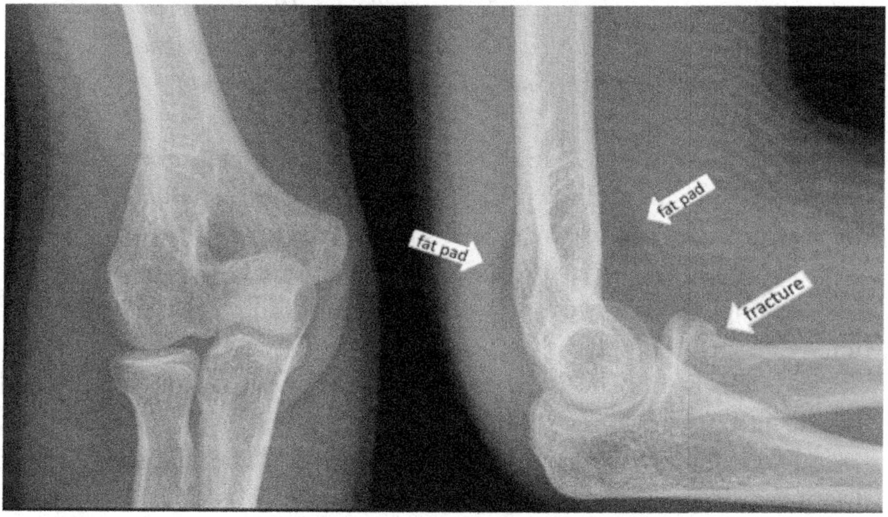

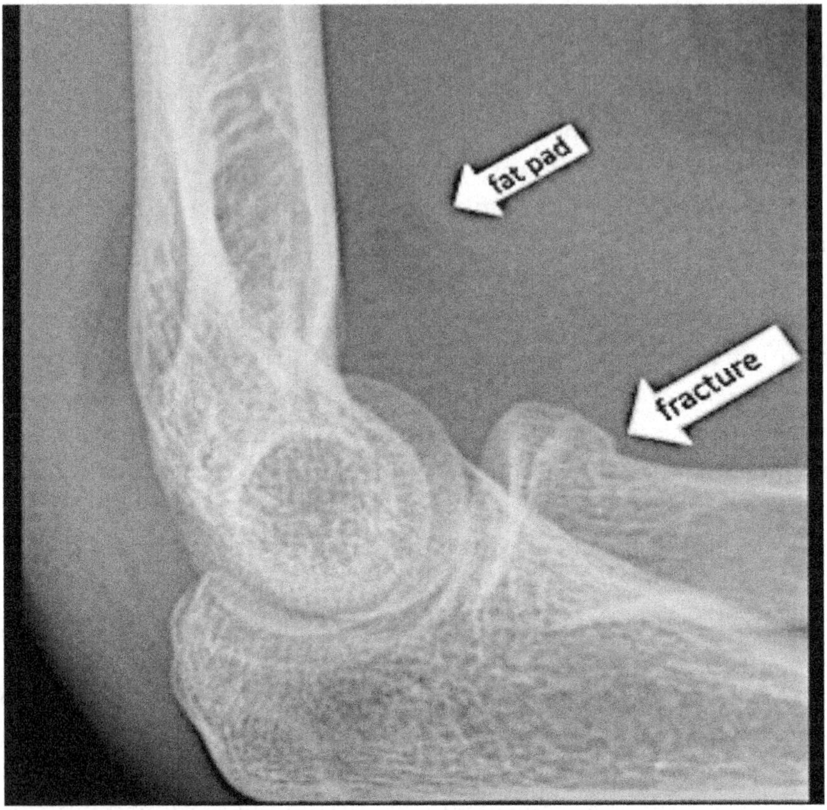

Correct. This is a radial head fracture! Great call! There are also elevated anterior and posterior fat pads, which indicate a joint effusion. Please review the images also with your attending of the day when he comes back from the conference.
The phone buzzed again. *Sure, will do! Thank you so much!*

Lili leaned back in her chair. The work never stopped. She closed her eyes for a moment and must have dozed off. When she heard a voice, she was not sure if it was real or if she had imagined it.

"Hello Lili, what a surprise to see you here!"

Lili opened her eyes and saw Dr. Robert Hill standing in front of her.

"Hello Robert, how is your shoulder?" she asked. She noticed that his arm was still in a sling.

"Oh, thanks for asking!" he responded. "The pain has almost disappeared. I am receiving physiotherapy, which is time consuming.

But otherwise, I believe my convalescence is going well!"

"I am glad to hear that!" Lili said. She liked Robert's matter of fact, no nonsense approach. He seemed to be smart, honest and not deformed by office politics, if that were possible in the academic environment.

"What brought you here?" she asked. "I would have assumed that a busy scientist would not spend much time in luxurious cafés like this?"

"You might be right!" he laughed. "I cannot remember ever sitting at this café. I sometimes do get a coffee here after a meeting but then usually hurry to the lab."

"But you did not get a coffee today?" Lili asked, looking at his hands. The left arm was in a sling. The right hand held an envelope. Robert had followed her gaze.

"Well, I got most of my brain chips back today!" he said, with a big smile on his face.

"Wow! That is some news!" Lili said, genuinely surprised. "How did you get the chips back?"

"The dean just handed them to me!" Robert explained, holding up the envelope in his hand. "Apparently, someone dropped them in his mailbox here overnight."

"Someone dropped them in his mailbox?" Lili asked. It seemed that the series of bizarre events today continued.

"Yes!" Robert said. He could hardly contain his relief and excitement. "These represent years of hard research, millions of dollars in research funding and a major advancement for humanity. I am so glad we have them back and could avoid a major scandal! That could have jeopardized our entire program!"

"I am very happy for you," Lili said. "Who brought the chips back? And how?" She thought about Susan. *Was she back?* Lili peeked on the two phones in her purse. But there was still no new text message on either one.

"Well, it might have been Annya," Robert explained. "The security cameras captured her walking up and down the promenade here last night. Dean Bennett said that he handed the security footage to Agent Weber this morning and the FBI is looking for her now."

"This can't be true!" Lili exclaimed. "Annya returned the brain chips? Where did she get them?"

"I do not know that. But cameras don't lie."

Lili looked at Robert in disbelief. "Do you think Annya was connected to the thieves? I cannot imagine that. She's the most honest person I know!"

"Well, I certainly do not know the circumstances. Perhaps there is a good explanation," Robert said, scratching his head. "All I know is that she was out there last night. I am her neighbor here at the SUEC village. My partner and I live in the apartment next to her. I did hear her leaving her apartment in the middle of the night and coming back about an hour later. So, I can confirm that she was outside her apartment somewhere during the night, when apparently my chips were returned."

"Wow! So, the chips were returned last night?" Lili tried to integrate this information with Santiago's story. *Why had Annya planted a chip in a suspect's cast hours later?* Even though she trusted Robert, her inner voice told her to not share this information right now. Annya was her friend and he considered her a suspect.

"Yes, according to the video, Annya returned the chips around three am," Robert explained. "Actually, Dean Bennett gave me four brain chips. The thieves stole five chips. So, one is still missing."

"Ah, so if Annya was somehow able to retrieve the chips, perhaps she is trying to get the fifth chip as well?"

"I really hope that's the case!" Robert responded. "I like her a lot! I just don't understand why she did not hand over the chips to me directly. That would've been much easier than walking to the SUEC mailbox in the middle of the night. Why would she drop the chips in the dean's mailbox? She surely knows that the octagon building is on constant camera surveillance."

"I don't know. Perhaps it has to do with the fifth chip. Would it be a major problem if one remains missing?"

"It depends," Robert said. "If the fifth chip were to just disappear, that would not be a major problem. We could produce another one. However, if the thieves use it and harm someone, that could shut down our entire research, millions of research dollars and perhaps billions of dollars from revenues when the chips are being marketed."

"I see." Lili felt a shiver down her back. That sounded like a reason to kill for. *I hope Susan is okay!* she prayed.

"Of course, the SUEC security team and the FBI checked all university emails and communications on the dark net. Undercover agents checked for transactions on the black market. But they did not find any signs that someone had offered a brain chip for purchase or that a transaction has taken place."

Lili looked at Robert. Since she was prohibited from doing any detective work, she did not want to share directly what she knew. But she could move the conversation into a certain direction so that he would develop his own idea. If the search team got the idea that Susan had the brain chip, they might be more motivated to find and rescue her.

"Would it be possible for the thief to have implanted a chip into their own brain?"

Robert looked at Lili. "I thought they were after money. Selling the brain chips would bring them a fortune."

"Do you think the payment would be much less if they sold four brain chips instead of five?"

"They can probably name any price."

"If they were just after money, they could have robbed a bank or a jewelry store. There must be a component of interest in brain-computer interfaces to even become aware of their existence and value."

Robert's forehead crinkled. "Perhaps they dissected one?"

"That is certainly a possibility. Although, nobody found fragments of a chip, right?"

"Perhaps they split them up between them?"

"That is also possible, but why is only one missing? Wouldn't they split them up more evenly? Similarly, if they wanted to hide the chips for a transaction at a later time, why would they hide four and not five? They must have done something special with one of the chips."

Robert's eyes widened. "One of the chips was implanted! Anything else just does not make sense!"

Lili smiled and nodded in agreement.

Robert looked at the envelope in his hand. "We have to find the thieves! One of them might have the fifth chip on them!"

"That is a brilliant idea!" Hopefully, he would tell as many as people as possible and they would intensify the search for the thieves.

Robert checked the time on his iPhone. "I have to go. In ten minutes, I have an interview with an internal candidate who applied to fill Juan's position. We do not want any public attention at this point. I just discussed with the dean that we will forego a job advertisement and fill the position internally, based on the unique qualifications of the candidate. Fortunately, he has an offer from another university, which will help us to justify an accelerated hiring process here."

"Good for you! Good luck with your interview!" Lili was intimately familiar with the urgency of the academic research environment. Research sponsors set tighter and tighter deadlines for progress reports. If you had an opening in a research lab, you had to fill it as quickly as possible to avoid delays. This favored everyone who was already in the system and made it difficult for outsiders to get in.

"It was good to see you, Lili!" Robert waved goodbye and hurried down the stairs of the terrace towards the promenade.

"It was good to see you too!" Lili called after him as his silhouette disappeared in the shadows of the beautiful redwood trees. She thought *I really hope they find Susan!*

- 38 -
Lili
A HIDDEN AGENDA

Wednesday, May 26, 2032, 9.30 am.

Lili finished her coffee and checked the time. She was five minutes early for the meeting with Dean Bennett, but she got up and made her way to the SUEC entrance desk again. She certainly did not want to be late for the meeting with the dean. Hopefully, he was in a better mood today since the brain chips had been returned – or at least four of them.

When she walked into the lobby, Aiko was sorting though some paperwork on her desk. "Hello, Aiko!" Lili said, flashing her teeth. "I am here for the meeting with Dean Bennett!"

Aiko looked up. "Hello, Lili! You remind me of my daughter, always a bit premature!" She faked a smile.

"Well, I did not want to be late." Lili tried to establish eye contact, but Aiko seemed to look past her.

"Oh, Dr. Houston!" she exclaimed with an upward glance. "How wonderful to see you!"

A middle-aged man in a perfectly ironed, expensive looking, dark gray suit stepped through the door. "Hello, Mrs. Tanaka. I am here for my appointment with Dr. Bennett."

"Dr. Houston, I am afraid, you are just a bit early," Aiko responded with a soft, lilting laugh. "This lady here" — she pointed at Lili — "has to meet with Dr. Bennett for just a few minutes. Would you mind waiting briefly in the lobby? We have freshly brewed coffee or tea for you at the bar. I will come get you as soon as Dr. Bennett is ready!"

"Sounds good to me. Thank you, Mrs. Tanaka!" The man walked past them into the lobby. Lili sighed. This was one of the many experiences she had every day with double standards.

"Do you mind if I walk up to his office now?" Lili asked.

Aiko looked briefly at her. "Of course, you know your way around, Lili. Suit yourself!" She responded with a waving gesture towards the lobby while her gaze went back to the paperwork on her desk.

"Thank you." Lili walked past her into the lobby.

Lili stopped briefly at the orchid garden to boost her mood and energy. She loved the simple, clean interior of the lobby and the sophisticated arrangement of the flowers. Clearly, a master of Phong Thuy, better known by its Chinese name, Feng Shui, had been involved in designing this space. Just looking at it calmed her mind. She specifically liked to look at the spider orchids, which were labeled *brassia caudata.* The bulbs were composed of large, spindly flowers with long, slender, yellow-green sepals and petals that were barred and blotched with brown, so that the delicate flowers looked like they were wearing a tiger-print dress. Lili marveled at the beauty of the flower arrangement, tried to absorb the tiger spirit and reset her mental balance. She took a deep breath and then walked up the stairs to Dr. Bennett's office. As she came closer, the door opened, and she heard Dr. Bennett's voice. "It was great meeting with you!"

"Thanks for your time, Dr. Bennett!" she heard another man's voice. "I am glad we could resolve all concerns!"

Apparently, Dr. Bennett was just finishing up another meeting. The men were still on the other side of the door. Lili could only hear them.

"I can assure you," Dr. Bennett continued, "you only heard gossip. The brain chips are safe and sound and our research is progressing as planned. You can visit Dr. Hill in the lab and see it for yourself."

"I am very glad to hear that!" the other man said with a commanding voice. "Perhaps the rumors came up because of the death of the lab employee. You should make sure to hire more emotionally stable personnel. We cannot tolerate any negative publicity."

"You can be assured that we will check the mental health of our employees more thoroughly in the future — and as a new requirement, we will include their spouses!" Dr. Bennett's responded in a subservient tone. "This was a very unfortunate tragedy, and I will do everything in my power to avoid anything like it in the future."

"I appreciate that!" the other man responded. "It is always great to see you, Ben! Let's wait a few months. That will also allow Dr. Hill to make further progress with his research, test it in human volunteers and publish the results. Then, we will make the announcement about the joined commercial development of the brain chips later next year and add another billion to SUECs endowment account!"

"We are immensely grateful for your generosity!" Dr. Bennett responded. "Your donation will spur important research on brain-computer interfaces and establish SUEC University as a leader in the world! We will unleash the unused capacity of our brains and create humans two point zero!"

"Our donations tomorrow will be the largest private donation to a university!" the other man responded proudly, "and this will only be the beginning of a very fruitful partnership! I will be happy to help you attracting more sponsors for great projects such as this one. Private sponsors are becoming more and more important for universities around the world. Mike Bloomberg donated one point eight billion dollars to Johns Hopkins University, Anil Agarwal donated a billion to the University in Odisha and Florence Irving donated six hundred million to Columbia University and New York-Presbyterian. If you want to play in the same league, you have to attract similar sponsorship."

Lili realized that she was overhearing sensitive information and walked back to the stairs as quietly as possible. She could barely hear the two men from here. She waited at the top of the stairs until the door of Dr. Bennett's office flung wide open and the two men appeared, still engaged in their conversation. Dr. Bennett saw Lili at the end of the hallway and waved at her. They walked towards each other, Lili taking small, slow steps to make the distance feel longer for them. They met close to the stairwell.

Dr. Bennett shook the hand of the other man. "Thanks again for a very productive meeting today!" he said to him.

"It was great meeting you too!" he responded. He nodded briefly at Lili, then walked down the stairs.

Dr. Bennett shifted his attention to Lili. "Hello Lili, thanks for coming by!" He gave her a friendly smile.

"Hello Dr. Bennett!" Lili said as politely as possible. Apparently, he did not remember how rudely he had treated her last night.

They walked back to his office. Dr. Bennett took a seat in an armchair behind his large desk and offered Lili a smaller seat in front of it. She felt small in this position. Perhaps that was the intention of the furniture arrangement.

"We have fantastic news!" he said, "The brain chips have been returned!"

Four of five! Lili thought. But she decided to avoid any debate. "Oh, that is wonderful! That must be a big relief!"

"It is indeed!" Dr. Bennett said cheerfully. "The FBI is still chasing the thieves. We hope that we will bring them to justice soon."

"That would be good!" Lili agreed.

"Lili, I have to remind you that our research on computer brain interfaces, including these brain chips, is highly confidential. You cannot talk about the chips or anything around their theft with anybody, including your closest family members."

"Of course!" Lili responded and thought. *This man has his own agenda. He will probably do anything to close this case as soon as possible.*

Dr. Bennett's friendly smile changed into a serious look. "Lili, I know you mean well. However, it has come to my attention that you did not follow my and Agent Weber's order to refrain from your own detective work."

"I am not sure what you mean, Dr. Bennett?" Lili responded with an innocent smile.

"Well, the FBI has been tracking your phone," he said. "This is standard procedure for anyone involved in a matter of national security."

Lili did not believe that statement.

Dr. Bennett continued, "Agent Weber informed me that you have been at the General Hospital twice and you have also exchanged text messages with a crime suspect, Amir Nielsson."

"Well, I am Stella's friend. As you know, her husband died some time ago and she does not have any close relatives here. She was afraid of her surgery and therefore, I visited her this morning," Lili explained. "I then went to the Radiology reading room. So, I did nothing out of the ordinary." *How genius that I had done that,* she thought.

"How do you know Amir Nielsson?" Dean Bennett asked.

"I don't know him at all," Lili said, trying to remember what exactly they had exchanged via text message. *Not much.* "You mean the nurse practitioner in the hospital, right?"

Dr. Bennett nodded, clearly annoyed about this cat and mouse game.

"Well, he offered to keep me informed about Stella," Lili lied. "If she encounters any medical problem, he will call or text me."

"Is that right?" Dr. Bennett asked.

Lili nodded with a sweet smile.

"Well, Amir Nielsson is not in the hospital anymore, so he cannot send you any updates. Agent Weber asked me to confiscate your phone," Dr. Bennett said with a triumphant voice. "Amir Nielsson may be one of the chip thieves and it seems that you are our only connection to him."

"If you confiscate my phone, you cannot track me anymore?"

"Since I just told you about it, I assume it would not be effective anymore from here," Dr. Bennett responded, "and at this time, it is more important to find Amir."

"I believe I left my phone in my car," Lili lied again, "and I need it for emergency calls from the hospital!"

Dr. Bennett looked at her. "Lili, look, you are a valuable physician scientist here at SUEC. I know you have nothing to do with this crime, apart from an unusual curiosity. I want to prevent you from getting arrested for collaborating with terrorists. I just told you that we tracked your phone and I assume you have it in your purse right here." He pointed at her purse. "I offer this for the last time. Hand over your phone! If you do not comply, then I will call the FBI and they will get it in a much less pleasant way."

Lili sighed, opened her purse and handed him the phone.

"I knew you would do the right thing," Dr. Bennett said, content. "Now let the adults do the work here. We will solve this problem and you will get your phone back in no time."

"Of course!" Lili said, getting up from her chair.

"I have one more question," Dr. Bennett asked.

The password? Lili wondered. She looked at him with a blank stare.

"I was also hoping to speak with Annya Segond but could not reach her. Do you know, where I can find her? It looks like she was involved in the theft of the brain chips."

Lili shrugged. "Sorry, I have no idea. I did not see her in the hospital this morning." *He probably already knew that.*

"Okay, thank you, Lili," Dr. Bennett responded. "We will find her!"

Why did that sound like a threat? Lili turned around and walked out of his office, down the stairs, through the lobby and past Aiko, who hardly noticed her. Her knees were shaking, and she realized that she was clutching her purse against her belly. As she stepped out of the octagon building, a little breeze went through her hair, gently erasing the sweat pearls on her temples. *Cameras along the promenade*, she remembered. She tried to relax as much as possible and walked down the promenade as fast as she could without raising suspicion. *How long would it take until Dr. Bennett realized that I gave him Stella's phone?* she thought.

Lili arrived at the parking lot and walked towards her car, when she heard a voice behind her. "Hello Lili, is that you?" She turned around and to her despair, saw Andrew, one of the security guards coming after her. Lili had known him for many years. They had started working at SUEC on the same day and had taken some of the same orientation classes. Andrew had some kind of crush on her. Whenever he saw her, he tried to involve her in a conversation and looked weirdly up and down her body. Perhaps it was just a habit as a security guard. But it made her feel uncomfortable and she tried to avoid him as much as possible. *Hopefully, it is just that!* she prayed.

"Hello Andy," Lili said with her most charming smile. "Great to see you!"

"Hello Lili, great to see you too!" he responded. "How are you?"

"I am doing well, thank you!" Lili said.

"Important business on campus?" he asked.

Lili did not want to mention the dean. "I was looking for Annya. But apparently, she's not at home."

"Interesting that you say that," Andrew responded, eager to catch her attention. "At our huddle this morning, Michael, the night guard, reported an unusual event. A stranger had parked at the SUEC parking lot and had walked up the promenade. When he came back, a woman was following him. Michael was quite sure that it was Dr. Segond. The man called after her, but she literally ran away."

"That is most peculiar indeed!" Lili exclaimed, "Did Michael report this incident?"

"Yes, we actually spent this morning reviewing the security cameras," Andrew explained. "We confirmed that the man walked up and down the promenade and apparently left an envelope in the mailbox of the main university building. We informed the dean and he said that this was just a sponsor, who had left a cheque for the university."

"That is an unusual time to deposit a donation!" Lili said, shaking her head about this amateurish excuse.

"Yes, and it was even more peculiar that the dean asked us to separate the videos of the man and the woman and give them to him as separate files!" Andrew said. "That did not seem right to me, Lili! But of course, it is not my place to question my superiors."

"I am really glad you brought this up," Lili said.

"I heard that the FBI had issued a search for Annya, and I cannot help but think that it is somehow related to this event," Andrew added.

"I will let her know when I see her," Lili said.

"Thank you!" Andrew responded. He paused for a while. Then he looked at Lili. "Actually, I made a copy of the videos." He produced a flash drive from his pocket and handed it to her.

Lili's jaw dropped for the second time today. "Andrew, you are amazing! Thank you!" she said, deeply impressed. If anybody ever accused Annya, she would have the evidence of what was really going on. Lili put the flash drive into her purse.

Andrew smiled. "Anything for you, Lili! Stay safe!"

Lili turned around and walked towards her car. She thought, *a man delivered the brain chips last night! Why did the dean accuse Annya instead? Why did Andrew tell me this story? Had he also received a warrant for me? If he did, he did not act on it.* Lili opened the car door, got in, fumbled for the key, started the car and drove off.

She made sure to leave the university campus, then stopped on the side of the road and checked her phone. She had a text message from Amir! The time above the message stated "5.55 am. *How could I have missed that? That was before I went to see Stella!* She thought. She had checked the phone several times since then and had not seen any message. That was weird. *Was it possible that the FBI had intercepted this message and delayed its delivery?* Perhaps that was the reason why Dr. Bennett had wanted her phone. He had known about this message! But if the FBI already had access to her texts, why would they need to confiscate Lili's phone? There was only one explanation. Dr. Bennett was *not* working with the FBI. He needed the texts for his own agenda! He had withheld the information about the man who brought the brain chips back and accused Annya instead. Lili had just learned that the brain chips were worth billions of dollars. And Dr. Bennett had just told the sponsor that the chips had never been stolen in the first place. He needed to fix his problem urgently!

Lili read Amir's text message. *Redwood Road 21, San Mateo. OMW.*

My God, that was five hours ago! She entered the address into the navigation system and prepared to get there as quickly as possible.

- 39 -
Amir
THE FIRE

Wednesday, May 25, 2032, 9.30 am.

Amir heard the hardwood floor snap as the crackling flames took over the living room of the cabin. From his place on the floor of the loft, he saw sparks of fire sputtered in all directions. Amir tried to calm his panicking mind. Working for years in the ER had prepared him to think clearly in times of adrenaline rushes. For now, the loft was above the fire. But the only way out was on the ground floor. He had to get down there and find a way out, either through the door or perhaps through a window. Amir looked through the front window. If he could get past Boris! He saw Boris outside, leaning against his car, crutches on each side, arms folded in front of his chest, watching the growing fire with a look of deep satisfaction. Amir considered calling for help. But it was probably pointless. *I am supposed to die here!* He thought, shivering despite the growing heat.

Suddenly, another car approached the cabin. Boris quickly ducked behind his Mercedes, pulling the crutches down as well. The second car arrived and parked besides the Mercedes. A man got out, holding a gun in his extended hands. He looked around the Mercedes, but Boris quickly moved out of his way. The man walked by the Mercedes and approached the cabin slowly. Boris got up behind him. Amir tried to shout a warning, but his voice got lost in the crackling sound of the growing fire. Boris swung his crutch into the air like a golf club and crashed it into the man's lower leg. The man cried out in pain and fell to the ground, holding his left lower leg. Boris quickly jumped around, opened the driver's door of his car, threw both crutches on the passenger seat, jumped in, started the car, backed out and raced away. The man lay on the ground, agonized.

Amir's attention was drawn to the growing heat in the cabin. He looked down at the fire. The flames in the cabin grew quickly. Harsh smoke was spiraling towards him and started to block his vision. His hands and feet were still tied. Amir saw the edge of the mattress at the base of the ladder. The mattress was still where he had placed it for Susan. Amir rolled to the base of the ladder and sat on the highest step, with his feet dangling down. Then, he slowly slid down the ladder. Suddenly, a pungent smell spread through the air, slowly turning into the smell of almonds. Amir felt his whole body tensing. *Cyanide!* He remembered from his emergency class that a smell of roasted almonds in a fire indicated a lethal poison from burning plastics or chemicals. Even the smallest amount of cyanide can cause severe illnesses. If you cannot get out of the room, you must get low to the floor, to minimize the exposure to cyanide gas which rises up. Amir jumped onto the mattress. Fortunately, he landed on his feet first. Since his arms and feet were tied, he lost balance and fell on the mattress.

That went well, he encouraged himself. *Now I need to find a way out.* Amir looked around to find the best possible exit. The raging flames had taken over most of the cabin. The exit door was completely blocked by blazes of fire. Amir could hardly see through the raging flames. The flames had not yet reached the area around the ladder. But they were quickly coming closer, spreading an unbearable heat. Amir thought about the many burn victims he had seen over the years. *Horrible! He had to find a way out of here!*

Amir looked around. To his right was a window. He could possibly fit through it, but how could he open it with tied hands and feet? Plus, he had to keep his head close to the floor to avoid the poisoning smoke as much as possible. Suddenly, he heard dull blows at the door, as if somebody was knocking very hard. Then, he realized that somebody was jumping against the door. He heard the door shudder to the ground. The flames doubled in size. A man stumbled into a cloud of smoke at the entrance, trying to orient himself. He had lifted his injured leg and had grabbed a broom to support his left side. Amir kept moving to the far-right end of the room, trying to escape the blazing flames. "I am here!" he shouted.

The man turned towards Amir. He looked familiar. But the blinding smoke obscured his face. A wall of flames separated them. Amir could not imagine that either of them could walk through this inferno, certainly not twice, back and forth.

"I will get you out of here," the man shouted back.

Amir recognized the voice. It was FBI agent Angus Weber!

"Can you open the window here?" Amir shouted back, pointing at the window above him. "Perhaps you can pull me though it!"

"Step back from the window as far as you can!" the man shouted back. Angus disappeared from the entrance area. Amir looked around. The flames had started to light up the mattress on which he had landed a few minutes ago. There was no more room to retreat to. So, he cowered under the window, face to the ground. A few seconds later, Amir heard a loud crash. Pieces of glass rained on him. A few cut the skin of his neck and arms. Blood started to drip down his body, but the adrenaline masked the pain. Amir shook his body to shake off the shards as much as possible. Then he got up and took a deep breath from the fresh air that came in from the open window. Angus looked directly at him from the other side.

"My hands and feet are tied," Amir shouted.

Angus nodded. He removed shards from the windowsill and placed his leather jacket on the lower part of the broken window frame. Then, he grabbed Amir under his armpits and pulled him up. Amir felt a second wave of relief as his head reached the other side of the wall. He saw that Angus was standing on one leg only, leaning with his left shoulder against the cabin and holding the injured leg above the ground. Angus made a little pause, as Amir's belly rested on the window frame. Amir heard him breathing heavily. Then, Angus grabbed the circumference of Amir's body and pulled him out of the cabin. They both fell backwards onto the sandy ground of the clearing around the burning cabin. They saw a blaze taking over the roof of the cabin. Angus slowly pulled Amir further away from the cabin as rampaging smoke from the burning roof fogged up the air. Angus slowly limped to his car, which was parked in front of the house, briefly leaped in, then turned around and came back with a Swiss Army knife. He quickly untied Amir's hands and feet.

"Thank you! You saved my life!" Amir exclaimed, trying to shout over the rumbling fire.

"You are welcome!" Angus shouted back, smiling at him. "Is Susan in the cabin?"

"No, she ran away!" Amir responded.

"Is anybody else in there?" Angus asked.

"Kaleo's body is in the kitchen, close to the entrance!" Amir shouted, "But he is dead!"

"Are you absolutely sure that he is dead?" Angus asked.

"Yes, sir!" Amir responded, "I work in the ICU and I am trained to determine who is alive or dead. I am so sorry we could not rescue him as well."

"What were you doing here?" Angus asked.

"Susan was held hostage here," Amir explained with a sense of pride. "I freed her and covered her back while she ran away.

Angus looked at the thin man with wide eyes, startled.

"I guess I do not look exactly like James Bond." Amir echoed the thoughts behind those dark-blue eyes.

"That is impressive indeed!" Angus said. They both smiled.

Amir felt a deep desire to break Angus's stereotypes and impress him further.

"And I got the fifth chip!" he said, fumbling the brain chip with his left hand out of the right pocket of his jeans.

Angus' jaw dropped. "Unbelievable!" he said, taking the chip and observing it carefully. He produced a small plastic bag from the front pocket of his shirt, sealed the chip in the bag and put it back into the front pocket. "Thank you for your service, Mr. Nielsson," he said. "I will return the chip to the university."

They were interrupted by sirens, which approached rapidly. A red firetruck raced down the small unpaved road to the cabin and came to a stop in front of them with squealing tires. A fireman opened the window of the driver's door and shouted at Angus and Amir. "Hello, please move your car out of the way immediately!"

"Of course!" Angus responded. He got into his car and drove it out of the way. The fire truck slowly approached the burning cabin and parked on the right side of the building. Fortunately, the clearing around the cabin provided enough space for the truck and a barrier towards the forest. The fire had not yet spread to the adjacent trees. Four firemen exited the truck. One of them ran to the cabin and smashed the front and west windows. The second firefighter put a mask on, positioned the nozzle of the hose towards the cabin and called for water. The third straightened the hose and removed kinks, while the fourth operated the water pump. Within seconds, a strong stream of water came down on the fire, while the nozzleman slowly made his way through the entrance into the cabin, carefully sweeping the stream of water on the flames inside. Meanwhile, a second firetruck arrived and stopped in front of the cabin. A second group of firefighters jumped out of the truck and joined the first team. They stretched a second hose line from the second engine to the loft area where the fire had extended as well.

Angus and Amir were sitting on the ground, watching the firefighters from a distance. The crew was very effective. The flames were slowly fading and turning into a large dark-gray cloud above the cabin. After a while, they heard another siren approaching. An ambulance raced towards the cabin and stopped beside them. Two paramedics jumped out. One of them ran to the firefighters. Amir saw him talking with one of the firefighters, who walked into the cabin and came back with a corpse in his extended arms. Amir recognized Kaleo and felt tears running down his cheeks. Kaleo's lifeless arms and legs were hanging down from the extended arms of the fireman. Kaleo's cloths were burned and hardly recognizable. Kaleo's head was hanging backwards, and his hair was burned, but his face was surprisingly preserved. Amir could not reconcile that he had spoken with Kaleo less than twenty-four hours ago. The firefighter carefully placed Kaleo's body on the ground and the paramedic started to examine him.

Meanwhile, the second paramedic approached Amir and Angus, taking their history and examining them carefully. After a while, a third paramedic joined him. They carried over a stretcher, stabilized Angus' broken leg with a splint and carried him into the ambulance. Then, they provided another splint for Amir's swollen hand. The paramedics wanted to bring the second stretcher over. But Amir refused to lie down on it. He explained to the paramedics that he was a nurse practitioner and that he had broken his hand, not his legs. He could walk just fine. After a lively debate, the paramedics slowly walked him to the ambulance and Amir settled on the second stretcher inside. One of the paramedics provided an oxygen mask and oral pain medication to both Amir and Angus. The second paramedic joined him in the back cabin and the third paramedic jumped into the driver's seat.

The ambulance was nearly ready to take off when a black van arrived. It stopped in some distance and five men jumped out. Four of them ran towards the cabin, while the fifth ran towards the ambulance, holding an FBI ID in the air and requesting access to the back cabin. It was Terrel Wright.

"Hello Terrel, we really missed you!" Angus said with a smirk.

"Angus, what happened to you?" Terrel responded, looking at Angus's splinted leg. "Can I not let you alone for an hour?"

"I had a fight with Mr. Bond here!" Angus said, pointing at Amir.

"I doubt that," Terrel responded, grinning as well. He looked at Amir's swollen and bruised hand. "I would be interested to see the face that met this hand! As far as I can see, it was not yours, Angus. What happened?"

"Well, Mr. Nielsson freed Susan Pellegrini and punched the kidnapper. The kidnapper killed Kaleo Kahale, one of the chip thieves. He tried to kill Mr. Nielsson as well. He tied him up in the cabin and set it on fire. I arrived and tried to arrest the man. But we got into a fight, and he broke my leg. Then, he escaped in a dark gray Mercedes."

"I am glad you both got out of this alive!" Terrel responded. "Sorry, we are late to the party. We picked up Susan Pellegrini on our way here."

"Thank God, she is safe!" Amir exclaimed.

"She was standing in the middle of the road, waving with both arms," Terrel explained., "It was good that we found her. She was very disturbed. I wanted to take her with us to the cabin here, but she got a panic attack when I even mentioned it. I ordered another van and one of our FBI agents escorted her to the hospital. I am afraid, that took some time."

"Where did you take her?" Amir asked.

"I am sorry, this is classified information," Terrel responded. "You are not an immediate family member and I have yet to understand your involvement here."

"Amir risked his live to save Susan," Angus weighed in. "I think it will positively affect his recovery, if he receives a little more information."

Terrel looked at both men. They clearly had just experienced a major trauma. "Well, we thought it would be best for Susan to be reunited with her mother," he explained.

"Thank you!" Amir exclaimed, "I am so relieved to hear that!"

"Perhaps you can return the favor," Amir responded. "We have yet to find the killer and his commander. Did you notice anything that could help us find them?"

"The name of the killer is Boris," Amir responded. "I do not know his last name. Susan saw how Boris killed Kaleo."

"We know his full name and have issued a search warrant for him," Terrel explained. "We have a major taskforce looking for him."

"His boss is Dr. Bennet!" Amir added. "I overheard a phone call, where Boris stated that he had retrieved the chips for Dr. Bennett. He also mentioned that he awaited payment from Dr. Bennett and that he was about to burn both me and Kaleo with the cabin. Dr. Bennett did nothing to prevent that plan."

Angus and Terrel stared at Amir. "The dean?" Angus finally said. "Are you sure you heard that correctly? That is quite an accusation!"

"I am absolutely sure and will be happy to repeat that in court when we bring that bastard to justice!" Amir exclaimed. "Boris told him that he would burn me with the cabin, and he did nothing to prevent that!"

Terrel looked at Amir, thinking. Then he waved one of his FBI team members to come over. A young Asian man approached them, introducing himself as Agent Lamong Saetang. "Hello Lamong," Terrel said. "Can you please accompany Mr. Nielsson to the hospital? He is an important witness for our case here and I want to make sure he will be safe until he can deliver his deposition. This is very important! I will have to stay here to secure all evidence. We will rely on you to keep the witness safe!"

"Of course!" Lamong answered, pride and devotion on his face for being assigned this important task. He jumped into the cabin of the ambulance and took a seat besides Amir.

"Thank you!" Amir said, looking at Lamong. He only realized now how exhausted he was. He had been so anxious about Susan, he was horrified by Kaleo's death, he had punched a professional killer in the face and he had escaped a burning cabin. Susan was with her mother, and he had a personal protector. Amir sighed and closed his eyes for a moment. The doors of the back cabin were shut, the ambulance took off and Amir fell into a deep sleep.

- 40 -
Boris
THE FIFTH CHIP

Wednesday, May 26, 2032, 9.30 am.

Boris raced down the unpaved road, away from the cabin and towards the I-280 highway. The car jumped up and down as the wheels were caught in various potholes along his path. Boris cursed. Was there a buzzing tone from his burner phone? The only two people who had this number were Bogdan and Dean Bennett. Boris had reached a paved road. He turned to the right and drove towards the highway. He stopped at an intersection with a red traffic light. He reached for the phone and checked it for messages. There was a text message from Ben Bennett. *EM from Robert Hill. One of the thieves might have the fifth chip implanted.* Boris slammed his fist onto the dashboard. It was immediately clear to him what had happened. Kaleo would have given him the fifth chip if he had it. *The little bitch had it the whole time! That's why she acted so weird! And then she ran away with his brain chip! He had been fooled by a girl - again!* Boris felt the blood rushing up into his face. He texted back. *Where is the girl?*

The phone buzzed again. *With mom at SFGH*

The traffic light turned green and a grass-green Audi behind Boris honked. Boris opened the window and showed his middle finger. The car drove around him, the driver pointing his index finger to his forehead. Boris felt an itch to take out his gun and teach this disrespectful guy a lesson. But he had to focus on Susan now. He texted back. *OMW!* Then, he hit the gas and raced past the Audi towards the highway ramp to San Francisco.

***

Boris arrived at the San Francisco General Hospital. He knew that the hospital had a metal detector at the entrance and surveillance cameras throughout the property. It would be difficult to walk in with a gun. In addition, he needed to keep a low profile in order to pick up his money from SUEC before he left the Bay Area. Therefore, he decided to wait for Susan outside. She had to come out eventually. As usual, he parked at the sidewalk three blocks down from the hospital. He opened the glove compartment and took out a baseball cap, a pair of sunglasses and a silencer. The ball cap was specifically designed for Boris's operations. It contained a carefully covered steel helmet, which provided protection in high-risk situations.

Boris put on the cap and added the sunglasses. With that, nobody would recognize him easily. Then, he took the Glock from the pocket of his jacket and put the silencer on the gun. He placed the gun back into the pocket of his jacket so that he could easily reach the trigger. He then carefully adjusted the position of the muzzle so that it pointed forwards. He would shoot her through the jacket. If the situation would allow it, he would remove the chip right there. More likely, chaos would break out and he would have to leave immediately. In that case, he would find a way into the morgue and remove the chip there. Boris got out of the car, took out his crutches and made his way to the hospital. An elderly woman passed by and looked at him with pity.

The crutches are a great disguise! he thought. *Anybody who sees me will think that I am a patient!* Boris looked around. There was a bus stop close by that provided a great view of the hospital entrance. Boris decided that this was a good place to wait. The people around him would provide a great shield. He stopped at a grocery store and bought a sandwich and an iced tea. He then continued to limp to the bus stop. The elderly woman who had passed him just a few minutes ago was sitting on a bench there. Boris sat down beside her and unpacked his sandwich.

The woman looked at his injured leg and asked. "Did you break your leg?"

Boris nodded and took another bite of his sandwich. Hopefully, he could avoid a conversation.

But the women continued. "My grandson got a fracture as well. I just visited him in the ER. He fell on his racket during a tennis match and injured his thumb. His parents are both working and my daughter – his mother – asked me to stop by to make sure he is okay. He is perfectly fine, but he will have to wait some more in the ER. I got tired and decided to go home. He will join me there later."

Boris opened his iced tea and took a sip.

The woman opened the image gallery on her iPhone. "I took a photo of his x-ray. The emergency physician said that there's a fracture. He called it skiers' fracture. But of course, my Brandon does not ski around this time of the year. And I cannot see anything. Do you see a fracture here?" She held the iPhone in front of Boris's face. He could not resist to look.

"It's a gamekeeper's fracture," Boris said, chewing.

"Oh, you know it?"

"Yes, I happen to be an x-ray technician. There is a small avulsion fracture at the corner of the base of the proximal phalanx of the thumb." Boris pointed out the injury.

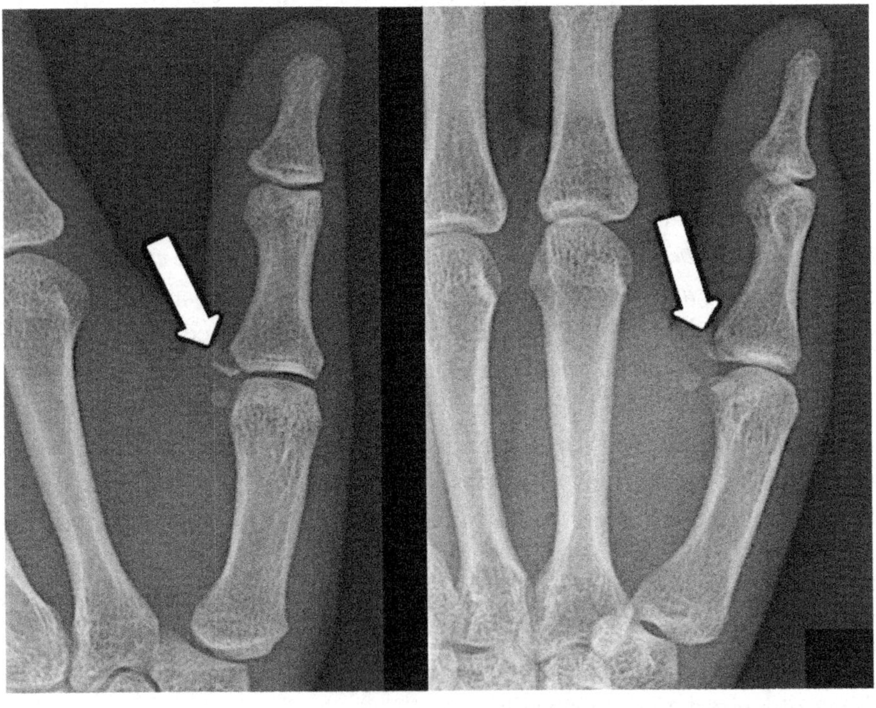

"Why do you call it gamekeepers' thumb?" she asked.

Boris looked at her. "It got the name from the typical injury of the thumb caused when a gamekeeper broke the neck of game, using their thumb, index finger and the ground."

The woman's jaw dropped. "Disgusting!"

Boris shrugged. "You asked, you got the answer."

The woman turned around briskly. She moved to the other end of the bench, took a book out of her purse and started to read."

Boris sighed. He had managed to lose her. He reached for his own iPhone. Dammit! It was not in his pocket. He must have left it in his car. This could turn into a very boring morning. He looked at the hospital entrance, waiting.

- 41 -
Amir
WEBER FRACTURE

Wednesday, May 26, 2032, 10.30 am.

Amir woke up when the FBI van arrived at the hospital. He had wondered if they would drive to the San Francisco General Hospital or SUEC hospital. To Amir's delight, the ambulance was stopping in front of the emergency room of the San Francisco General. *Susan is here!* he thought. A great joy overwhelmed him. Four porters came out to carry him and Angus into the ER on their stretchers. Amir felt very uncomfortable. He was pretty sure that he had broken his fist on Boris's face. But he could surely walk. He knew everyone in the ER, and he did not want to be embarrassed by an entrance on a stretcher. But this time, the security personnel would not compromise. The security guard explained the hospital policies to Amir, which he knew too well. All patients who arrived with the ambulance were carried into the exam rooms to avoid any additional accidents. Amir tried to be a "good" patient and not interfere with the intake protocols. He would have preferred to just go straight to the x-ray suite and see which bones were broken. But the system had to take its usual course.

Dr. Williams came to see Amir in the exam room. "Hello Amir, long time no see! I had no idea that you are getting involved in bar fights!"

Amir waved with his swollen hand. "Hello, Calvin! It was my first major fight in a long time. I guess it didn't go so well."

Dr. Williams inspected Amir's hand with a serious look on his face. "I am afraid, there is almost certainly a fracture here," he pointed at Amir's fifth finger. "I will order an x-ray."

Amir smiled. "That seems like a good idea."

"That will take a few minutes. I will see another patient and then be back." Dr. Williams left the room.

Shortly afterwards, an x-ray technician came in to take medical images of Amir's hand. Amir looked over her shoulder as the electronic image appeared on her screen. *Surgery or no surgery – that is the question*, he thought.

Dr. Williams came back into the room and also stepped towards the computer and inspected the radiograph. "The frontal radiograph shows a typical transverse fracture through the neck of the fifth metacarpal, with volar angulation of the distal fragment. The lateral radiograph demonstrates significant palmar angulation of the distal fragment. This is a Boxer's fracture."

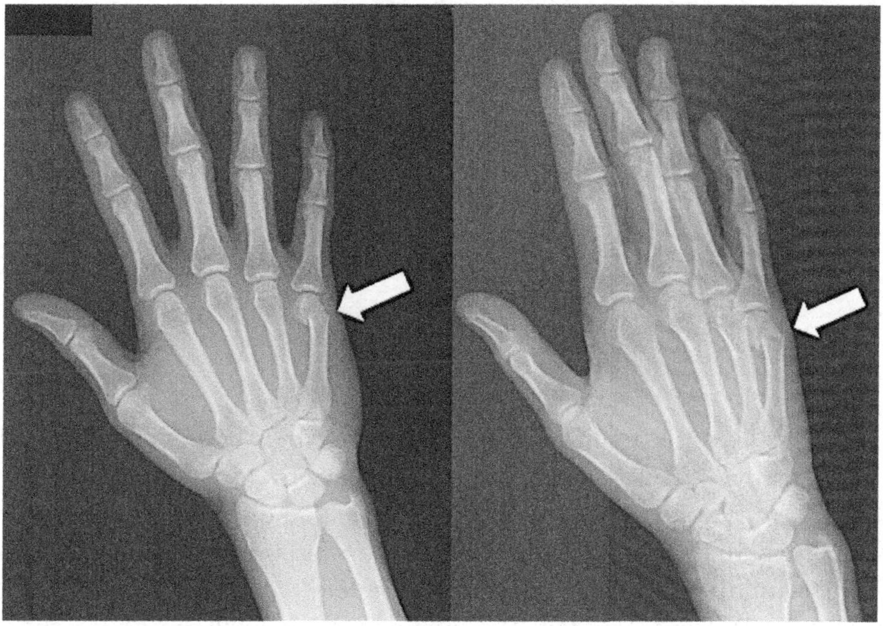

Amir looked at the radiographs on the computer screen and smiled. "Nomen is omen! I have a typical injury of a boxer!"

"Yes, indeed! A Boxer's fracture is an impaction injury that almost always results from a direct blow with a clenched fist against a hard surface, often time another person."

Dr. Williams magnified the radiograph so that Amir could see the injury better. He placed an arrow at the fracture site.

"How do you treat it?" Amir asked.

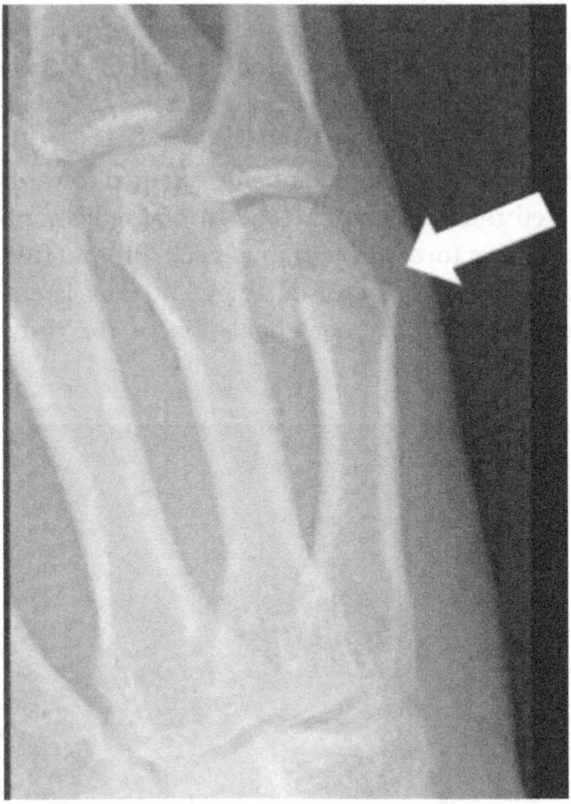

"A Boxer's fracture is relatively unstable. It could be treated conservatively. But K-wire fixation us usually preferred."

Amir looked at Dr. Williams. "I would like to try a conservative approach first. We could do a follow up radiograph in one or two weeks and then decide if a surgery is needed?"

Dr. Williams nodded. "Your choice, Amir. I will prescribe a short arm gutter-splint, with flexion of the metacarpophalangeal joint and schedule a follow up exam in two weeks. We also checked your oxygen saturation, and it was normal. Based on that and since you do not seem to have any breathing problems right now, I will not order a chest x-ray to evaluate the lungs."

Amir nodded. "That sounds good. I would like to minimize radiation exposure, if possible."

A nurse practitioner came in and placed the splint. Lamong had been patiently waiting during all exams and procedures. Both Amir and

Lamong were very happy when Amir was finally discharged.

Amir, with Lamong in tow, immediately made his way to the orthopedic surgery ward, where he expected to find Susan and Stella. As he walked down the hallway in the ER, he noticed Angus Weber laying alone in another exam room. He remembered how scary the medical environment could be if you were completely on your own. Amir entered the exam room, Lamong following him. "Hello, Angus, how are you doing?" he asked casually.

"Thanks for asking, Amir," Angus responded., "I have been diagnosed with a Weber fracture." He pointed at a computer screen, which showed a radiograph of his lower leg. Amir stepped closer and saw a fracture through the left lower fibula, the bone of the outer leg.

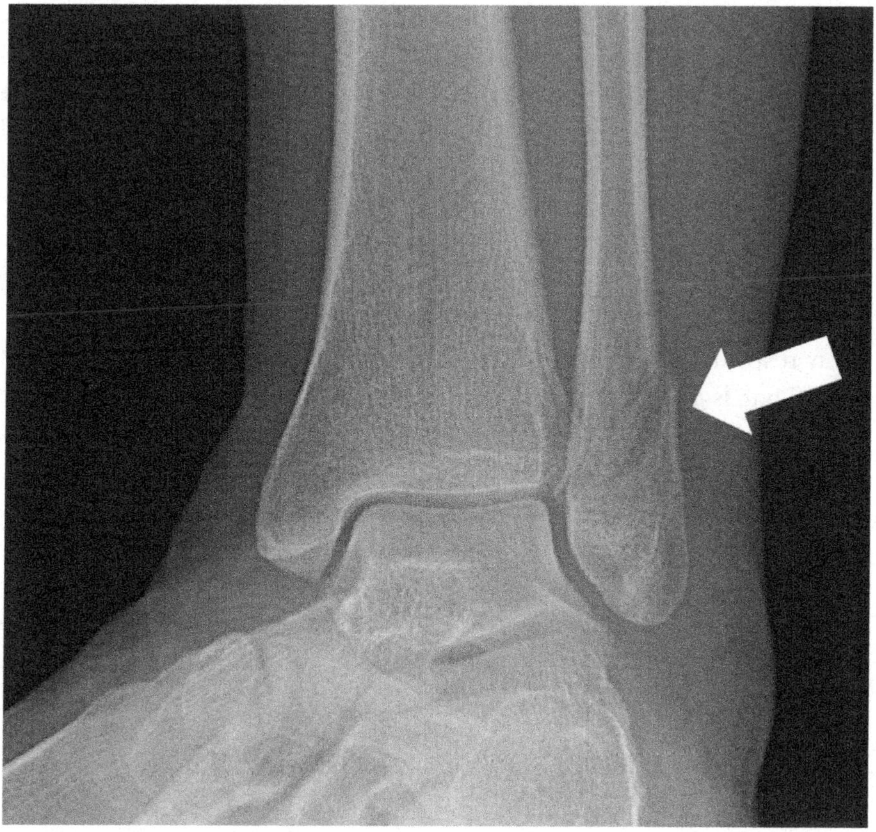

"Do you know why this is a Weber B fracture and not A or C?" Angus asked. "What does the B mean? Is it bad or good?

"Perhaps I can help out with this question," Dr. Williams said as he walked into the room. "A Weber B fracture is a fracture through the fibula at the level of the syndesmosis."

"What is the syndesmosis?" Angus asked.

"The syndesmosis is a connection between the lower fibula and tibia, or shinbone. It is the area where those bones are held closely together by ligaments." He pointed to the syndesmosis of Angus' ankle. "There are three types of Weber fractures, based on the level of the fracture line. A Weber A fracture is a transverse fracture through the fibula below the level of the syndesmosis. It is usually stable if the medial malleolus – the bony protrusion of the inner ankle – is intact. A Weber B fracture is a fracture through the fibula at the level of the syndesmosis. It is often a spiral fracture, as in your case here. The deltoid ligament over the medial ankle may be torn as well. This fracture has variable stability, dependent on the integrity of the medial structures. A Weber C fracture is a fracture through the fibula above the level of the syndesmosis. There is often a widened distal tibiofibular space and there is often an associated injury of the deltoid ligament and fracture of the medial malleolus. "

"Agent Weber has a Weber fracture!" Amir noted, smiling.

"I am aware of the irony," Angus responded with a serious voice.

"I am very sorry that you suffered this injury, Agent Weber," Amir responded, "but on the positive side, your shinbone did not get hurt. That is the most important bone of your lower leg. It has the main weight-bearing function." Then, he turned to Dr. Williams. "What is the treatment plan?"

Dr. Williams looked from Amir to Angus. "Mr. Weber, do you feel comfortable discussing your treatment plan with Mr. Nielsson being present?"

"Yes, of course, no problem," Angus responded. "I like his positive attitude. I feel a little better already, knowing that my shinbone is fine!"

"Well, I agree with the comment about your shinbone," Dr. Williams continued, "however, the fracture of your fibula still needs medical attention. I would like to consult our surgeons to understand if they would advise to place orthopedic hardware to stabilize the ankle joint."

Angus nodded. "Of course, that sounds good to me!"

"I already called our orthopedic surgery colleagues. They have availability in the OR this afternoon. I also took the liberty to ask them to reserve the spot for you, if they feel that you need a surgery. If you agree, we could do the surgery later today. Due to the circumstances of your accident, we would like to keep you in the hospital overnight. Then, we will train you in using your crutches early tomorrow morning and if all is well, you can go home right afterwards."

Angus nodded again. "If a surgery is needed, I would appreciate if it could be done as soon as possible."

"Of course!" Dr. Williams responded. "I will check where our orthopedic surgery colleagues are and lead them to you." He walked out of the exam room.

Amir turned to Angus. "Do you have a family member who could come to support you here?"

"I am afraid I live in Washington DC, close to the FBI headquarters," Angus responded. "I am actually divorced. So, there's no spouse coming. But my son studies bioengineering at Stanford University, and he will come by later this afternoon."

"Hello Lamong, would you mind staying with Agent Weber here until I get back?" Amir asked, looking at the young FBI agent who had waited at the entrance to the exam room. "I know it can be daunting to be alone in a hospital, especially if a surgery as planned. You could make sure that Agent Weber has everything he needs until his son arrives."

Lamong looked from Amir to Angus.

Angus said. "It would be great if you could stay for a while, Lamong. Just in case I need assistance with anything. I am clearly not able to walk now. If I receive any urgent messages about our case, then you could help addressing them. Amir should be fine here in the hospital. But if he leaves the building, you will accompany him again."

"Of course, sir!" Lamong responded dutifully.

Amir continued. "I have to leave now, but I will come back again in an hour or so to check on you and pick up Lamong. Hopefully, your son will arrive soon thereafter."

"That is very kind of you," Angus responded. "I think I'm fine for the moment, especially with Lamong's help! What do you need to do so urgently?"

"Well, I want to find Susan and see for myself that she is safe.

Hopefully, she is with her mother upstairs on the orthopedic surgery ward. As far as I understand Dr. Williams, we might find you in a room on the same ward very soon." Amir smiled.

"Okay, perhaps see you there," Angus responded, smiling as well.

It is interesting how a traumatic experience can bond people, Amir thought. His impression of Angus Weber had completely changed, and he was sure that Angus' impression of him had changed as well. They were friends now. Amir left the exam room, walked down the hallway, up the stairs and to the orthopedic surgery ward.

***

From the moment he had found himself tied up in the cabin, Amir had been looking forwards to this moment. He walked down the hallway of the orthopedic surgery ward to Stella's room, where he hoped to find Susan. He had known Susan for almost his entire life. But he was anxious and nervous to see her again after they had exchanged that passionate kiss in the cabin. Amir heard his heart pounding in his ears as he opened the door. There she was, sitting at the bedside, holding her mother's hand. The women had been engaged in a conversation and they both looked up as Amir stepped in.

"Amir, it is so good to see you!" Stella exclaimed with a beaming smile.

Susan had jumped up from her seat. Amir noted that she had a new sling around her casted right arm. "I am so glad that you are safe!" she cried. "You saved my life, Amir!"

Amir felt a warm feeling expanding his chest. "Susan, I am so happy that you made it to safety! I heard from Terrel Wright that he picked you up. What a great luck! Just a little later, Boris drove down that same road. I cannot imagine what could've happened if he had found you instead of Terrel!"

Susan came closer and Amir hugged her tightly.

"I am safe now!" she said.

Stella called from her bed. "That is all that matters! Amir, you brought my daughter back! I cannot express in words how grateful I am! She is everything to me!"

"Of course, Mrs. Pellegrini!" Amir responded. "Susan is

everything to me as well!"

He looked into Susan's beautiful eyes and whispered in her ear. "And I am so relieved that your brain is working normally again!"

"I did not tell my mother the chip-on-my-brain part," she whispered back. "I thought it might cause less trouble for her if we keep that part to our ourselves."

"Do you feel any remaining side effects from the brain chip?" Amir asked anxiously.

"The last hours in the cabin were pure horror!" Susan responded. "All of a sudden, I was transported to never-never land. I saw deep, dark holes opening all around me, trying to suck me into a deep, cold abyss. There were snakes on the floor, encircling me on my chair and preventing me from running away. Long arms and hands were coming out of the walls, trying to pull me into the darkness. I thought I was going nuts!"

"You are safe now," Amir whispered.

Susan's eyes slowly filled with tears. "I am so sorry that I caused all this trouble, Amir!" she said loudly, so that Stella could hear it as well. "Kaleo is dead because of me! If we had never broken into Dr. Hill's lab, he would still be alive now!"

Amir's eyes filled with tears as well. "None of us could foresee the events that happened today. Boris killed Kaleo, not you. Always remember that."

Susan swallowed and looked to the ground.

"He was a very brave young man," Stella added. "He fetched me when I was tied to the chair in the apartment and this maniac threw me to the ground. And then he came for you, Susan. He must have loved you very much!"

"It is still hard to comprehend that Kaleo is dead," Amir said, looking from Stella to Susan. "Just two nights ago, we were eating pizza together and made plans for the future." He felt the same knot-in-the-pit-of-the-stomach sensation that he always felt when he thought about the fatal car accident of his parents.

"I will miss him so much!" Susan responded, tears running down her cheeks.

Amir looked at her in silence, not knowing what else to say or how to comfort her.

"Please come over here and have a seat," Stella called, patting the bed besides her. And when Amir looked at her, she added. "Both of you! I know, it is terrible that Kaleo was killed. But I am also so glad, that you both got out of there alive! We will figure everything else out. It will take some time. But we can do it!"

Amir and Susan both walked over to Stella's bed.

"How is your leg, Mrs. Pellegrini?" Amir asked, trying to change the subject.

"Oh, I'm doing fine," Stella responded. "The surgery was really quick and not as bad as I thought. The fracture was secured with a plate and several screws. The leg is still anesthetized and I do not feel any pain now. And I feel so happy that I have my daughter back!" Stella squeezed her daughter's hand and smiled at her.

"Now, I want to know everything about your escape!"

Susan and Amir sat down. Susan settled on the bed besides her mother. Amir sat down on the chair beside Stella's bed. And then they talked. They told Stella about the cabin, how Amir had released Susan, how Boris suddenly arrived, how Susan managed to escape, how Amir got into a fist fight, was tied up in the burning loft and rescued by Angus Weber.

At the end of the story, Susan sighed. "I am so glad to have you both back! You were this close to being killed!" She showed a non-existing gap between her thumb and index finger.

"From what I heard, you could have been killed as well!" Amir responded.

"We all got our scars, but we are alive! God gave us a second chance! We are family and we belong together!" Susan squeezed both Amir and Susan's hand. They talked a little longer and then Stella fell asleep. Susan wiped away the sweat on her forehead with a paper towel. Then she looked at Amir. "I just realized how hungry I am!"

Amir nodded. "Same here. There is a little café just a few meters down the street. Let's go there!"

- 42 -
Boris
THE ATTACK

Wednesday, May 26, 2032, 11.30 am.

Boris was patiently waiting at the bus stop in front of the San Francisco General. He knew that Susan was in the hospital. She would come out eventually. And he was lucky. After about two hours of waiting in front of the hospital, he saw a young woman with a long, brunette ponytail and a cast around her right arm exiting the main entrance. That was Susan! She was accompanied by a thin young man with fair hair and a cast around his right hand — Amir! *He had made it out of the cabin!*

Boris adjusted his sunglasses and examined them carefully. Amir had a cast as well! Amir and Susan were engaged in a lively conversation, not noticing much around them. Susan had swollen eyes and Amir supported her with his free left arm. Was there another man following them? Boris watched the couple for a few more seconds. But they were surrounded by people, similar to his situation at the bus stop. Boris was surrounded by many waiting people who shielded him from being spotted. Similarly, many other people were exiting the hospital building and partially obscured his view of Susan and Amir. It was not clear, if the man behind them simply had the same route out of the building. Boris' gut instinct told him that he somehow belonged to the couple, although he walked behind them and did not talk with them. Boris grunted. He did not like unknown variables during his operations. He watched the couple for a few more seconds. They were completely self-absorbed and unguarded. He decided that the man probably did not matter. Boris slowly got up from his seat, pulled the baseball hat down to cover his face and strolled down the street. From the corner of his eyes, he carefully watched Susan and Amir. They did not notice him or anyone else around them. They slowly walked towards a coffee shop and disappeared inside. The man behind them followed them into the coffee shop. Boris found a bench a few meters down the street. He sat down, placed the crutches beside him, grabbed the gun in his pocket and adjusted the muzzle so that it pointed to the entrance of the coffee shop. He would shoot through his jacket, without taking the gun out of his pocket.

***

After about ten more minutes, the couple walked out of the coffee shop, holding paper cups. Amir also carried a bag with the same hand that held his coffee, probably with more food items. Boris pointed at Susan and pulled the trigger. He heard a high-pitched sound. *Had the silencer come off?* The second man was still behind the couple. In the fraction of a second, the man leaped forwards and jumped in front of Susan. He let out a cry as the bullet hit his chest. Susan screamed in horror, while Amir instantly ducked down behind a parked car. The man fell to the ground. Chaos broke out, with screaming people running in all directions. Amir had dropped the coffee and bag and reached out to Susan. He pulled her towards him, dragging her behind the parked car. A bullet could penetrate it. Only the driver's side of a police car had reinforced doors. But Boris could not see them behind the car and aim at them directly.

After pulling the trigger, Boris felt a sharp pain in his right ear lobe. He reached for his ear. It was wet. He looked at his hand. It was full of blood! *What on earth had happened?* Boris looked around. Was there a gun barrel beside the corner of the building across the street? He heard another high-pitched sound, followed by a metallic "clang" sound and a sharp pain at his right temple. Something had hit the base cap and fell to the ground. A bullet! He was under attack!

Boris jumped to his feet. He grabbed both crutches with his left hand and pulled out his gun with his right hand. He shot towards the shooter on the other side of the street. The gun barrel retreated. He ran as fast as he could towards his car. People along the way were screaming, watching the man with the cast sprinting towards a dark gray Mercedes and jumping in. Two more bullets hit the rear window. Boris started the car; he took a U-turn with squealing wheels and sped away. Several people took photos of him and the car with their cell phones.

He heard police sirens in the distance. He would have to get rid of his car as quickly as possible. Boris turned into a small alley. This was his lucky day! He saw an unattended, running, black Honda Civic a few meters down the road. The owner was retrieving money at an adjacent ATM. Boris stopped the car, got out, ran to the Honda, jumped in, hit the gas pedal and raced away. The owner threw his arms into the air, yelling profanities at him. But he soon disappeared in the rear mirror. Boris sighed. This was not quite over yet. The police would be soon on his heels. But they would always be one step behind. He would change cars a few more times, then walk the rest of the way. Under other circumstances, he would switch to public transportation or Uber. But the cast at his leg was too revealing. He would have to find another way. He always did.

- 43 -
Lili
THE EVIDENCE

Wednesday, May 25, 2032, 11.30 am.

The GPS in Lili's car showed that she was getting close to the address that she had entered from Amir's text message. She had passed the town of San Mateo and drove down a road in the countryside, crossing through forested hillsides, ranches, sweeping grasslands, cattle, vegetable farms and pumpkin patches. The melodic female voice in the GPS directed her to turn right into a small road. The red target pin on the GPS map was only four minutes away. Lili followed the road which led towards a dense, shady forest. Her car jumped up and down as she tried to maneuver around several potholes. She noticed a dark cloud over the trees, possibly indicating a fire close by. She wondered for a moment if she should turn around. But her curiosity won. She had to find Amir and help to rescue Susan!

Lili continued to drive down the road, now passing towering pine trees and eucalyptus trees. After a short drive through the woods, she saw bright rays of sunlight in the distance, probably a clearing. A strong odor of wood smoke seeped through the half-open car window. The road took a slight turn towards the clearing. As she turned the corner, she saw the charred log cabin. Two large firetrucks, two FBI vans and a police car had parked in front of it. Multiple people were swarming around the house. Lili saw firefighters with their red helmets and bulky tan coats with yellow reflective stripes. Two firefighters walked around the cabin with a fire hose, carefully inspecting the logs and niches. The cabin was not burning any more. It was covered in soot and surrounded by puddles of water. In front of the house was a group of FBI agents, also geared up in helmets and bulletproof vests with the FBI crest on them. Several teams of firefighters and FBI agents were walking in and out of the cabin. Others secured the perimeter around the cabin with tape. *Was there a dead body in front of the cabin?* There was clearly a human body lying on the porch. Lili could not see much detail, but it seemed to be a man and he did not move. Two FBI agents were in the process of placing him into a white body bag. *Who is this?*

Lili's heart started to race. The man was half burned, and she did not recognize him from the distance. She wanted to drive onto the clearing. But a police officer appeared in front of her car and stopped her with raised palms. He apparently had the task of keeping civilians away from the scene. As she drove closer, Lili recognized him. It was the same cop who had stopped her for speeding last night! She sighed and stopped the car.

"Sorry, ma'am, you need to turn around. This property is closed."

Lili rolled down the car window. "Hello officer, I wanted to check on two of my friends who might be here, Susan Pellegrini and Amir Nielsen."

The agent looked at her with a stern, penetrating gaze. He had recognized her as well. "What did you say your name was?"

"I did not mention it so far. My name is Dr. Lili Pham."

"I caught you speeding on Fell Street last night! You promised to stay out of trouble. And here you are at a crime scene!"

"I am sorry, officer, this is a very unfortunate coincidence."

"I have to ask you to step out of your car, Mrs. Pham." The police officer said with a serious voice, reaching for the weapon at his belt.

Oh crap! Lili thought, starting to feel very uncomfortable. *How stupid of me to mention Susan's name,* she thought. This police officer was clearly armed, and she got the feeling that he treated her like a suspect.

"Please step out of your car, Mrs. Pham," he repeated.

Her instincts told her to keep the door between herself and this man. But she did not want him to think that she was a threat. Lili opened the driver's door and slowly stepped out of the car, trying to appear as non-threatening as possible.

"Let me see your hands," the cop asked with an aggressive tone.

Lili showed him the palms of her hands. *What did he think? That I am a kidnapper and intentionally drove into the arms of a man with a big Police sign on his jacket?* The situation would have been somewhat comical if she hadn't seen the man's steady grip at his gun.

"Is Terrel Wright here?" she asked. "Can I speak with him?"

The police officer watched her with a piercing gaze, while pointing to the police car and one of the FBI vans, which parked side-by-side at the upper end of the clearing. "Please come over here," he said.

They walked over to the police car while he was talking with a lowered voice to someone on his walkie talkie.

They arrived at the car. There was a folded chair in front of it.

"You can sit down here, if you like," the cop said.

Sitting down was the last thing Lili wanted to do now. She wanted to walk over to the body bag and see who was inside. *Was it the kidnapper?* She wanted to know where Susan was — and Amir. *Were they safe?* But the cop clearly was not up for negotiation. He looked tired and Lili did not want to overstretch his patience. She sat down, glaring at him.

"How do you know this cabin?" he asked.

"I received the address from Amir Nielsson. He sent me the address early this morning, but it only appeared on my cell phone shortly before noon. Apparently, the FBI intercepted my phone and caused the delay."

"Is that so?" the cop asked, raising his eyebrows. "Why would the FBI intercept your phone?"

"They might have thought that I know where Amir is," Lili responded. "He was a friend of Susan Pellegrini, the kidnapped girl, and he disappeared yesterday. Are they safe now?"

"How did you know about a kidnapped girl?" the police officer asked, ignoring her question. "Did you inform the police about a kidnapping incident?"

This conversation was clearly not going very well. "Her mother asked us to not say anything," Lili explained. "The kidnapper had threatened her that her daughter would be harmed, if we told anybody."

"The mother was supposed to stay quiet, but she told you and the man who sent you the address?" the police officer asked. "That sounds as fabulous as the tire story you told me last night!"

"Well, her mother did tell me to stay quiet. And Kaleo and Amir, Susan's friends, came here to rescue her."

"Do you realize that this story is hard to believe?"

"It is the truth!" Lili tried to contain her raising annoyance.

The man looked at her. "Do you know what I think? You worked together with the kidnapper. He escaped and let you run into the trap!"

"If I had kidnapped the girl, why would I drive into this place, which is clearly swamped with feds?" Lili asked.

"Well, you clearly did not see me when you arrived. I think you locked the girl in the cabin, and it caught fire. Perhaps you did want to rescue her, if only to secure your ransom."

The police officer looked up as an FBI agent approached the van.

"Hello, Lili!" Terrel called from a distance, walking towards Lili with long strides. "What on earth are you doing here?"

"Hello Terrel, it is so great to see you!" Lili jumped up from her chair with a sigh of relief. She could have kissed him for saving her from this impossible situation. "I received the address from Amir Nielsson. He texted me that he was looking for Susan here. Did you find her?"

Terrel had arrived and shook the hand of the police officer.

"It is okay. I know this lady," Terrel explained. "She is a radiologist at SUEC hospital and has helped us with the investigation of this case."

"With all due respect, my interview with her indicates that she is a suspect!" the police officer responded. "She knows details that only the kidnapper can know. I would like to put her under arrest. Our citizens deserve justice!"

It occurred to Lili that an arrest of a suspect would look very good for all involved. Was she collateral damage? A chill went down her spine.

"This is a classified operation," Terrel responded with an authoritarian voice. "A manhunt is ongoing, and we will not jeopardize it with any publicity whatsoever. Dr. Pham is a member of our team. That's why she is informed about details of this operation."

The two men looked at each other, sizing up each other's power. Terrel was clearly the more senior and higher ranked officer. Lili wondered if this entire encounter would have happened if Terrel had been white. After a moment of awkward silence, the police officer laughed. "No worries, Terrel, she is all yours!" He clapped Terrel on his shoulder, turned around and walked away.

Lili let out a sigh of relief. "My God, I am so glad you came to rescue me!"

"My pleasure!" Terrel said, smiling.

"That man scared me more than the kidnapper!" Lili exclaimed.

"I am sorry for the inconvenience, Lili. But this guy is harmless. He is young and this is probably his first major case. Did you notice how nervous he was? He was probably more nervous than you! He is just eager to prove himself. He will learn and do better in the future."

Lili looked at Terrel with admiration. He had a big heart and was a role model for integrity and generosity. "Did you find Susan and Amir?" she asked.

"No worries, she and Amir are safe," Terrel said. "I wonder why he sent you this address?"

"I was his insurance," Lili responded. "If I didn't hear from him, I would call the police. That's why I'm here."

Terrel shook his head. "I am not sure I can follow your train of thought. Why did you think it would be helpful for you to come here? Do you have no concern for your personal safety? Imagine if the kidnapper had still been here! You could've been killed!"

"Well, I wanted to make sure that there was indeed an emergency before I got in trouble for exchanging texts with a crime suspect. You just saw how that was received." Lili's head started to boil over. "Is the kidnapper not here anymore? Who is the dead man in the bag? You said Susan and Amir are safe. I hope the dead man is not…." She could not finish the sentence and looked anxiously at Terrel.

"I am afraid it is Kaleo," Terrel responded.

Lili swallowed, processing the information. They both stood in silence for a moment. Lili saw two FBI agents in the distance lifting the man in the body bag, carrying the body over to the van and loading it into the cabin. The policemen were rolling up the fire hose. The action here was coming to an end.

"I wished we had arrived earlier," Lili finally said. "Perhaps we could have saved him."

"There is no point in brooding about the past. You cannot undo it," Terrel said softly. "You can only change the future. Let's make sure nobody else gets hurt."

"I was surprised that you were still here and not chasing the kidnapper," Lili said.

"Our team is taking care of that, and we will get to him," Terrel explained. "I was looking for evidence that would allow me to take out the mastermind of this operation, the man who planned all this. Boris was just executing orders."

"Did you find the evidence?" Lili asked.

"Well, Amir overheard a conversation that gave away the identity of Boris's boss. But this man is very powerful. He could easily argue that Amir misheard or misunderstood something. It is not enough for me to arrest him."

"What do you need?" Lili suddenly was glad she had come here. She already knew who the boss was, and she had the key to bring him down in her pocket. She grinned in anticipation.

"I was looking for something more tangible," Terrel explained, "evidence that cannot be easily discussed away. Perhaps a letter, fingerprints, money that can be traced back. I was hoping that they burned the cabin down because there was some key evidence here. But it looks like the mastermind of this plot was very careful. My team turned the place upside down and we did not find anything. "

"Perhaps I can help out with that," Lili produced a memory stick from her pocket and handed it over to Terrel.

He looked at it, turning it around. "What is it?" He asked.

"It contains a video file that shows a man walking up to SUEC and delivering the package with the brain chips into the mailbox of the octagon building," Lili explained.

"Wow!" Terrel was impressed. "You do qualify as an FBI agent, Lili! How did you shoot that video?"

"It was recorded by the video cameras of the university. A friend of mine, who is a security guard at SUEC, gave it to me. This morning, Dr. Bennett asked him to download a video that showed Annya walking up and down the promenade in her jogging outfit. He handed it to the FBI with the explanation that she had been involved in the chip theft. He knew about the second video and actively hid it."

"Yes, we received the video which shows Dr. Segond walking down the promenade in front of the octagon building in the middle of the night. But I found it odd that she should have delivered the brain chips. Dr. Segond is an employee who lives on campus. It would've been much less conspicuous if she had just handed over the chips during a personal encounter in Dean Bennett's office rather than in the middle of the night."

"Yes, indeed! She would not be so stupid. She knows that there are surveillance cameras along the promenade."

"So, she was framed!" Terrel looked at Lili, processing the information. "But why did she run away? We cannot find her anywhere."

"That is a mystery to me as well," Lili responded. She contemplated for a moment if she should tell him about the GPS chip in the cast. But she decided against it. She did not want to bring her trouble.

"Well, the important part here is that that there is another video, which shows a man delivering the envelope with the brain chips to the SUEC building. And there are several witnesses who can testify that Dean Bennett requested to withhold this second video from the FBI. At the very least, this is obstruction of justice. And if you can identify the man and he confirms that Dr. Bennett hired him, then you have the mastermind!"

"Let's see the video," Terrel said. "Would you like to come with me?" He walked over to the FBI van. Lili followed him. Terrel opened the sliding side door and stepped into the cabin. Lili was intrigued. She had always wanted to see an FBI van from the inside. She followed Terrel into the van and looked around. The cabin of the van was completely sealed off from natural light. The seemingly tinted windows were glazed with paint. Multiple small neon lights were set up within the walls and roof of the cabin and illuminated the small space with an artificial light. A faint scent of chlorine filled the cabin. Someone had probably disinfected the interior recently. There were three ergonomic seats facing a minimalist desk with multiple computer workstations and monitors. Terrel sat down in front of one of the workstations and put the memory stick into the computer. A virus detection software scanned the file. Lili sat down beside Terrel. The monitor in front of them provided a 360-degree capture of the surroundings of the van. Lili could see one of the firetrucks backing out of the clearing and leaving towards the road, where her car was parked. She wondered for a moment if they would be able to pass by, but then saw that they were entering the road without problems. Terrel had followed her gaze. "We have pretty cool cameras and audio surveillance systems in these vans," he explained. "They include built-in surveillance radar for all-weather tracking of targets. There is also a drone operation workstation." He pointed to another monitor. Lili was thoroughly impressed.

The virus detection software gave off a soft tone and a little text window popped up, indicating that the Universal Serial Bus drive had been scanned. *Interesting,* Lili thought, *until today, I had not known what USB means.* Terrel double clicked the USB drive and a video file appeared. He opened it and played it at accelerated speed. Different segments of videos showed a man walking up the SUEC promenade and dropping an envelope into the mailbox at the door of the octagon building. Terrel activated more software on the workstation. They looked at a spinning circle.

"This will take a little a while," Terrel explained.

"What is this?" Lili asked.

"It is a face detection software. Even though it was dark, some of the video images got a pretty good shot of the face of the man. If he is in our criminal database, then we will know shortly who he is."

Lili took a breath. "There is another incident that I would like to report."

"What is that?" Terrel asked, his eyebrows raised.

"Well, earlier today, I was summoned to Dr. Bennett's office. That's how I ran into the security guard. Dr. Bennett asked me to hand over my iPhone. I found that very peculiar. I wanted to refuse, but he threatened me."

"What did he want with the phone?"

"He did not say. I really needed my phone because I was waiting for a message from Amir. Earlier today, Stella gave me her phone to watch while she was in surgery. So, I gave Dr. Bennett Stella's phone. "

"What a smart move," Terrel chuckled. "Either he wanted to see your messages – and in that case you effectively intervened – or he wanted to send a message to someone, pretending that he was you. If that is the case, then we have to consider if he could also accomplish that plan with Stella's phone."

"Well, if he wanted to contact Amir or Susan, they are already with Stella," Lili thought out loud. "But if he wanted to contact Annya, perhaps it could work."

"Do you have Stella's phone number?" Terrel asked.

"Sure!" Lili looked it up on her phone and wrote it down for him on a piece of paper that she found on the desk.

"I will ask our communication specialists to check, if any calls or messages were sent from her phone." Terrel typed a note into a messaging system on his computer.

"Oh, that's what you did with my phone this morning?"

"I don't know about that. We do take privacy very seriously. But in a matter of national security, we can obtain information from a cell phone. It is possible that Angus did that."

"You can do that without getting hold of the phone?"

"Of course. Your iPhone sends your text message over electromagnetic waves that your service provider is licensed to use. I saw that you use AT&T. If you send a message to someone who uses a different network, let's say T-Mobile, then AT&T uses an intercarrier to transfer messages between networks. If needed, the FBI can intercept text messages or calls from all these networks. We can also check your browsing history and GPS location."

"I'll keep that in mind when I use my phone next time!"

"No worries. We use it much less frequently than you might think. We are not interested in your daily drama. Accessing personal communications is one of the FBI's most sensitive techniques and is strictly controlled by federal laws. We have to establish probable cause that the obtained information will provide evidence of a felony violation of federal law."

Another tone interrupted our conversation and another pop-up window appeared on the computer screen. On the left of the screen, they saw the man in the video with a red circle around his face on multiple frames. On the right side of the screen, they saw a mug shot of a man with name, demographics and criminal history underneath.

Terrel looked at Lili. "Bingo! It is Boris Sokolov. This video will be sufficient evidence for us to connect him to Dr. Bennett. At the very least, we can arrest him for withholding important information. Once we have caught Boris, we can hopefully get his confession that Dr. Bennett hired him. Lili, you did your country a great service!"

Lili flushed. "Thank you!" She felt proud and satisfied to bring this man to justice. "Dr. Bennett probably got stressed out by the theft of the brain chips and the upcoming donor symposium. He wanted to get the chips back at all costs."

"Well, three people were murdered and two people were almost killed, including a minor. He will be held responsible in court, whether he ordered the killings or tolerated them."

"I hope so!"

"Lili, I have to report recent events to Angus. Can you wait here for a moment? I want to make a quick phone call outside and then be back."

Lili nodded. "Of course, no problem."

Terrel opened the sliding door of the van, stepped out, took his cell phone out of his pocket, pushed a button to dial a number and started talking on the phone, pacing back and forth in front of the van.

Lili looked around inside the cabin. There was another pop-up window on Terrel's screen, indicating a new incoming message. She stared at it for a while, wondering what it was. She looked at Terrel. He was deeply engaged in his conversation. Lili hovered the mouse over the message and read it.

"A text message was sent from Stella Pellegrini's phone to Annya Segond's phone. *FBI is looking for you. I have proof that you are innocent. Come to Café Marco in SF at 2 pm today. CU there!"*

Annya will believe that Stella had asked her to meet at the café in San Francisco, Lili thought. *She is being set up!* She looked at Terrel again. He was still talking on the phone.

Lili quickly took her phone out of her pocket and sent Annya a WhatsApp message. *Hi Annya, DO NOT GO TO THE CAFÉ. IT'S A TRAP! Lili.* She prayed that Annya would receive it before it was intercepted or deleted. But this was the only thing she could do at this point. She put her phone back into her pocket.

Terrel had hung up the phone as well and came back to the van. He followed her gaze. "I see that you got some more detective work done while I was gone," he said with a faint smile.

"Sorry, I could not help but read this message. Annya will think that Stella had asked her to meet at the café in San Francisco."

He nodded.

Lili wondered. "But why would she go to such a meeting if she is hiding somewhere? And why is she hiding in the first place?"

"Perhaps she is hiding because she knew that she was being set up."

"Do you think the meeting at the café is a trap?"

"I am pretty sure that is the case. Earlier this morning, we received an anonymous tip that Annya will be at this café at two pm today. We already have a team there waiting for her and whoever wants to meet her."

"I have known Annya for many years; she is not a criminal!"

"I hope you are right. But the nicest people can have a dark side. If there's something that we are missing, she will get a chance to explain it to us."

"Of course." Lili respected Terrel. But she did not share the same confidence in the justice system. There were too many people who played out their politics and got away with it. She hoped that Annya had received her message.

"What did Angus say?" she tried to change the subject.

"He agreed that we have enough evidence to arrest Dr. Bennett," Terrel said. "We will try to do that as discreetly as possible. We do not want to cause any negative publicity for the university shortly before the donor symposium. SUEC is the crown jewel in our country. The upcoming donations will have a major impact on ground-breaking innovations of national interest. Research at SUEC will fuel our economy and ensure our technological leadership in the world."

"It seems that the chip theft occurred at the worst possible moment."

"Well, it is never the right time for a national security threat. But you could argue that the timing was good because we had mobilized a special forces team to ensure the safety of all involved at the upcoming event. At any other time, we probably would not have been able to mobilize an entire team so instantly." Terrel looked at her again. "Lili, I was wondering if you could accompany me to the dean's office. I would prefer not to show my badge at the SUEC entrance and security checks so that we can hopefully catch Dr. Bennett by surprise. You could just introduce me as a visitor. SUEC employees are allowed to show visitors around, right?"

"Sure, I would be happy to assist!" Lili said. "How do you know you will find him in his office?"

"Well, I thought you might be able to call his secretary and ask if he is there?"

"But then she might tell him, and he might walk away?"

"You are right. Do you think we could ask her to make sure that he will be there when we come?"

"I am not sure, how persuasive I can be. But I am pretty sure you will be very convincing. Currently, Aiko Tanaka is at the front desk. You might remember her from the ER."

"Oh, the lady who showed me around and introduced me to you? Of course, I remember her! She was so sweet!"

"Well, there might be different points of view on that matter. But she has a knack for detective stories, and she is obsessed with the FBI. I believe, if you would ask her to assist you as an FBI agent, she will do everything to help out."

"Okay, let's try that. Do you have her phone number?"

"Sure!" Lili showed it to him on her phone. Terrel dialed the number of the SUEC front desk. After a brief moment, he said in a deep, well-modulated voice. "Hello Mrs. Tanaka, this is Agent Wright from the FBI. You might remember me. You showed me around in the ER recently."

Lili could hear Aiko's excitement through the phone.

"Hello, Mr. Wright!" she responded. "Of course, I remember you very well! Would you like to speak with Dr. Bennett?"

"No, I actually wanted to talk with you, Mrs. Tanaka. Can you help me in a matter of national security? If anyone is standing near you now, please let me know and we can talk later."

Aiko lowered her voice. "No, no, no, there's nobody here! Please let me know how I can assist the FBI!"

Lili could not suppress a smile. Her reaction was exactly as she had predicted.

"Well, we have reasons to believe that Dr. Bennett got involved in a felony that may affect our national security. I want to invite him for questioning, without causing much publicity for him or the university."

"Really? Dr. Bennett is the most distinguished professor I know. He broke the law?" Aiko's voice was toneless and strong at the same time. It could be well heard through the iPhone. Hopefully, there was really nobody close by in the lobby.

"Well, as you can imagine, this is a delicate matter. Your help is very important," Terrel continued. "I am on my way to you now and expect to arrive within an hour or less. To make this as discreet as possible, I would prefer to meet Dr. Bennett in his office. In the meantime, can you please make sure that he does not leave the building."

"Yes, sir!" Aiko whispered. "You can count on me!"

"Okay, see you soon!" Terrel responded.

"At your service, sir!"

Terrel looked at Lili. "That went surprisingly well! I hope she can prevent a runaway!"

"If Aiko is on a mission, nothing can stop her!" Lili responded. "You found the perfect undercover agent!"

Terrel smiled and reached for his jacket. "Okay, let's go! I parked my car not too far from yours. I suggest we drive there with two cars. Then, I can take Dr. Bennett with me, and you can go wherever you need to go."

"Of course!"

They walked over to their cars. Terrel had parked a little closer to the clearing. He got into his Ford SUV, slowly passed Lili's car and waited for her. Lili got into her X3 BMW, started the car and followed him. They both drove towards the interstate 280 and Redwood City.

- 44 -
Annya
RIB FRACTURE

Wednesday, May 25, 2032, 12.00 pm.

Annya had located Boris through the GPS chip in his cast and the tracking system on her phone. When she arrived at Potrero Avenue in San Francisco, he was ambling around in front of the general hospital. Annya followed Boris from a distance. He sat down on a bench. His head moved in all directions, but his gaze always seemed to linger for a few extra seconds on a café a few meters down the street. *What was he up to?* Annya strolled down the sidewalk on the other side of the street, carefully observing the situation. She walked around the corner of a brick building with a large roof, which provided covering shade. She leaned against the wall of the building, pulled her cell phone out of her pursue and pretended to read, while keeping her eye on Boris. Suddenly he jumped up from his seat. The hand in his leather jacket moved up, pointing towards three people who were exiting the café. One of them was Stella's daughter! *He was shooting at her!*

An Asian man jumped in front of Susan, got hit and fell to the ground. Boris aimed at the young woman again. Annya pulled her own gun out of her purse and shot at Boris. *Damn, she hadn't practiced much lately!* Boris grabbed at his ear and looked at his hand. It was covered in blood. He looked around in surprise. Annya shot at him again. He ducked down, grabbed his crutches and ran down the sidewalk, away from the scene. People started screaming and running all over the street. Some cars stopped, others collided, others behind them started honking. Annya tried to follow Boris, but she got caught in the chaos. She could see him jumping into a car and racing off. She saw some people taking photos. That would work for a general citizen. But Boris was a professional. He surely had registered his car under a fake name, and he would get rid of the car in no time. Annya looked at her GPS tracker. The GPS signal slowly moved away from the scene and towards the Mission district. She could follow him later. Annya looked over to Stella's daughter. She and another man kneeled beside the Asian man who had been hit by Boris's gunshot. Annya considered the situation. It would probably take a few minutes until the police arrived. If the man was seriously injured, she as an emergency physician could possibly save his life. She ran across the street. When she arrived, the man had slowly sat up, holding his chest.

Annya introduced herself. "Hello, I am an emergency physician. Are you hurt?"

The man looked at her with a penetrating gaze. "Thank you for your concern, ma'am. I am FBI Special Agent Lamong Saetang. I am fine. I am wearing a bulletproof vest."

What a relief! Annya sighed. "I am glad to hear that!" She looked at Susan and Amir. "That was quite a shock. Are you okay?"

Susan and Amir both nodded, although they looked very distressed. Susan was trembling and Amir was holding her tight, his free left arm was wrapped around her. He appeared very pale; his lips pressed together in agony. Annya heard police sirens in the background.

Susan pointed at Annya. "I know you! You work at SUEC hospital, and you live on campus!"

Annya smiled at Susan. "Yes, I am a physician at SUEC hospital. I came by the hospital here to see a colleague and saw this accident."

"It was an attack!" Susan exclaimed, clenching her free left wrist.

"Well, I am really glad that you were protected by this brave man!" Annya responded. Then she looked at Lamong. He seemed to take short, shallow breaths while clutching his right chest.

Annya pointed at his left chest. "A bulletproof vest can save your life, but it does not prevent injury from gunshots. At the very minimum, you got some decent bruises here."

Lamong nodded, carefully exhaling. "That is very possible. It hurts quite a bit."

Annya watched him carefully. "The impact could have also cracked some ribs. If the blow was hard enough to fracture a rib, then there could also be an injury to the lung or other parts of your body. You should get checked out at the hospital. It is right there!" She pointed at the hospital behind them.

Lamong nodded again. "I will surely do that!"

Annya saw two paramedics running towards them. The police sirens were coming closer. She got up.

"I have to leave now," she said as calmly as possible.

Lamong grabbed her wrist. "I am sorry, ma'am. You need to stay and provide a statement. You saw what happened."

Annya looked at Lamong, Susan and Amir. She did not want a scene in the middle of the street. She wanted to leave without a major fight. She grabbed into her purse, flashed her badge for a brief instant and put it back.

"I am a specialized skills officer of the CIA's National Clandestine Service. I have to follow the suspect, to prevent him from assaulting anyone else."

Susan's jaw dropped and Amir stared at Annya in surprise. Lamong let go of Annya's wrist, but he looked at her with a tilted head. "A few minutes ago, you said that you are an ER physician. Now you are a CIA agent? How come I am not aware of you or your operation? The CIA is not in the business of spying on domestic citizens. Its concentration is on foreign intelligence."

Annya got up. "This man is connected with the KGB, and he wanted to sell information of national interest to them. That's how I got involved."

Lamong shook his head. "But the CIA does not pursue suspects. The agency's primary function is foreign intelligence gathering. The CIA does not carry out manhunts in a domestic capacity. That is our job!"

The paramedics arrived and a police car was coming down the street, making its way through the chaos of swirling pedestrians and congested traffic.

"I am sorry, I have to leave now!" Annya waved goodbye. She turned around and looked at one of the paramedics. "This man needs a chest x-ray with forty-five-degree oblique views. He might have a rib fracture." Then, she stepped into a group of spectators that had watched them from a secure distance. Whoever this woman was, Susan wanted to thank her. But Annya had already disappeared in the crowd.

A few minutes later, three police cars and two FBI vans arrived at the scene. The police officers secured the area and started to interview witnesses. When there is a hot pursuit, the law enforcement team races after a suspect. But in a manhunt, the search must slow down. The SWAT officers carefully approached each building, car and tree with the anticipation that Boris could be waiting behind it with a weapon. Meanwhile, the paramedics escorted Lamong to the ER. He had refused to lie down on a stretcher. He enjoyed walking down the street past spectators, who were applauding as he passed them. Susan and Amir followed, flanked on each side by police officers. The small procession made its way back to the hospital, where Angus Weber waited for them at the entrance.

"Congratulations on this excellent work, Lamong! You saved two lives today!"

Lamong beamed with pride, while still holding his chest.

"Thank you, Agent Weber! I am glad I could be of service!"

Stella came through the ER as fast as her crutches would take her, tears running through down her cheeks. "Susan, I am so glad you are well!" she cried as she embraced her daughter. Then she turned to Lamong and gave him a big kiss on his cheek. "Thank you for saving my daughter! I will be forever in your debt!"

"I am glad, I could help, Mrs. Pellegrini!" Lamong smiled at her. Then, he pointed at Amir. "This man got her out of the gunfire. You should thank him as well."

Amir looked to the ground in embarrassment as both Stella and Susan embraced him. "Thank you, Amir!" Stella exclaimed, "you have been our guardian angel all along!"

Dr. Williams stepped towards the party. "I am glad you are all doing well – more or less. Please come in and please remember that this is an emergency room. Mr. Saetang, you can please go to exam room three so that I can examine you and order an x-ray if needed. Mr. Weber, your anesthesiologist just arrived and would be eager to talk with you. The sooner we get your leg operated on, the sooner you will be back on your feet. Amir, can you please guide Mrs. Pellegrini and her daughter back to the orthopedic surgery ward. The team there can decide if Mrs. Pellegrini is ready to be discharged. She surely can ambulate without any problems."

The group dissolved according to Dr. Williams's directions. Lamong entered the exam room. He had trouble removing his jacket, bulletproof vest and shirt. The bullet was still stuck in his vest. Lamong carefully removed a plastic bag from his pocket and placed the bullet in it for ballistic analysis. He held his hand against the lower part of his right chest to support it. Above his hand, there was indeed a large bruise of the chest wall. Dr. Williams examined the area and then ordered a chest x-ray. An x-ray technician came in shortly afterwards and took a radiograph. Dr. Williams reviewed the x-rays with Lamong. He pointed at Lamong's right ninth rib. "You have indeed a rib fracture, Mr. Saetang! You can see it here, that is the fracture line. There is also a small right pleural effusion."

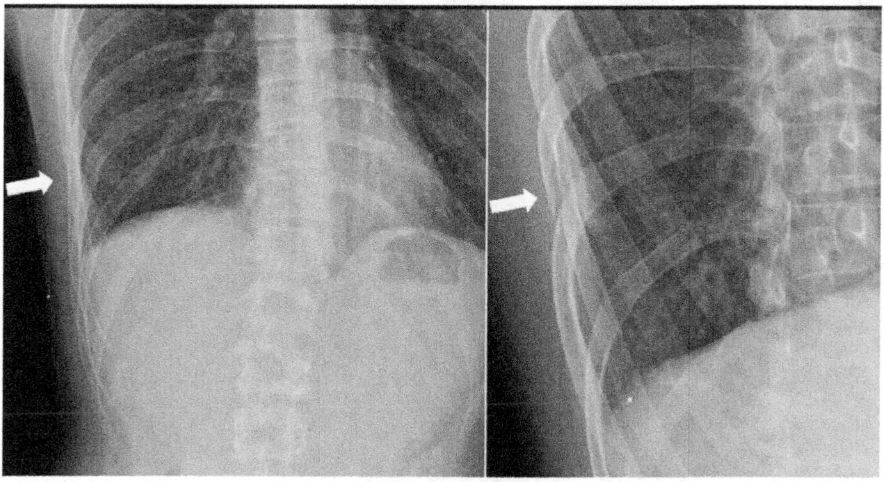

Lamong leaned forward and inspected the radiograph. "I don't see it, Dr. Williams. Can you please point it out to me some more?"

Dr. Williams chuckled. "This is a common problem, even for physicians. These rib fractures can be very subtle. They often occur at the lateral circumference of the rib, where they are difficult to see on a frontal radiograph. Therefore, we often obtain additional oblique views, where the patient turns such that the injured area of the rib is better aligned with the x-ray beam. A normal rib should have one continuous bowed outline. Your injured rib here shows a step off. That is a clear fracture." Dr. Williams magnified the radiographs and pointed out the abnormality with an arrow.

"Thank you for explaining this to me. I can see it now! It seems to be such a small injury. But it hurts a lot!"

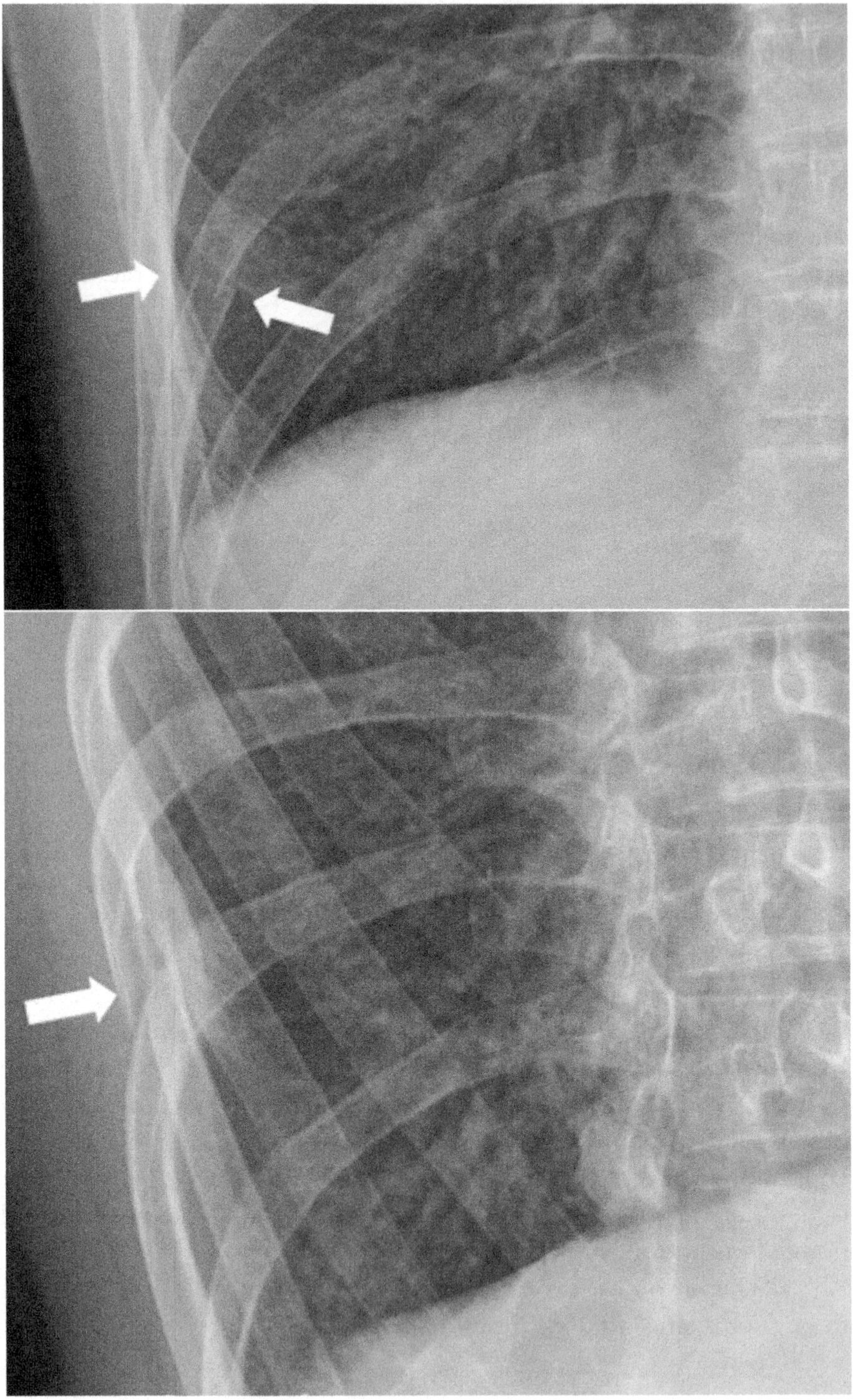

"Well, the chest cavity is lined by a thin membrane, the pleura. Normally, the pleura produces a small amount of fluid, which serves as a lubricant to the lungs as they move back and forth against the chest wall when you breathe. When the ribs break, blood and fluid will accumulate in the pleural space, which irritates nerves in the area and causes pain."

"How long will it take to heal?"

"Unlike bones of the arms and legs, broken ribs cannot be placed in a cast. You need to help minimizing the risk that the two fragments could come apart before they heal. Usually, we just wait for the fracture to heal. This can take up to six weeks. I can prescribe pain medication such as acetaminophen to relieve the pain while the rib heals."

"That might be helpful, thank you!"

"I would strongly recommend that you leave the pursuit of shooters to your colleagues for the next few weeks. Perhaps you can be helpful in a more remote fashion."

"I am afraid, you may be right. I cannot tolerate any sudden movements. My colleagues will have to take it from here."

"I am glad we're on the same page. I will prescribe some pain medication and then you are free to go. Our team will prepare the discharge paperwork."

Lamong nodded. "Thank you for your help, Dr. Williams!"

Dr. Williams bowed slightly and left the room.

***

Annya followed Boris' path through San Francisco. He seemed to take a zig zag tour through the city, perpetually slowing down and speeding up, which was possibly a reflection of stealing different cars and changing them along the way. Annya smiled wryly. She was glad that she had decided to take charge and become personally involved. Boris had outsmarted the FBI and escaped too many times. She would end this nightmare once and for all. As she looked at her phone, she noticed a text message. It was from Lili.

Hi Annya, DO NOT GO TO THE CAFÉ. IT'S A TRAP!

Annya smiled. She was prepared for that.

- 45 -
Ben
THE FIGHT

Wednesday, May 25, 2032, 1.00 pm.

Dean Bennett opened the lower drawer of his desk. He took out a bottle of whisky and poured some into his coffee. He rarely drank alcohol during the day. But now he needed a drink. Perhaps it would make him feel better. When he had been informed of the theft on Monday, he had felt an urgency to act. He had worked for years to orchestrate this once-in-a-lifetime donation to the university and he did not trust the FBI to resolve the brain chip issue in three days. Law enforcement had to follow rules and procedures, and those took time. But he needed this problem to evaporate before the symposium tomorrow. Too much was at stakes. The future of the university, a $30 billion donation and a hefty bonus for himself! He would not allow a bunch of saboteurs to destroy this historical feat.

So, he had hired Boris Sokolow. The underground world routinely produced results on short notice and Boris had an excellent reputation for attending to his clients' needs discreetly and efficiently. Dean Bennett was surely not proud of the consequences. But tough times required difficult decisions. When he heard that the scientist and his wife had been killed, he knew that Boris had taken his calling too far. But he had to admit that Boris had efficiently turned a security breach at SUEC to gossip about a family drama. This man was a maven indeed.

Dean Bennett took another sip from his Irish coffee. He thought of his favorite quote that had always motivated him in times of difficulties. *No matter how much falls on us, we keep plowing ahead!* Of course, he felt bad for his assistant when he heard that her daughter had been kidnapped. But this stupid child had brought this on herself. Why did she steal university property from a highly classified science lab? Why did her boyfriend attack a professional killer? How on earth did he think that would help anyone? Now he was dead, and Dean Bennett had to meet with the family to extend his condolences. As if he had all the time in the world. Fortunately, the death had happened outside of the university and was already reported to be an accident. Boris had again done a good job keeping the university out of this.

Dean Bennett let another sip run down his throat. A pleasant warm sensation extended from his stomach through his body. His spinning mind relaxed a little. He looked through the curved window onto the valley below him. Beautiful. He imagined the entry in history books. *With an unprecedented coordination of twelve billionaires towards the largest donation in human history, Dean Ben Bennett catapulted SUEC to the top of the world!* Why could people not stand back and let him do his work? Why had Lili Pham and Annya Segond had to play detective? They were great worker bees — and pleasant to look at. But they just wasted an enormous amount of time and energy creating problems rather than solving them!

Bennett sighed. He clearly had to climb a steep mountain here. Not only was he protecting SUEC, but he also had to save these women from their own stupidity. He had confiscated Lili's phone and asked the FBI to arrest Annya because he wanted to save them from being killed. He could not rationally explain another dead body to the donors. But the foolishness of these women was hopeless. Even when he clearly told them to stay away, overconfidence and a silly degree of curiosity led them to waste their energy on pointless ideas. If they did not listen, it was their fault if they got hurt. He would blame them for any dirt that they dug up.

The burner phone rang. Dean Bennett took another sip of coffee and answered it. "Hello Boris, what's up?"

"I am afraid I could not retrieve the fifth chip."

"That is unfortunate. Can you try again?"

"Someone was shooting at me. I believe it was a woman."

Speaking of stupidity…. Dean Bennett shook his head. "I am sorry to hear that. I don't know this for sure, but I guess this was Annya."

"Annya who?"

"Annya Segond."

"Segond?" Boris chuckled. "That is the name of a fracture! Is this a fake name?"

Dean Bennett thought about it for a moment. "That never occurred to me. But now that you bring it up, that is certainly possible. She snooped around the promenade last night and she disappeared this morning."

"She is a university employee?"

"Yes, she is one of our ER physicians."

"Interesting, I saw a woman at the promenade last night. Perhaps that was her. I was also at the ER early this morning, to get treated for a foot problem. I did not see a lady physician there. I would surely remember that."

"Our security cameras captured a video of her walking up the promenade. I gave it to the FBI. They are now looking for her as a possible suspect."

"Excellent! The FBI has a target and is busy. But who is this woman? Do you have a photo? I just googled her name and I'm getting nothing!"

"We do not post photos of our faculty online for security and privacy reasons. Let me see if I can find a photo in my files." Dean Bennett opened the personnel folder on his computer and looked through the files. "Ah, I found one. It may be two or three years old, but she looks pretty much the same now. I will send it to you with a text message."

The other end went silent.

"Boris, are you still on the line?"

"This is impossible!"

"What is impossible?"

"This is my ex-wife, Anastasia Ivanov! But she was shot about twenty years ago. She is supposed to be dead!"

"Well, I can assure you that this woman is very much alive. And I want to keep it this way. Perhaps you know her sister or some other relative who looks like her."

"Perhaps. Or perhaps not. You said she went missing?"

"Yes, she disappeared from the hospital this morning. We do not know why she left or where she is now. But we sent her a message through the phone of a friend and asked her to come to Café Carlos in San Francisco at two pm today. The FBI is waiting there for her."

"Perhaps I should have a look as well. I would really like to know if it is my wife. Imagine, I have been grieving her death for twenty years and she is actually alive and well! That's a bummer!"

Dean Bennett scratched his head. "I am not sure I understand. If this is indeed your wife, why would she shoot you?"

"Well, let me just say we did not exactly part on friendly terms."

Dean Bennett sighed. *A personal vendetta.* "Boris, I worked very hard to lead the FBI away from you. Do not put our mission in danger! I want no more shootings and no more dead people!"

"Keep cool, professor! Nobody will link you with anything unless you confess yourself!"

"Just to make this very clear. I purchased a *discreet* operation, not a massacre. No more killings or accidents!"

"Of course, professor! You tell me when the job is done! You can just give me my compensation and I will be gone for good!"

Dean Bennett cleared his throat. "Well, Boris, you brought me four brain chips instead of five. Therefore, I will pay eighty per cent of the discussed price. And for every by dead body, I will subtract one hundred K."

Boris' voice became cold. "You will do nothing like that, Dr. Bennett. I will tell you what the compensation is. The operation became much more complex than discussed initially and the price went up. I want the Rembrandt painting in your office. You will wrap it nicely for me and Bogdan will pick it up later this afternoon."

"Bogdan is in the custody of the FBI."

"They have nothing to keep him for. They will let him go after twenty-four hours. Once he's out, he will stop by your office to pick up the painting. He will hand it over to me and you will never see me again."

Dean Bennett thought about this. Perhaps it was not a bad idea. There would be no monetary transaction that the FBI could track back to him. Nobody would ask questions if he modernized his office and put up a new painting. "When will Bogdan come by my office?"

"Later this afternoon. You do not need to be there. In fact, it is better if you're not. If anyone does notice a missing painting, you can always say it was stolen."

"What if the FBI follows him?"

"They likely will, and they know that he knows. They want him to lead them to me. If they do not see me, they are likely instructed to not interfere. They will not anticipate that he is so bold as to carry away a Rembrandt under their eyes. If any of the FBI agents does ask him what he is carrying, he will tell them that he has been fired and is moving out. That will also explain if he carries any items. If they want a confirmation, he will ask them to call you."

Dean Bennett sighed. "It seems like you thought of everything!"

"This is not my first rodeo, sir!"

"OK, Boris, you will get your painting. All in all, the operation has been completed almost successfully."

"You should practice gratefulness, professor. Nobody else would have brought you the brain chips back in two days. I look forwards to receiving the painting. And just so that we are very clear here. For every extra day that I wait for my compensation, there will be a dead body."

"You will get your painting. And I said no more dead bodies!"

Dean Bennett hung up the phone. He was annoyed. Boris had delivered less than discussed but negotiated a much higher compensation than initially planned. In addition, he, Ben Bennett, had offered valuable information to Boris and received nothing in return. And then he had to endure this condescending tone! Dean Bennett turned his swivel chair around and looked out of the window. This view always calmed his boiling nerves. But what was that now? Could he not relax for even a minute? He saw Lili Pham and Terrel Wright coming up the promenade. Something was not right about them. They could not see him through the multicolored glass façade of the octagon building. Terrel looked very serious, while Lili's gaze was triumphant, almost jubilant. The expression on her face made him feel uneasy. *Payback time!*

Dean Bennett got up from his seat. Did the FBI have evidence against him? What could it be? An intercepted communication with Boris? That was unlikely since he always used a secure phone and turned on a noise diffuser in his office when he talked with Boris. Or his order to send Annya's video from last night to the FBI? His order to confiscate Lili's phone? He would create a story to explain these actions. He had not touched anyone or anything. Any other concerns relied on assumptions which could be explained away. He was a master of creating alternate realities. But he could not do that instantaneously. He needed time to think up a watertight story. In addition, he would be in a much more powerful place tomorrow, when he had sealed the deal for the university. Dean Bennett quickly walked out of his office, down the hall, down the stairs and through the lobby to the exit. He had to avoid the FBI until the symposium tomorrow morning. He was not sure how he would manage that, but he would approach this as every big project. One step at a time. For now, he needed to leave and avoid an encounter with Terrel Wright.

As Dean Bennett made his way through the lobby, the administrative assistant at the entrance turned around and looked at him. *What was her name again?* He did not remember. She was temporarily helping while Stella was on sick leave. He liked the frail, bony old lady. She was hard-working, polite and efficient. But now, she stepped into his path with a vile grin on her wrinkled face.

"Hello, I have to urgently talk with a donor outside!" he called from a distance.

The lady did not move. "I'm sorry, Dr. Bennett. You need to please wait here for a few minutes. I was asked by the FBI to make sure that you will be present here when they come for a brief discussion. They need important information from you for a case of national security."

Dean Bennett looked at the old lady. *Was this a joke? Did everyone think they could order him around today?* "I will be happy to talk with them. They can find me outside on the terrace!" He continued to walk towards the old woman and the exit behind her. If this bitch would not step away, he would simply run her over. He would later say that she stepped into his way and ask her to check her glasses. He surely could not employ entrance staff who had problems with their vision! Perhaps he would discipline her and prescribe a mandatory course in courtesy. That would teach her a lesson!

As he walked towards the woman, Dean Bennett extended his right arm and front-kicked her to shove her out of the way. But to his surprise, she did not move an inch. As if she were glued to the floor. Aiko looked at him with an alert, confident gaze and slightly bowed towards him. Dean Bennett was surprised and undecided how to react.

He looked at her, trying to make sense of this woman who seemed to be an easy target but stood her ground, totally calm and unafraid. Was a woman preventing him from leaving the building? His anger boiled up again. He had to get out of this building now! Dean Bennett grabbed Aiko's left wrist with his right hand and tried to pull her out of the way. Aiko quickly kicked his lower leg. He led out a cry of pain. A second later, Aiko grabbed the thumb which encircled her wrist and pulled it backwards, into an unnatural angle. Dean Bennett went down on his knees. They both heard a bone crack.

- 46 -
Lili
BENNETT'S FRACTURE

Wednesday, May 25, 2032, 1.00 pm.

Lili and Terrel arrived at the SUEC parking lot. At the entrance gate, Lili checked in with her SUEC faculty ID and registered Terrel as her guest. Then, they walked up the promenade to the octagonal university building. They passed by the café where Lili had been waiting earlier this morning and walked towards the main entrance of the building. When they opened the door to the lobby, they saw Aiko blocking the narrow area beside the entrance desk, where people checked in and checked out. Aiko was standing with her back towards the entrance, facing the lobby area and slightly bowing towards a big, overweight man, who was rushing towards her. It was the dean! Lili saw his impressive outline on both sides and above Aiko's small figure, coming closer. He was running towards Aiko, raising his arms to punch her out of the way. But the thin woman did not move. She continued to block the exit. As the dean ran towards her, she moved her feet slightly apart, bent her knees, hunched her shoulders, tucked her chin and raised her arms slightly. The two figures clashed. Aiko quickly grabbed the dean's thumb and a second later, the dean was on the ground. He cried out in pain.

Lili's jaw dropped. "Wow! What on earth was that?"

The dean was lying on the ground, looking at Terrel. "Agent Wright, you need to arrest this woman immediately. She assaulted me!"

Aiko put her hands into the pockets of her wool blazer and sent Terrel a concerned look.

Terrel shrugged. "Sorry, Dr. Bennett. Local fights are not part of my jurisdiction. Those are taken care of by the police. However, if you decide to file a complaint, I would be happy to serve as a witness. As far as I could see, you attacked the woman first and she acted in self-defense."

Lili nodded. "I can confirm that!" Then she turned to Aiko. "Aiko, you overwhelmed a man three times your size! I had no idea that you are trained in martial arts. I am amazed by your hidden talents!"

Aiko smirked. "Well, I grew up in a gang-infested neighborhood. My father taught me Shotokan karate since I was six years old. He wanted to make sure that I could defend myself. Later, I continued my training with a local dojo."

Terrel raised his eyebrows. "I was in a karate club as well when I was a kid. But I did not learn to twist any thumbs!"

"Well, martial arts that are taught at most modern sport clubs look fancy, but they do more harm than good in a real-life situation. The moves that I learned are from my family. Traditional karate resembled full contact, bare fists, no mouth guard, no pads, fighting."

Lili looked at Aiko and saw an entirely different woman in front of her. Every wrinkle in her face told a story of her struggle and survival. Lili felt remorseful for their petty little word fights. "I'm so sorry you had such a rough childhood, Aiko!"

Aiko looked at her with her calm, confident gaze. "I had a happy childhood, Lili. And a very loving family! There were just more predators out there than today. And don't get me wrong. Our family members did not fight on a regular basis. In fact, we were not allowed to hit anyone first. Shotokan is practical and designed for self-defense. If someone attacked me, I could end a fight in a few seconds by striking their weakest point."

"I'm sure you are an expert on that!" They both smiled.

Terrel offered his hand to the dean, who was still sitting on the ground, inspecting his severely bruised thumb. The dean extended his uninjured left hand and Terrel pulled him up.

"Dr. Bennett, you are under arrest for public corruption, white-collar crime and hiring a hitman."

The dean looked at him in surprise. "You cannot do that. You do not have any proof of these allegations."

Terrel responded coldly. "Don't worry, I have plenty of evidence."

The dean raised his uninjured index finger. "You know that we have a very important donor event tomorrow, where we expect a donation of thirty billion dollars. Thirty billion! You want to interfere with that? You will piss off a lot of people."

Terrel shrugged. "I am just doing my job, Dr. Bennett. I am concerned about our national security and the safety of SUEC employees. You committed federal offenses and will be brought to justice. But if you cooperate with the FBI, our office will let you give your speech at the symposium tomorrow. You will announce and accept the donations — and then we will take you back into custody."

"Why would I cooperate with you if I end up in jail anyways?"

"You will get your trial. If the FBI can report that you cooperated with us, that will likely have a very positive effect on the outcome. This is of course your decision. We can also take you in custody now, explain to the donors that you experienced a sudden illness, perhaps Covid, and introduce your successor at the symposium tomorrow. Your choice."

Dean Bennett hit the entrance table with his uninjured left fist. "I planned this symposium for the past five years! I will announce this historic donation! I am innocent! I have cooperated with the FBI all along and will continue to do so, even if you treat me so badly now."

"I'm glad we have an agreement," Terrel said.

Lili thanked the stars. She knew from their earlier conversation that Terrel had slightly overstepped his authority. He had strict instructions to not interfere in any way with the donation event tomorrow.

Dean Bennett pointed at his swollen thumb. "What about my hand? I'm pretty sure this crazy woman broke my thumb!"

"We will stop over at the hospital and get you a cast there, or whatever is needed."

Terrel turned to Lili. "Lili, I would appreciate your help. I'm sure we need a radiograph. Can you handle this as discreetly as possible?"

Lili nodded. "Sure, I will give our team a heads up and I can also provide a read out right away."

Terrel looked back at Aiko. "Aiko, can you please call the ER staff at the hospital and let them know that Dean Bennett will arrive in about thirty minutes? It would be great if we could bypass the waiting room. Hopefully, they can accommodate us without stirring any public attention."

"Sure, I will call them right away."

"Thank you for your service, Aiko. And please get checked out at the hospital as well, to make sure that you did not suffer any injuries. I would also appreciate if you would share the result with me so that I can include it in my report of the incident."

Aiko smiled proudly, slightly bowing her head. "I am fine. But if that is helpful, I will stop by the hospital on my way home."

Terrel looked at Dean Bennett. "Okay, let's go. And just in case this idea came into your head. I run much faster than you!"

The Dean grumbled something.

Lili chuckled. She admired Terrel's confidence and thought of *her* favorite quote. *The arch of the universe is long, but it always bends towards justice!* What a day! She could not wait to tell Mark about it!

Terrel, Dean Bennett and Lili left the building, Terrel gently holding the Dean's left upper arm. They walked down the promenade to the parking lot. They passed by a few students and researchers, who politely greeted the dean. Nobody appeared to notice anything unusual. That was part of the plan.

***

They arrived at the hospital thirty minutes later. A security guard picked them up at the entrance and led them through a back door into the building and to an exam room. Santiago arrived shortly afterwards. He examined the thumb and ordered an x-ray. An x-ray tech came in and took several radiographs of the hand and thumb from different angles. Lili walked over to the PACS viewing station and had a look at the x-ray. Dean Bennett, Terrel and Santiago looked over her shoulder. She pointed to the first metacarpal bone. "There is a Bennett fracture."

Dean Bennett raced his eyebrows. "A Bennett fracture?"

She smirked. "Yes, it looks like you got a fracture with your very own name!"

Terrel asked. "What is a Bennett fracture?"

Lili pointed to the fracture. "A Bennett fracture is a two-piece fracture of the first metacarpal bone, that is the bone that connects one of the small bones of the hand, the trapezium, with the lower bone of the thumb. A Bennett fracture typically extends into the joint space between the first metacarpal bone and the trapezium."

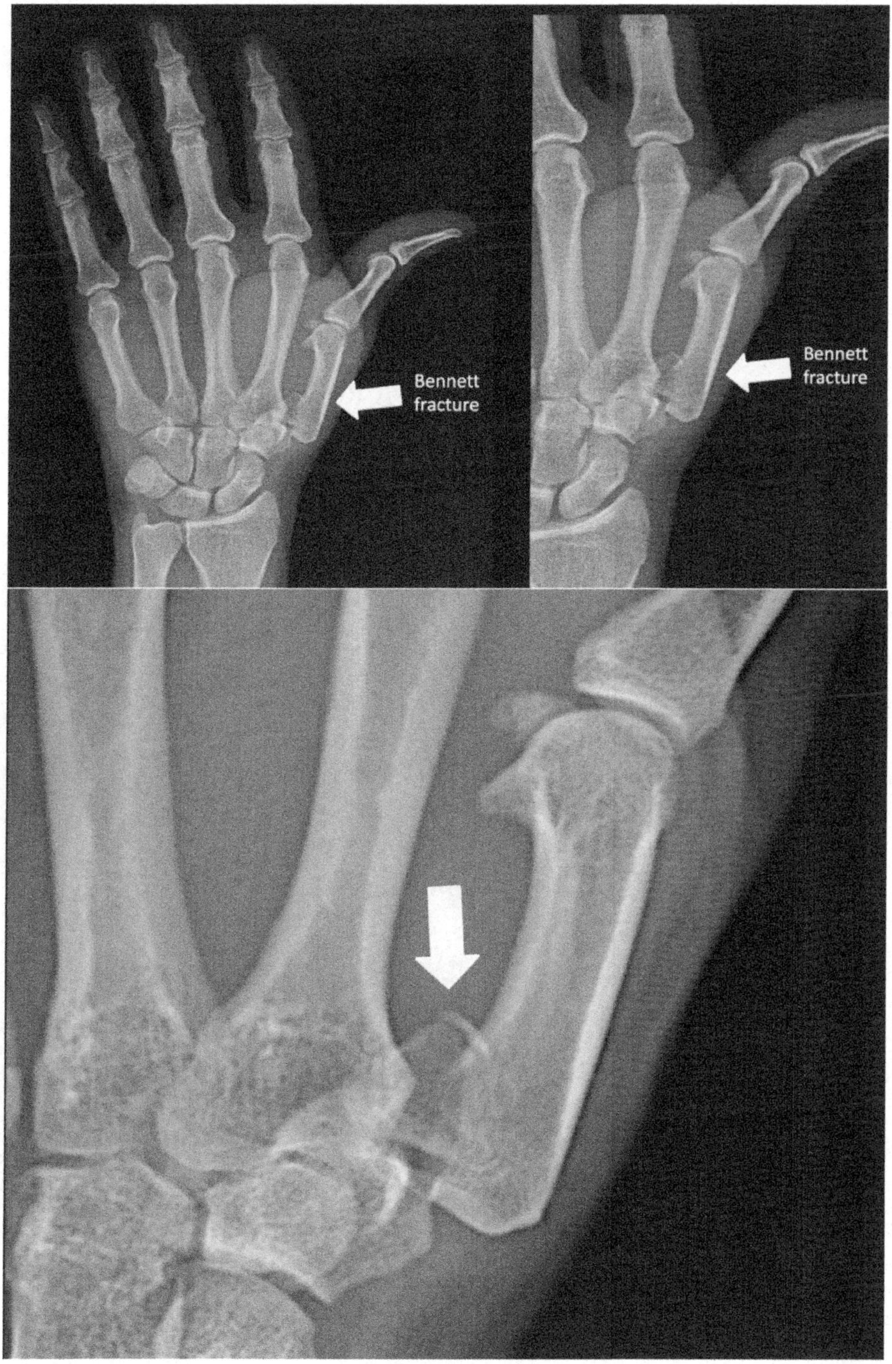

Santiago looked at the images as well. “Isn’t this a Rolando fracture?”
Lili smiled. “You remember this very well, Santiago! Dean Bennett has a Bennett fracture, an oblique or L-shaped fracture of the first metacarpal bone. A Bennett fracture is composed of two pieces. A small fragment of the first metacarpal bone and the remaining first metacarpal bone. You are right that a Rolando fracture is a fracture in the same area. However, a Rolando fracture is a three-piece fracture. The fracture line in a Rolando fracture has more of a T-shape. I have an example here.” Lili brought up one of her teaching cases, where the name of the patient had been removed for teaching purposes.

“See this example here,” she said. “As you can see, this fracture is composed of three bone fragments. A Rolando fracture.”

Santiago looked at the images and nodded. “Thank you for explaining this to me, Lili! Now I see the difference!”

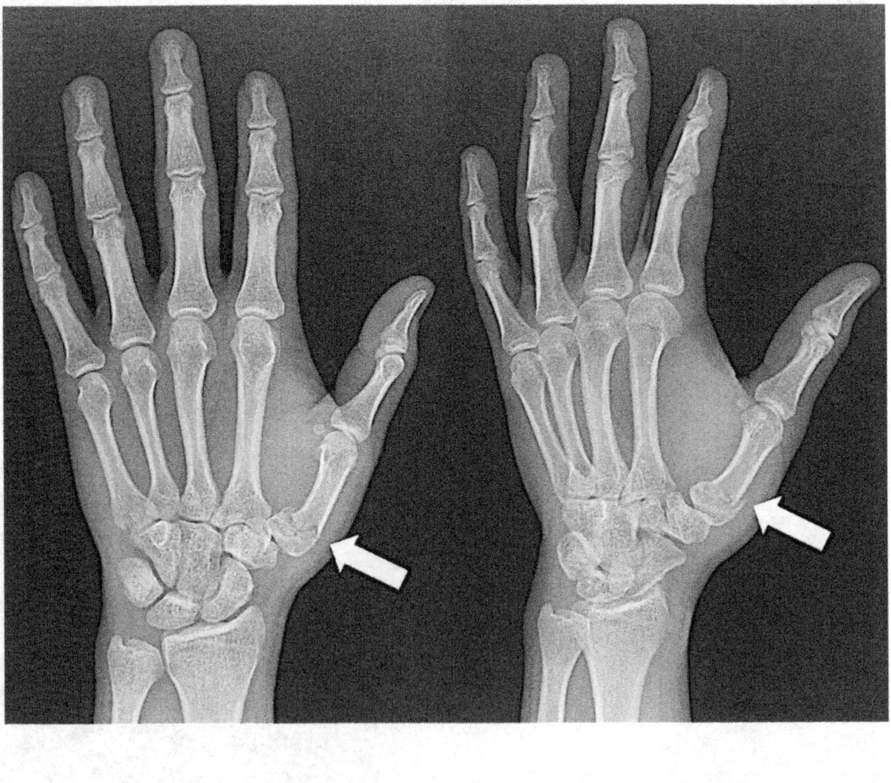

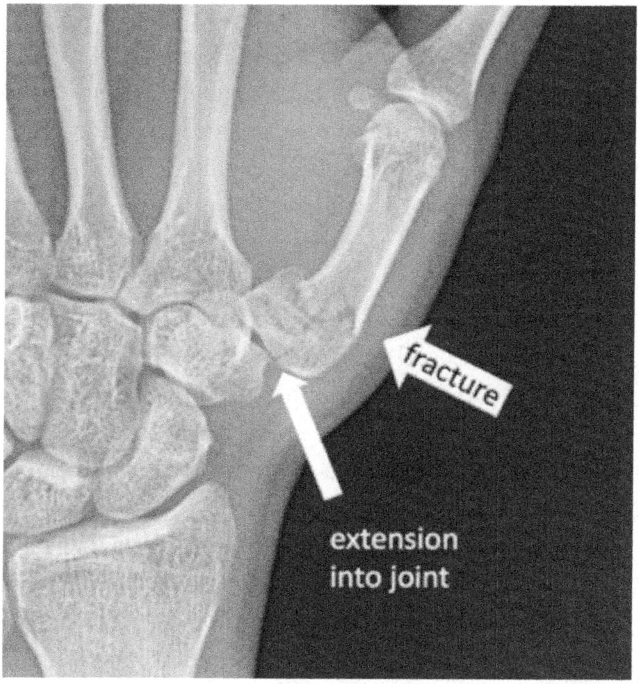

Dean Bennett asked, "Do I need a cast?"

Santiago answered. "I will arrange for a consultation with our orthopedic surgeons. Usually, if there is a displacement of more than 1 mm, they prefer to secure it with an orthopedic screw. But they will have to take a look and they will make the ultimate recommendation."

Dean Bennett shook his head. "I have to lead a very important symposium tomorrow!"

Santiago looked to Terral for help. He responded politely. "Well, Dr. Bennett, your thumb is severely swollen. Our surgeons will likely want to wait for the swelling to improve before they secure the bone with a screw. I will provide you with a thumb spica splint for now and we can make an appointment later this week for the surgery."

Dean Bennett nodded. "That should work!"

Santiago exhaled. "Okay, I am glad we are on the same page. I will get the thumb spica splint for you and ask the orthopedic surgeon to have a quick look as well to confirm our plan. I will come back in a few minutes with an appointment for the surgery. This can be done in an outpatient setting. You do not need to be hospitalized for this."

Dean Bennett nodded. "Okay!"

Santiago left the room and Terrel turned to Dean Bennett. "I'm glad we could resolve this. Once we are done here, I will take you into custody until tomorrow. This is for your own safety and to prevent any further criminal operations. We have an FBI facility close by. My colleagues will take good care of you. I will bring you there now, pick you up tomorrow morning and drive you to the symposium. Do you need anything from your office?"

Dr Bennett nodded. "I need the painting in my office!"

Terrel looked at him with raised eyebrows. "Excuse me?"

"Sorry, this might sound trivial under the circumstances. But it is possible that one of our staff will come and pick it up. It looks quite antiquated. We wanted to exchange it with a more modern painting, to give my office a fresh look!"

Terrel shook his head. "I am sorry, Dr. Bennett. That will have to wait. Nobody can enter your office for the next several days. The FBI will seal and guard your office, to make sure all evidence there is secured. I was asking about more immediate needs, any items that you might need for the event tomorrow?"

"Well, I need my suit and my speech, they are both in my office."

"Where are these items exactly?"

"The suit is hanging on a coat rack behind the office door. The speech had been printed on SUEC stationery, which is on my desk."

Terrel reached for his phone and typed a text message. Then he looked up at Ben Bennett. "I have asked one of my men to get these items for you.

"Thank you!" Ben Bennett said politely.

Terrel turned to Lili. "Thank you for your help today, Lili!"

"Always my pleasure!" she wished both men a good day – realizing the irony – and retreated to the Radiology reading room.

- 47 -
Boris
THE SHOT

Wednesday, May 25, 2032, 2.00 pm.

Against his usual routine, Boris had parked directly across the street from the café. He felt like he had been waiting here forever. After leaving the shooting scene at the General Hospital, he had changed cars seven times and exchanged the license plates of the last one, a marine blue Chevrolet Malibu. He had put on large, round, diamante sunglasses and a wig with long, blonde hair, which he hoped would make him look like a woman – at least from a distance. *Partner look with Anastasia!* he thought. He pulled down the sleeves of his shirt to cover his hairy forearms. If anyone noticed that he was actually a man, that would probably not raise many eyebrows in San Francisco. People would definitely not recognize him. But he needed to be cautious. FBI agents were likely everywhere, scanning the area. But they were busy looking for a redhead. And as far as he was concerned, it was worth the risk. In fact, he loved the thrill! If this was really Anastasia, then he would make sure that she got her bullet this time. She had betrayed him and he, Boris Sokolov, would not let her get away with it. Leaning back in his seat, Boris carefully observed the café from a safe distance. In case anyone recognized him, he could quickly drive away.

Boris was still thinking about the fifth chip. He wanted it. Over the past two days, it had never occurred to him that Susan could have it. She had walked around with it in front of his nose! She had made a fool out of him! That bothered him — a lot. Boris's thoughts wandered. He could not stand these bitches. They were at the core of every bad thing that ever happened to him. He wanted Anastasia dead…and Susan.

Suddenly, Boris's swirling mind produced a great idea. Perhaps he could kill two birds with one stone. He had to get Susan here as well. If both Anastasia and Susan were to come here, he could open fire and kill both women. If Susan was still wearing the chip, then she had not told anyone about it. Boris could wait if needed to retrieve it. When the dust had settled, he could go to the morgue and cut the chip out of her pretty head. He would bring flowers for Anastasia's grave as well. Boris grinned. It seemed difficult to get all the players together. But he was ready for the challenge.!

He pulled up his phone and sent a text message to Susan. *Hi Susan, the FBI lied to you. Kaleo is not dead. I will tell you the truth. Meet me at Café Carlos. Annya*

He added Annya's photo. Now he only had to wait. He was pretty sure that Susan would take the bait. She would come and find Anastasia for him. And then he could shoot them both.

Boris lit up a cigarette and inhaled deeply. These bitches would not fool him anymore. He was in charge now! Boris exhaled slowly and watched the stress of the morning vanish into thin smoke. As the nicotine reached his brain, he felt a sense of heightened alertness, increased focus and deep satisfaction.

Boris's phone rang. There were only two people in the world who had this number: his brother and his mother.

It was Bogdan. "Hey Boris, the FBI just released me. I followed your instructions to just repeat over and over that I don't know anything. And then they let me go!"

"I'm glad to hear that, Bogdan. They had no other choice. They have no evidence against you. You work as a security guard at SUEC. There are a million explanations for how some of your DNA could get into a lab there. Maybe the professor had a crush on you and came too close in the cafeteria, who knows?"

Bogdad laughed. "You always keep me safe!"

"Yes, brother, and I will make you a millionaire as well. Then you won't need these shabby jobs anymore!"

"I actually liked my job at SUEC! I was paid by the university to keep the competition out and I was paid by the KGB to get sensitive information. Easy job – generous double payment! I am quite sad that I got fired!"

"I am sorry, Bogdan. But once we have completed this coup, you don't need to work at all anymore – at least not for the next few years."

"Do you want to pay me a pension?"

"Well, sort of. The dean agreed to give us the Rembrandt in his office as compensation for our troubles. He will not report it missing, so it will take a long time until someone notices. If at all."

"That is great! You will split it with me?"

"Of course! I love my little brother! I checked with one of my friends from the black market. It is worth about twenty-five million US dollars. If we wait a little bit and invest a few million dollars to sell it discreetly at a discount, we should each get at least ten million out of this."

"Wow, that sounds pretty good to me!"

"Yeah, you just need to help me with one more thing."

"What is that? You know that the FBI is on my heels right now?"

"Yes, and they know that you know. This is exactly why they won't expect you to do anything major. They want to catch me. They will just follow you from a distance and watch out for me."

"You are so smart! What do you want me to do?"

"You need to go to the dean's office, detach the painting from the security alarm, retrieve it, wrap it in some old paper, carry it to your car and drive away. Dean Bennett said that he would wrap it for us. But I would not count on that. If it is still hanging on the wall, I trust that you can disable the alarm and carry it to your car. You can add a box with office supplies, so that it looks like you are moving out of your office after being fired. It is a perfect disguise. I doubt that anyone will ask you about it. It just looks like some old stuff. But if anyone recognizes it, you can just say that the dean asked you to move it. He will confirm."

"Okay, boss. I'm on my way."

"Thank you, brother! We will soon sit on a beach and celebrate the occasion with a nice champagne!"

Boris sighed. His brother was not the sharpest knife in the drawer. But Boris loved him dearly. Bogdan had such a deep trust in him. Like a little puppy. Boris surely did not want to create any trouble for him. He just made strategic decisions when he sent him out into the field. Bogdan was the only one who could realistically retrieve the painting right now. Boris hoped that he would not disappoint Bogdan's trust in him one day.

From the corner of his eye, Boris saw some movement at the café across the street. It was a beautiful, sunny Californian afternoon and all tables in front of the café were taken. Several waiters walked from table to table, taking orders, distributing drinks and dishes or collecting bills. It was busy. However, three people all looked at once to the right. A young man with dark sunglasses at one of the tables, an athletic woman who was walking with a stroller on the sidewalk in front of the café and a middle-aged man who was apparently repairing his bike all turned their heads at the same time, as if they were choreographed. Boris noted their surprised faces and followed their gaze. There she was! Susan walked with long strides towards the café, looking from one table to another, presumably looking for Anastasia. Boris smiled. His plan was working. He started the car, fetched his leather jacket from the backseat and placed it over his legs. Then, he opened the glove compartment, got out the Glock and placed it under the jacket, with his finger on the trigger. He opened the driver's door window. As soon as Anastasia showed up, he would act.

Susan had arrived at the café and was now walking in between the tables, inspecting the faces of different customers, clearly searching for someone. She walked into the café, disappeared for a while inside, then came out again and did another round between the tables outside. She talked to the waiters, holding her cell phone up, probably showing the photo of Anastasia. The waiters shook their heads. Susan stood in front of the café, looking around, apparently undecided what to do.

Boris realized that he would have to make a decision. He might not get them both after all. Anastasia was too smart to just show up in the open. She might not come at all, and he could lose this great target line on Susan. If he could not get them both at once, then he wanted to get as least one of them. He looked over to the café. Susan just turned around, inspecting the café guests one more time, while presenting her back to Boris. He lifted the muzzle of the gun just slightly above the lower frame of the car window and aimed at Susan. He was about to pull the trigger when he heard a loud bang. The passenger window of his car smashed, and a bullet landed on the dashboard. Boris eyes widened. He was under attack — again. Had the FBI spotted him?

He stamped his foot on the gas and raced away. He saw a woman with long red hair jumping from behind a tree onto the sidewalk. It was Anastasia! She had a gun in her hands, extended her arms, aimed at the car and shot again. The car wobbled. The young man at the café table had jumped up as well and was also aiming a gun at his car. Boris heard police sirens in a distance. He noted a police car in the rear window. He doubled his speed and raced towards the pier. A second police car joined the first one behind him. Boris took several turns at high speed until he could see the bay. The sirens came closer. He aimed for the water. As he reached the shoreline, the car took off, flew through the air and landed with a crash in the water.

- 48 -
Susan
THE SAFE HOUSE

Wednesday, May 25, 2032, 2.30 pm.

Susan looked for Annya at Café Carlos. But she could not find her. Why had Annya texted her that Kaleo was alive? Was it a cruel joke? Susan had seen his dead body. But then, she had been under the influence of the brain chip, and she had seen other horrible things in that cabin that were not real. She was still trying to figure out which of her experiences in that cabin had been real and which were hallucinations. She could still feel the rope that tied her to the chair in that loft. She could still see the look on Kaleo's face when he looked up to her and told her that he loved her. She could still feel the gag in her mouth that prevented her from shouting that she had the fifth chip. She *wished* it had been all just a bad, bad dream! But then she remembered the bang of the gunshot. Her brain played it over and over again. She heard it right now behind her. *Was it real?*

Susan jerked around. She wasn't quite sure where the sound had come from. But she instantly ducked down. She saw a man at one of the tables jumping up and pulling a gun. Several people in front of the café started screaming and ran away. A woman with a stroller on the sidewalk pulled a gun out of the stroller as well. And on the other side of the street was Annya, who had pretended to be a CIA agent.

Susan was not sure if she was awake or if she was having a flashback. Was this all real? Who were these people shooting at? Susan heard smashing glass and squealing tires. A car on the other side of the street raced away. Annya walked into the street, aimed at the car and sent several shots after it. One of her bullets hit the car, but the car kept going. Susan heard police sirens in the distance, slowly coming closer. Several of the café guests had run into the building, others had ducked under their tables, pulled out their cell phones and taken videos of the scene. The young man with the gun walked towards Susan. Was he another killer? Susan screamed. She jerked up, turned around and wanted to run away. But Annya was suddenly in front of her and embraced her with both arms. Susan screamed louder.

"You are safe now, Susan!" Annya said with a soothing voice.

Susan slowly calmed down. Annya let go of her. Susan looked at Annya. "Who are you?"

"I already told you. I am a CIA agent."

"You don't look like a CIA agent."

"Why would you say that? Because I am a woman? CIA agents do not look special in any way, and they do not wear a uniform. We do not want to grab attention; we want to blend in and become invisible to the public. We are everywhere and nowhere. We help keep you safe."

"Were you spying on me?"

"No, I did not spy on you. The CIA does not spy on United States citizens. Our job is on foreign intelligence. You walked into me, not the other way around!

"No, that's not true! You asked me to come here!" Susan pulled up her cell phone and showed Annya the text message.

Annya gasped. "I am sorry, Susan. But this was a trap. I did not write this."

"Of course!" was all that Susan could say. Tears were running down her cheeks.

Annya sighed. She stroked Susan's head and said softly, "Dealing with trauma can take up a lot of space in your brain, with little room for anything else. Anything that triggers a flashback can impair your judgment and get you in danger."

Susan sobbed. "I know that. I just *wanted* this text message to be true! I want Kaleo to be alive!"

The man in front of them cleared his throat. He looked at Annya. "Dr. Ivanov – or Segond, whichever you prefer, I am FBI Special Agent Rogers. I have a phone call here for you." He handed Annya his cell phone.

"Hello Anastasia," she heard Angus Weber's voice. "You caused quite a turmoil today!"

"Hello Angus, it is great to hear your voice. I had expected you to come in person. Without you here, things are sort of getting out of hand!"

Angus chuckled. "I'm sorry, I'm compromised currently. I broke my leg and will have it repaired later this afternoon so that I can attend the symposium tomorrow. But I heard that you had things pretty much under control, Anastasia! You saved Susan's life twice!"

Annya looked at Susan. "Yes, I'm glad she is safe, at least for now."

Angus voice turned more serious. "Anastasia, I want to thank you for saving Susan's life. I am very grateful for that! However, you are acting outside of your jurisdiction. Your task is foreign intelligence gathering at SUEC. The CIA has no law enforcement power. You are not authorized to pursue suspects or carry out arrests. That's our job!"

"Well, I expanded my radius when it became clear that we are dealing with my ex-husband, Boris Sokolov. He is extremely dangerous. He is closely connected with the KGB, and he is a professional killer. Very few people know him as well as I do."

"You are emotionally compromised when it comes to your ex-husband, Anastasia. That makes you vulnerable. We have an entire team on this. Boris sent a text message to Susan that asked her to look for you. He wanted to kill you both at the same time. You are in great danger. I would like to take both you and Susan to a safe house."

"I think it is an excellent idea to bring Susan to a safe house. Perhaps add her mother and her friend, Amir. Boris previously used the mother to get to her. And he opened a fire in front of the hospital on both Susan and Amir. So, all three should be put into a safe place until we have Boris, alive or dead."

"That is my concern. You want to make this a personal vendetta. We have a safe house close by and I can put all four of you there until Boris is in custody. I don't want any more dead bodies."

"I prevented dead bodies today, Angus. When your people were still drinking coffee at the café, Boris had his gun on Susan. If I had not intervened, she would be dead now. I know him! I can best predict his next moves."

"Well, you can always predict from the safe house."

Annya shrugged. "I guess we've exchanged our arguments."

She looked at the FBI agent in front of her. "Could you please hold the phone for a moment. My nose is running."

The agent took the phone. They heard Agent Weber's voice. "Anastasia, are you there?"

Annya put her hand into her jacket, apparently searching for a tissue. Then, she quickly pulled her hand out and threw something on the ground. Suddenly, everyone was standing in a large smoke cloud.

Susan coughed and exclaimed. "I cannot see anything."

The agent in front of her cursed. "Damn it! A smoke grenade!" He tried to grab Annya, but he reached into an empty space. He then grabbed Susan's arm and pulled her towards the right side of the café, out of the cloud. The few spectators who were still at the café screamed and similarly tried to find a way out of the smoke.

Susan heard Agent Weber shouting through the phone. "Hold Anastasia! Hold Anastasia! Do not let her run away!"

But she was already gone.

- 49 -
Boris
THE BOMB

Wednesday, May 25, 2032, 2.30 pm.

After fleeing from the shooting scene, Boris raced towards the shoreline of the San Francisco Bay. The car took off, flew through the air and landed with a crash in the water. It sank quickly. Boris gasped as ice cold water embraced him. Fortunately, the windows were already down. Boris extracted himself through the window and allowed the current to take him away, towards the Golden Gate Bridge. The wig on his head dislodged and floated away. Boris stayed underwater as long as possible. He noted a seal close by. He dived up briefly besides him, then dived down again and continued his way down the Bay. If anyone had seen his head and looked at it again, he would only see the seal. The seal looked at Boris with great interest and followed him. A few others joined them. This gave him great cover to come up for air a few more times. At Crissy Field, Boris felt safe enough to swim towards the beach.

Boris got out of the water. Several people strolling down the waterfront stopped and watched him. A fully dressed man with a cast on his leg walking out of the water onto the beach. A man asked him if he needed help. Boris mumbled something that his kayak had capsized and that he was fine otherwise. After seeing that he was okay, most of the spectators walked away. A homeless man offered him a blanket, which he gratefully accepted. Boris's whole body shivered and trembled. A young woman with a child, perhaps two years old, sat on the beach a few meters away. The woman watched Boris as he tried to dry his wet clothes with the blanket. Boris grinned at her. She looked away.

The plaster cast was soaked and heavy. He had to get rid of it as soon as possible. One of the ends had loosened in the water. Boris sat down on the sand. He grabbed the loose end and pulled on it. He could unwrap the layers. He unwrapped the cast slowly, carefully avoiding any further pressure on his foot, which was hurting a lot. He finished the last part with sheer force and released his ice-cold foot from the wet undercast padding. As he pulled out his sore foot, a small, shimmering, silver item dropped into the sand.

What was that? Boris picked it up with his thumb and index finger and inspected it closely. *Son of a bitch!* That guy in the hospital had planted a GPS chip in his cast. And Dean Bennett had mentioned that Anastasia worked in the ER. She was behind this! That's why she had found him so easily. Boris slammed his fist into the sandy ground. That bitch would get to know Boris Sokolov!

Boris sat for a while at the beach, catching his breath, shivering under his blanket and contemplating his options. Even the homeless guy had pity in his eyes when he looked at him. Boris tried to focus and plan his next move. The FBI agents in and around the café had not known his location. Only Anastasia had known it. *Only Anastasia was tracking him.* He could exploit that. His initial reflex had been to throw the GPS chip away. But he could use the chip to lead Anastasia to wherever he wanted her to go. He put the GPS chip back into his pocket. Now that he knew that she was following the chip, he would find great use for it.

The mother and child got into some argument. The boy threw a tantrum and ran towards the sea. The mother ran after him, trying to fetch him before he reached the water. Boris quickly got up and walked to the blanket where the two had been sitting. He had spotted a large bag on it. He quickly reached into it, found a phone and purse, grabbed them and turned around. The mother was busy with her child and did not notice what was happening behind her back. But the homeless guy watched Boris with alert eyes. Boris opened the purse, took out sixty dollars, left a twenty-dollar bill behind and threw the purse to the guy, who caught it.

Boris stumbled up to the street. His foot hurt. He had to ignore this for now. The first order of business was to get away as far as possible. He saw a taxicab approaching. He limped to the street and waved. The cab stopped. He jumped in and asked the driver to take him to Redwood City. Bogdan and he had an extra apartment there, as a backup for times such as this. Boris took out the iPhone that he had just stolen from the woman at the beach. It took him two minutes to crack into the phone. He texted Bogdan. *Am compromised. Will go to #3.*

Number 3 was the secret name for their third apartment. Boris had apartment number one, Bogdan had apartment number two and Boris was now on his way to apartment number three. The phone announced an incoming text message with a "bing" tone. *Sorry. I will see you there.*

What would he do without his brother? Bogdan was the most loyal person in the world! Boris opened the window and held his arm into the warm summer wind. It felt good.

Someone cut in front of the taxi driver. The taxi driver cursed and honked. Boris took the occasion to throw the iPhone out of the window. He did not want to become the victim of another GPS chase.

The taxi driver had reached the interstate 280 and drove towards Redwood City. Boris asked the taxi driver to led him out at the city hall. Even though it was unlikely that the driver would remember him, he did not want to lead him to the apartment. This was his last refuge. His foot hurt. But he limped the six blocks to the apartment.

When he arrived, he realized that he didn't have the keys. He walked around the house and found the key under one of the stones in the garden. He sighed. Bogdan and he had debated whether it was a good idea to plant a key in the garden or not. For situations like this, it was helpful. Bogdan had not removed the key. He was not only his brother, but he was also his best friend. Boris opened the door and stepped into the apartment. Home at last. He took off his wet clothes, had a hot shower and put on dry clothes. He found pirozhki in the freezer and put some into the oven. There was beer in the fridge. Even though it was summer, Boris turned on the fireplace. He was still cold through and through from swimming in the bay. He took the hot pirozhki out of the oven, opened the beer and sat down on the couch in front of the burning flames. The warmth slowly penetrated his body, expanded into his extremities and finally reached his hands and feet. The fire felt good.

He must have dozed off. Boris woke up when he heard a key turning in the lock of the door. It was dark outside. Bogdan stepped in, walked towards the windows, closed the curtains and then turned the light on.

"Boris, what happened? You look like shit!"

"I was chased in San Francisco, jumped into the bay and swam to Crissy Field."

"Wow! That is quite a stunt!"

"No worries. I've survived worse. Did you make sure that the FBI did not follow you?"

"Yeah, that's why I am so late. It took me some time to lose them. I went into a wine bar and out through the back door. To make sure, I called an Uber for a drive to Sacramento. After a mile, I told the driver that I changed my mind and left. I left my iPhone inside the car. I hope the FBI guys will wait in front of the bar for a while and then chase the iPhone. If they intercepted the phone, then they might even drive to Sacramento."

Boris laughed. "Great job!"

"Yeah, I believe that part went well. However, I have bad news."

"More bad news than we already had today?"

"Don't get upset, Boris. I went to Dr. Bennett's office. But the entrance door was sealed, and an FBI agent was guarding the entrance. There was no way for me to get in without a major fight."

Boris felt the blood rushing into his face. "That bastard betrayed us! We are risking our lives here, while he cashes in billions! And then he thinks he can walk away with our money!"

"I know how you must feel, Boris. I also went to Dr. Hill's lab. But the FBI agents who followed me told me that the entire area around the lab is off limits now. Nobody gets within two hundred meters of the lab and the entrance is also guarded by the FBI. There is no way for us to get the brain chip design plans without causing a major fight, either."

"If the dean does not give us our payment, we will take it! I will figure out a way!"

"Boris, the most important part is that we are okay. I could have been locked up in jail and you could have drowned in the bay. We can start over somewhere else. We will always find some money. That has never been a problem. We will do just fine!"

Boris looked at Bogdan. "It is also our reputation that is at stake here. People will talk if we leave this unpunished. Also, I saw Anastasia today, my ex-wife. She's not dead!"

Bogdan's face hardened. "Are you sure? I thought you shot her dead?"

"Well, that's what I thought as well. Apparently, I didn't. I saw her today. There is only one woman like her, and I am one hundred per cent sure it was her. And in case you needed any confirmation, she shot at me."

Bogdan chuckled. "That bitch! We had a very lucrative business in Miami when you married her. Then, she cheated on you, she denounced us and we lost everything. She convinced my wife Lydia to leave me. If she is not dead yet, God help her! I will shoot her myself!"

"I think we should teach them all a lesson. The deceitful dean, the arrogant SUEC staff, the FBI agents, that little bitch that stole our brain chip and Anastasia."

"That is a long list. How would we do that?"

"I have all parts here to build a bomb. I can put it together tonight and you can plant it under the podium for the symposium."

"I would love to blast that entire crew into pieces! But I am not sure if I can get access to the SUEC campus. They fired me!"

"Your FBI surveillance team is busy searching for you elsewhere. You can go to the SUEC campus tonight, tell the night guard that you forgot something, go up to the terrace, plant the bomb, pick up something from your office, show it to the security guard at the exit to defuse any concerns and walk away."

Bogdan looked at Boris for a while, trying to understand the task at hand. After a while, he nodded. "Okay, let's teach them a lesson!"

"Yes, we will teach them some respect!" Boris felt energized. He took a swig from his beer.

"You got beer here?"

Boris nodded. "Yeah, there is more in the kitchen. Help yourself!"

Bogdan threw his jacket on the couch and walked over to the kitchen. Boris heard him opening the refrigerator. "There are also some leftover pirozhki in the oven!"

"Awesome! You're always prepared!" Boris heard the sound of China on the kitchen counter. He quickly fetched Bogdan's jacket and dropped Anastasia's GPS chip into the inside pocket. He felt a little bad about it. But if he told him, Anastasia would notice and stay away. *They have to meet as a surprise for both.* Boris thought, Bogdan was an excellent shot. Anastasia was not. She had missed him three times! And Anastasia was not a killer, either. She wanted revenge on Boris, but she had no unfinished business with Bogdan. In a chance encounter, Bogdan would win. Boris checked the outer pocket and made sure that Bogdan's gun was loaded.

Bogdan came back from the kitchen, chewing.

"Do you need a new gun?"

"No, I have one in the bedroom here. I just wanted to make sure that your gun is loaded, in case you meet Anastasia. She clearly is looking for us."

"Looking for you!"

"If she sees you, she will shoot at you, Bogdan. Remember that. You'll have to shoot her first!"

"I sure will! But I think she is after you! Check your own gun!"

"I will do that too. Be careful out there, Bogdan! You never know what you'll find behind the next corner!"

"Yes, sir! A toast to a successful big bang!" Bogdan raised his beer bottle.

"Cheers!" Boris looked at Bogdan, thinking.

"What's up, Boris?"

"Well, I just thought. If a bomb goes off on the terrace beside the SUEC building, then it is very well possible that the FBI agent in front of Dr. Bennett's office gets hurt."

"I couldn't care less. What's your point?"

"You could still get our painting tomorrow morning. You can decommission the FBI agent who watches the office door. If someone finds him later, they will think it was the bomb."

"Yeah, I really want the painting. If everyone else is busy watching twelve billionaires on the terrace, it should be easy to get into the office and walk away with the painting. So, you want me to plant the bomb and get the painting? What is your part?"

"I will build the bomb right now and I will kill Dean Bennett tomorrow myself. This is important to retain the respect of our community!"

"How will you kill the dean among hundreds of FBI officers? They will kill you first! And if they don't kill you first, then they will kill you second. Either way, you will be dead!"

"Not if we orchestrate the event well. I will text the dean that there is a bomb under the terrace. That man has never cared about anybody but himself. He will not tell anybody. But he will run away, likely seeking shelter in the forest behind the terrace. That's where I will wait for him."

"But the bomb will kill him for you? Why do you want to shoot him? He cannot be more dead."

"You never know who gets hit by a bomb and who does not. Dean Bennett is the kind of man who will get out of this somehow. I want to shoot him by myself, to make sure he does not survive."

"But won't someone from the FBI notice? You will have them all on your heels."

"Not if we time this well. Let's say we program the bomb to go off at eleven am. You'll get the painting at ten am and will be on your way to Redwood City at ten-thirty. I will inform the dean around the same time. Once he runs into the woods, I will shoot him there. The bomb will go off shortly afterwards and the FBI agents will be busy saving as many billionaires as possible. I can take my sweet time walking back to my car and driving away. We will meet here and leave right away. Make sure your car is fully fueled and you have packed all the stuff that you want to take with you. Don't forget the painting. We will drive cross country and then take a ship to South America."

"I would love to stop over in Florida again. I really liked it there!"

"Of course, Bogdan, we can stop over wherever you want. Perhaps we find you a new woman in Florida. You have been lonely for too long! Now let's start with step one. Putting the bomb together. Do you want to give me a hand?"

Bogdan nodded.

Boris got up and walked down the stairs to the basement. Bogdan followed him.

***

Annya stood in the darkness across of the street, watching Boris and Bogdan through a small gap between the curtains that covered the windows of the living room. She debated with herself if she should go in. But she was realistic enough to conclude that she could not win against both of them. They were both trained shooters, while her skills were rusty. In addition, she was really tired, which would impair her ability to react quickly in a fight. She had hardly slept last night, worked in the ER this morning, planted a GPS chip in Boris's cast and tried to shoot him twice – unfortunately unsuccessfully. Next time, she would do better. She had to recharge her senses to 100 per cent capacity. Anya's stomach grumbled. She saw the two men enjoying some snacks and beers on the couch. Boris had a rough day as well and probably needed to unwind. It was unlikely that he would cause another shooting scene tonight. Annya decided to get some sleep. Tomorrow was another day. She turned around, walked towards the train station and took the Caltrain to Palo Alto. She would spend the night at the Sheraton there. She did not dare to go back to her apartment. The FBI was probably waiting there for her.

- 50 -
Lili
THE CELEBRATION

Thursday, May 27, 2032, 10.00 am.

Lili walked up the stairs to the visitors' terrace of the octagon building. The organizers had set up a stage there, with a podium, two large flower arrangements and several amplifiers on each side. It was a beautiful California morning. The fog had just settled, and the golden sun illuminated the octagon building and its terrace in a dazzling light. The loudspeakers emitted the harp solo from Donizetti's opera *Lucia di Lammermoor*, which created a mystical and soothing atmosphere. Rows of chairs were neatly arranged facing the stage. Lili calculated that there were 288 guests, not many for an epic event such as this. The center aisle was covered by a red carpet and led up the stairs to the stage. A team of photographers were busy positioning their cameras to both sides of the red carpet and the stairs that led up to the stage.

People in elegant suits and extravagant dresses were stepping on the terrace from different directions, some chatting with each other, others greeting new arrivals, others taking photos of the venue and the breathtaking view over the valley, and yet others wandering around and looking for their seats. SUEC employees in silver-shimmering jeans and T-shirts with SUEC logos were handing out champagne flutes and Erlenmeyer flask-shaped bottles with rose water. Others supervised humanoid robots, who were walking through the chattering audience with trays of beautifully decorated snacks, offering diamond-shaped pastries, bacon-wrapped dates, golden smokies, cheese-filled pretzels, baked mushrooms, shrimp-mango skewers and baked jalapeno poppers. Lili took one of the delicate golden pastries with a napkin. It was still warm, probably freshly baked, and smelled delicious. She took a bite. It was crunchy on the outside and fluffy on the inside, with a taste of almonds, melted chocolate and a hint of apricot. She sighed. This was as close to heaven as it could get!

Lili walked down the aisle and looked for her seat number. 78. It was a seat in the third last row, close to the middle aisle. A man was already sitting at the outer edge of the same row. As she came closer, she recognized Terrel. He had taken a seat at the outer border of the seating area. Lili figured that this would make it easy for him to get up if needed. He held a leash that led to a large goldendoodle, who was lying on the floor in front of him. The dog's large paws and head were sticking out of the row and several people stopped by to pat him. The dog clearly enjoyed the attention, wagging his tail. Lili waved at Terrel, and he waved back. She walked over to him.

"Hello, Terrel, great to see you!"

"Great to see you as well, Lili!"

"Did you arrest the killer?"

"This is classified information. All I can say is that our operation is still ongoing. That's why we are here."

"I take that as a no."

"I hope *you* had an uneventful rest of the day yesterday?"

"Yes, I am pleased to report that I did not encounter any further kidnappings, burning houses or karate fights!"

Terrel chuckled. "I am glad to hear that! Did Aiko come to see you to have her hand checked out? I hope she did not get hurt in the fight yesterday?"

Lili sat down on the empty seat besides Terrel. "Yes, she did come to see me. I took a snapshot of her radiographs; in case I saw you today. Aiko agreed that I could provide you with her radiographs for your report, if you need them." Lili opened her iPhone and showed the images to Terrel.

"Oh, she did get injured!" Terrel exclaimed. "Her finger joints look very abnormal!"

"Well, you are correct that the radiograph is abnormal. However, the changes shown here are not due to the fight yesterday," Lili explained. "Aiko has a severe erosive osteoarthritis of her hands. That is a degenerative joint disease that occurs due to cartilage degeneration, especially in elderly female patients. As you can see, there are similar changes in both hands."

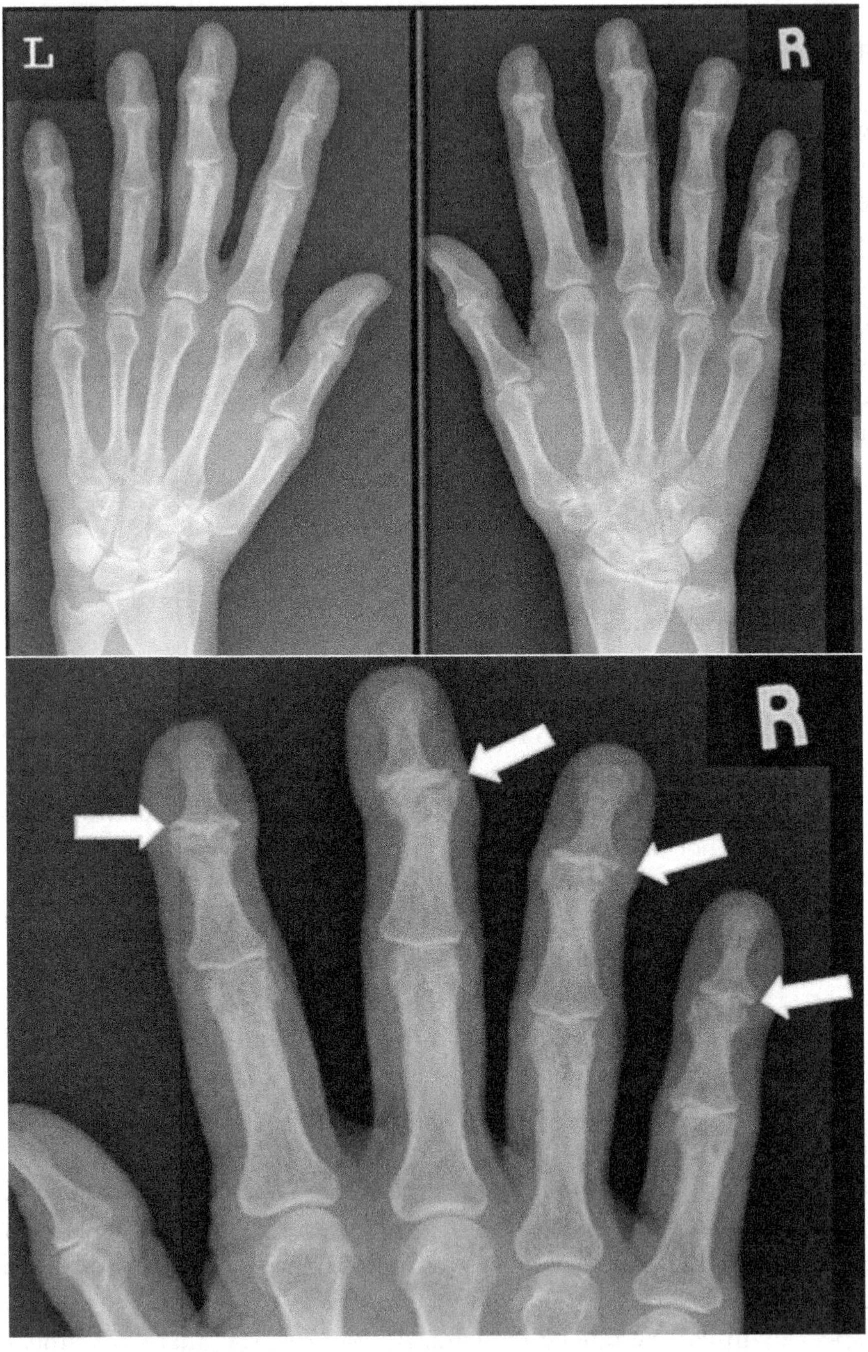
L
R
R

"How do you know it is an osteoarthritis?" Terrel asked.

Lili magnified the radiograph of the right hand in order to show the important changes better. "Osteoarthritis typically involves the distal interphalangeal joints and to a lesser degree the proximal interphalangeal joints. The joint space is severely narrowed. The bone under the injured cartilage degenerates as well, leading to bone erosions, which start at the center of the joint, where the cartilage is very thick. That leads to a typical "gull wing" appearance of the bone destruction."

Terrel looked with interest at the radiograph. He shook his head. "You radiologists have a lot of imagination! I think I can see a flying seagull here at the last joint of the index finger!"

"Yes, some also call these erosions seagull or sawtooth erosions. The ends of the affected bones often protrude beyond the margins of the joint. We call them marginal osteophyte proliferations."

"Fascinating!" Terrel inspected the radiographs some more. "How do you know this is not a rheumatoid arthritis? That typically causes changes of the finger joints as well, right?"

"Yes, indeed!" Lili looked through her online teaching file. And brought up radiographs from a patient with rheumatoid arthritis.

"See this case here. Rheumatoid arthritis often starts in the wrist joints and then involves the joints of the small joints of the hands, the so-called carpal bones. In this case here, there are extensive erosions of the styloid process of the ulna. This is often where we see the earliest changes." Lili pointed at the destructed styloid process of the ulna. "There are also extensive erosions of the distal ulna and radius and extensive erosions of all of the carpal bones. Some of the carpal joints have developed an ankylosis, which means that they have fused. This can lead to joint stiffness and severely impact the functionality of the hand. When the bones are fused, the hand cannot move as usual."

"Wow, when you compare this to Aiko's wrist, these are very severe changes!" Terrel said. "But the fingers are not as affected."

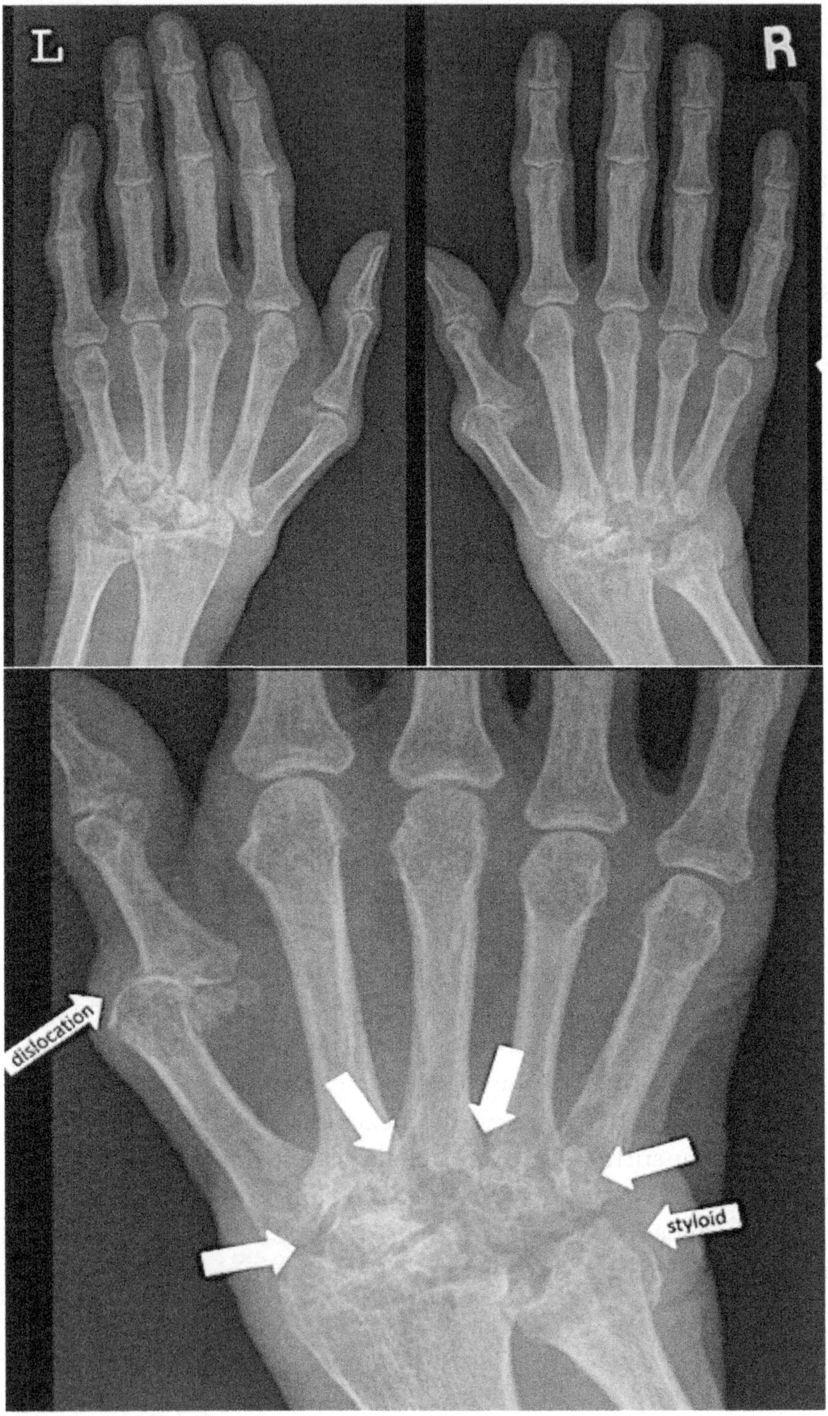
L
R
dislocation
styloid

Lili nodded. "The finger joints are not as severely affected in this particular patient. But they are also often affected. But rheumatoid arthritis favors the more proximal joints and the erosions usually begin at the articular margins. The forces of tendon imbalance and capsular contraction ultimately result in joint subluxations. This patient here has a luxation of the metacarpophalangeal joint of the thumb." She pointed at the abnormality.

They were interrupted by a familiar voice.

"Hello, Lili and Terrel, are you reviewing classified materials at a party?"

Lili looked up and saw Angus Weber standing in front of them, leaning on his crutches. His right leg was in an orthopedic shoe. The goldendoodle jumped up and greeted Angus by nuzzling his injured leg and wagging his tail.

"Hello, Angus!" Terrel greeted him cheerfully. "Would you like to sit down?"

Lili got up as well. "Hello Agent Weber! I can assure you that all images we reviewed here were de-identified."

"I am glad to hear that!" he said. He passed by Terrel and sat beside him, on the chair that Lili had just vacated. He extended his injured leg and placed the two crutches beside him. Terrel leaned forward and placed his upright briefcase under Angus's leg, to elevate it.

"Thank you, Terrel," Angus said. "That makes this much more comfortable! My leg still swells as soon as I put it to the ground!"

Angus nodded. The goldendoodle settled in front of both men.

"I should probably take my seat as well." Lili excused herself. She still did not feel comfortable in Agent Weber's presence. He seemed to have something to criticize about her every time she met him. She wished both agents a good day, turned around and walked over to her seat at the other end of the row.

As she arrived at her seat, Lili heard a familiar voice behind her. "Hello, Lili, great to see you again!"

She turned around and saw Robert Hill and his partner, Atharv Patel, walking towards her.

"Hello Robert and Atharv, great to see you indeed!"

Atharv looked at her with a mischievous smile. "Lili, did you bring your significant other? I am very curious to meet him! I heard he is very handsome!"

Lili laughed. "I am afraid Mark has an important conference with the National Institutes of Health today about one of his own research grants. He leads the emergency imaging service at UCSF, and he has his own government-funded research enterprise, which keeps him very busy!"

That was not the whole truth. Mark was busy and he would probably not have been interested in joining her here. But she was embarrassed to share that she had received only one invitation. In fact, it was not clear to her why she had been invited. She saw multiple SUEC executives and the most famous SUEC scientists in the audience. But these were clearly all above her pay grade.

Atharv shook his head. "Well, we must find out when he will not be busy so that Robert and I can get to know him! Perhaps we can go to dinner sometime!"

Lili laughed as well. "We would love to do that!"

Robert pointed at the napkin in her hand. "Did you notice that the program is printed on the napkins?"

Lili looked closer at the bamboo napkin in her hand. It had a uniform green color on the outside, with a SUEC logo on the front and a list of donors and their businesses on the back. When she flipped it open, the napkin indeed contained the program list on the inside. The bamboo material was sturdy enough that little fat droplets from the outer side had not penetrated it. "What a great idea!"

"Yes, every detail has been planned to perfection! This is such a historical event!" Robert Hill raised his champagne glass and Atharv and Lili clinked theirs with his.

The harp music stopped, and a powerful gong sound interrupted their conversation. Lili looked up and saw a beautifully carved instrument at the right side of the podium. It consisted of a central circular bronze disk, which was suspended vertically by a golden cord and connected to an ornately carved ebony frame. One of the SUEC employees had hit the metal disk with a large hammer, which produced a sustained vibrating sound with a series of overtones. People intuitively understood the sign and scrambled around to take their seats.

Lili looked around. Apparently, the killer was still on the loose. What if he was somewhere here? She looked towards Angus and Terrel. They studied the program as well.

Robert followed her gaze. "No worries, Lili, we are safe here. For an event such as this, there is an army of security personnel."

Lili looked around and lowered her voice. "I can see at least two dozen SUEC security guards circling around the terrace. But apart from Angus and Terrel, I did not see any FBI agents."

The people to her left looked at them for a moment. When they turned their attention back to the podium, Robert quickly put his index finger on his mouth. He said calmly. "Why would FBI agents be here? There's really no reason for that at a university symposium."

Lili nodded. "Of course!"

Atharv came closer and whispered into her ear. "There are about fifty FBI agents here. But they are disguised as regular people. For all we know, the man to your left could be one of them. Or some of the waiters. Or even one of the presumed SUEC security guards. By dressing as regular people, they can better pick up any unusual activities."

"I'm really glad that these agents are keeping us safe!" Lili whispered back.

A second, louder gong sent sonic percussions around the terrace. Lili could feel the sound physically passing through her body. The rustling noise of moving bodies and chatter slowly faded. A few late guests rushed to their seats. When the third gong filled the terrace, it was so quiet that she could hear her own heartbeat. The audience looked expectantly towards the stage.

At first, nothing happened, which increased the anticipation. Once the venue had gone absolutely silent, a procession appeared behind them. The choreography reminded Lili of an Academy Awards celebration. First, twelve SUEC employees in their silver-shimmering jeans and T-shirts walked down the middle aisle and on the stage. They parted in front of the podium. Six of them walked to the right and six to the left. They carried silver trumpets, lifted these simultaneously and played a fanfare. Lili was amazed by the pure, hearty sound and found in the program that these were Bach Stradivarius Artisan trumpets. While the trumpets were playing, Dean Bennett walked down the aisle, up the stage and to the podium. He wore a black tuxedo and a broad smile, holding his head high and waving at the audience. The attendants gave him a roaring applause. Dean Bennett was followed by twelve pairs of people. Most were male-female couples, others were same-sex couples and two looked like parent-child pairs. Lili assumed that these were the donors. They were all dressed in extravagant outfits, with several minutes of distance between them, which gave them appropriate time to interact with the audience and pose for the photographers. Dean Bennett walked up to the podium and introduced each donor via the microphone as they walked down the red carpet. They waved at the spectators, posed for photographs and then took their seats in the front row.

Lili watched the procession in awe. The first couple looked rather traditional, the man wearing a dark blue tuxedo and the woman wearing a long, flame-red dress with a deep, plunging neckline and open shoulders. They waved at the applauding audience and posed for the photographers. Next came a male couple who both wore a metallic-white blazer with black collar, black lapels and black pocket square, matched with a white metallic shirt, black bowtie, black sunglasses and black trousers. Atharv whispered to Lili. "I would kill for that suit!" She smiled, although she felt a little uncomfortable joking about assassinations here. She looked around. Atharv had said that the FBI and security teams were all around them, although she could not spot anyone. Perhaps they were hiding in the trees and the octagon building. To their left and front was thick forest, to the right was the octagon building and behind them was the terrace and a steep slope towards the SUEC valley. This seemed to be a most secure spot for an exclusive event such as this. Nobody got into this area within a three-mile radius. Lili could not possibly imagine that a terrorist could get through the many layers of security here.

She focused back on the donor procession. A very elegant Indian couple had just passed by on the red carpet. The man wore a classic gold and maroon sherwani and the woman wore a beautiful pink satin saree, embroidered with gold ornaments and diamonds, emeralds, rubies, yellow sapphires and topaz. Fascinating!

Next came a black man in a light-gray and blue plaid suit with a teenage girl, his daughter according to the program. She wore a matching light-blue petticoat dress with embroidered multicolored aerophane roses. Several of the audience members got up to take a photo and SUEC employees rushed to them to remind them to remain seated.

Suddenly, the goldendoodle jumped up and barked at something in the forest in front of him. Lili looked over to Terrel who had gotten up from his seat. He talked briefly with Angus and then disappeared with the dog in the woods. None of the SUEC employees intervened. Some of the people around them looked annoyed, but most of the audience did not notice.

Lili looked to the dean on the podium. He should have been most concerned about Terrel walking into the forest, but he did not react at all. Perhaps the loud trumpets made it impossible for him to hear the dog. Dean Bennett continued to announce the arriving donors, while Terrel and the dog disappeared between the trees.

Lili felt an urge to follow them. But this was impossible. To her right was the red carpet and to her left were seven other people, likely all VIP's. It would cause a major turmoil, if she would try to step over their feet to get out of this row. It dawned on her that she might have been invited to this event to keep her in check. Even if she made it out of this row, the security team would likely prevent her from going any further. *What a brilliant move to place me in this audience, where I was essentially immobilized!* she thought.

- 51 -
Annya
THE CONFESSION

Thursday, May 26, 2032, 10.00 am.

Annya woke up at the Sheraton hotel at ten on Thursday morning. *My God!* she thought. *Did I sleep that long?* She jumped up, got dressed and looked for the location of the GPS chip on her cell phone. It was on the SUEC campus! Annya grabbed her few belongings, checked out on the hotel app, ran out of the building, waved for a taxi at the entrance and asked the driver to take her to the SUEC campus as quickly as possible. The donor symposium was going on there. If Boris was there as well, that meant trouble!

The cab made its way up the university avenue. Annya munched a power bar that she had found in her purse. She felt well rested and energized. Shortly before they reached the parking lot, Annya asked the driver to stop. She paid and got out. There were likely security personnel at the entrance to the university. She could not risk being arrested right now. Annya stepped into the thick forest. She remembered that there was an old logging trail that led up the hill in parallel to the right-sided university promenade. She made her way through dense underbrush and looked around. At first, she did not see the hint of a path between the dense, sometimes thorny, bushes. But after circling around for a few minutes, she finally found the remainders of the road that had been cut into the hillside a long time ago. Now shrubs and trees were growing up through it. But it would make it easier for her to walk up the hill within the cover of the redwood trees. Annya stepped on the path and walked up the hill as quickly as possible. She felt an unexplainable sense of urgency. In the three years that she had lived with Boris, she had learned a lot from him. If she could make her way up the hill through the forest, then he could too. And it seemed like he was already ahead of her. What was he up to? Annya checked her GPS tracking app. The GPS chip was slowly moving down the right side of promenade. Was Boris walking down the promenade in the open when likely hundreds of FBI agents were around? That seemed very much out of character. He was not that stupid! What was going on?

Annya walked up the hidden path until she was a few hundred meters below the location of the GPS chip, which was coming down the hill. She slowly worked her way back through bushes and thorns, towards the promenade. She hid behind a giant sequoia tree, unlocked the gun in her purse and carefully observed the path in front of her. She saw a large group of spectators standing under the visitors' terrace on the other side of the octagon building, trying to watch the donor celebration from a distance. The promenade on the right was unusually empty. Annya spotted the silhouette of a single man coming down the hill. He carried a large, rectangular packet under his right arm and came down the promenade with a bouncy gait, whistling "The Final Countdown." This was not Boris. Annya checked the GPS map on her phone. The GPS signal was clearly coming from the man. As he came closer, Annya recognized him. It was Bogdan — the walking proof that happiness and stupidity were closely related.

Why did Bogdan have the GPS chip? Apparently, he was not aware that he was being tracked, otherwise he would act more cautiously and scan his surroundings. Boris must have transferred the GPS chip to Bogdan without his knowledge and with the goal of keeping Annya away from whatever he was up to. Only Bogdan could tell her what this was. And the song that he was whistling made Annya very uneasy. She pulled her gun and put her finger on the trigger. Then, she called to him.

"Hello Bogdan, it is great to see you again!"

Bogdan stopped. He carefully leaned the package against a pine tree on the other side of the path. He looked towards the woods and spread his arms. "Hello Anastasia, long time no see!"

Annya was pretty sure that he could not actually see her. He scanned different trees, trying to figure out from where her voice was coming from. "Do you not want to give your brother-in-law a hug?"

"No, I don't think that would be safe for me, Bogdan. I know that you would shoot me if you could. I have a gun here as well. But remember, there are hundreds of FBI agents around us. The moment you start shooting, you will be arrested. And you won't get that little package of yours to the car."

Annya did not know if the package was of any value. But from the anxious gaze that Bogdan sent to it, she sensed that she had hit a nerve. She might miss the target in gun fights, but she was always on target in word fights.

Bogdan slowly stepped towards the forest. "What do you want, Anastasia? I do not have much time for a long discussion. I am busy."

"Do not walk any further, Bogdan. My gun is pointing at you."

Bogdan grinned. "You just told me that you will not shoot."

"I have a silencer."

He stopped. He scanned the trees, trying to make out her location.

Annya looked around as well, anxiously trying to find a place to hide. Bogdan was faster and stronger than her. She could only stop him for so long. She did not actually have a silencer. Eventually, Bogdan would realize that she was bluffing and come after her. Before that happened, she needed to find out where Boris was and find an escape route.

"Guess how I found you, Bogdan?"

"Am I a bloody mind-reader?"

"You have a GPS chip in your clothes somewhere. I placed it into Boris's cast. He must have removed it and placed it into your pants or jacket."

"Liar!"

"Check for yourself, Bogdan! Boris wanted to lead me away from him. He had no concern for you!"

Bogdan patted the pockets of his jeans, then his jacket.

Annya tried to reason with him. "Your brother controls and exploits you, Bogdan. He manipulates people because that gets him what he wants when he wants it. It is always about him, never about you."

Bogdan produced a shimmering silver microchip from the inside pocket of his jacket. His jaw dropped as he inspected it closely.

"See, I am telling the truth! You were played by your brother, Bogdan!" Annya had found what she was looking for. She grabbed a thorny bush at the trunk and pulled it out of the detritus of the dry forest floor. She bluffed again. "Boris did not know that the chip also includes a microphone. I heard your entire conversation last night!"

Bogdan laughed. "Then why are you not at the terrace right now, trying to save the party from the bomb?"

Not the sharpest knife... Annya's heart jumped. She tried to keep her cool composure. "I do not care about strangers. I am after Boris."

"No worries, he will be here in a few minutes. Then he can break your neck with his own hands! Boris is the smartest man in the world! He put the chip into my jacket so that I could fetch you while he is busy with the dean!"

Annya sighed. She had got the information she needed. She felt pity for Bogdan. He was only being used. But Bogdan had an unshakable trust in his brother. She wanted to give it one more try. "Bogdan, I have to leave now. But I want you to know that Boris deceived you all along. He told you that I estranged Lydia from you, but that is not true. Boris threatened that he would shoot her if she would not leave. Like he shot me. He needed you to come with him to the West Coast. Lydia did not want to leave so he had to eliminate her to get what he wanted. Remember. He manipulates people!"

Bogdan's' face turned traffic-light red. "You double-tonged snake! I will kill you myself!" He jumped towards the woods. Annya quickly ducked and entered a small hole at the base of the sequoia tree that led into a natural den inside the trunk. She covered the entrance with the thorny bush and held her breath. Inside the trunk, it was dark and cool. The noise outside was dampened. Annya heard Bogdan cursing outside, his voice and footsteps coming closer and fading away, coming closer again and fading away. Then, it was silent. Had he left? Annya felt almost sorry for Bogdan. He was not malicious like his brother; he was just very impressionable and easily influenced. He had a naïve way of thinking that made him an easy target for manipulators like Boris. So, perhaps it was higher justice that the *little* brother Boris had exploited so much would now be his downfall. Annya considered contacting Angus or Terrel. But she decided against it. They would track her down. She had just bought a new phone. If the FBI tracked it and knew that she was on campus, it would get difficult for her to find Boris. From the belly of the sequoia tree, Annya texted to Lili. *Lili, there is a bomb in the venue!*

- 52 -
Lili
TEN MINUTES

Thursday, May 26, 2032, 10.30 am.

The entrance of the donors at the SUEC symposium had been a major spectacle. Lili had never seen so much concentrated wealth and abundance. Now, all donors had taken their seats in the first row of the auditorium. Two pianos were moved to the center of the stage. Two SUEC students, a boy and a girl, walked up to the stage and bowed to the audience. The dean handed each of them a helmet-like device, which they put on their heads. Then, they sat down at the pianos and played "La Campanella" by Franz Liszt as a duet. Lili looked at the players in awe. They seemed to be perfectly synchronized. Were they robots or real people? According to the program, the helmets captured and synchronized their brain waves such that they played in perfect coordination. Lili closed her eyes for a moment and enjoyed the beautiful tune. Hearing the music from two slightly different directions gave it a new depth, like a newly discovered third dimension.

While the audience enjoyed the ingenious music, Lili closely observed the donors from a distance. The male couple couldn't take their eyes of each other, hardly paying attention to the performance on stage. By contrast, the mixed-gender couple besides them avoided any eye or body contact whatsoever. The woman inspected the floor in front of her and the man stared at the program in his hands. Some kind of drama. Sad. The girl with the beautiful dress was completely absorbed typing messages on her iPhone. Lili was not sure if she would notice a dinosaur crossing the stage. A man on the other side of the aisle slept in the first row, his head slowly tilting to the right, then jerking up to the midline and repeating the downwards slope in another direction. Clearly, money did not buy mindfulness.

The presentation ended and the audience provided enthusiastic applause. Dean Bennett entered the podium again. The applause soared. He wore an elegant, perfectly ironed dark tuxedo with a white shirt and a shimmering silver tie, which carried the SUEC logo. The thumb spica cast around his right hand matched perfectly with the color of his jacket. The dean took a handkerchief out of his pocket and patted his bald forehead. Every head in the audience, including the first row, was directed towards him. The dean smiled. He clearly enjoyed the moment. This was the pinnacle of his career! The long-awaited success of his hard work over the past several years! He welcomed everyone, thanked every donor personally again and then started his speech.

"Dear colleagues and friends,
It is my great pleasure and honor to celebrate the largest donation in history to a university with you. Thanks to the generous donations of twelve donors who are here with us today, we are delighted and honored to announce the unprecedented donation of thirty billion US dollars to SUEC!"

He was interrupted by a roaring applause by the audience. He waited a moment for the applause to fade until he continued.

"This groundbreaking donation will allow us to ignite a new era of innovation, research and education that will catapult SUEC to the top of the world! We are now the university with the largest endowment fund anywhere! After years of limited investments in academic institutions, we are taking the lead to re-establish the United States of America as a world leader in technology development and innovation!"

He waited for another round of applause.

"Orchestrating a historical event such as this is never easy. When we started to plan this event two years ago, it seemed impossible to bring all twelve donors together at the same time. At some point, I thought it would be easier to hold our symposium on the moon than here at SUEC. Lately, more of our donors seem to be in space at the same time then on planet Earth.

The audience laughed.

"Seriously, it has been an exciting journey to prepare for this moment and I am beyond grateful for the contributions of our amazing trainees, staff, faculty and industry collaborators who helped us creating a strategic plan that excited our donors, our university teams and the US government."

Another round of applause.

"Together, we managed setbacks, sometimes from a direction we least expected. No matter how we felt we got up, dressed up, showed up and did not ever give up. If we encountered a roadblock, we tried a little harder. And as you can see, it is impossible to stop someone who never gives up!"

The audience applauded again.

"To our donors. I am incredibly grateful for the immense opportunities that you have seeded here and the many doors that your donations will open for us. Together, we will create a better future for all of us, where we will preserve human health rather than treating disease! SUEC is a place where anything is possible — where Americans and immigrants alike can realize the American dream! Thank you for all your hard efforts and for daring greatly!"

People jumped up from their seats and provided standing ovations.

Lili's cell phone vibrated. She looked at the screen. There was an incoming text message. *Lili, there is a bomb in the venue! Annya.*

Lili stared at the audience and the scene on the stage. Everyone sat down again. The dean invited the donors to come up to the stage for a brief comment. The trumpets played again as the donors slowly walked up to the stage. SUEC employees directed them to form a half circle behind the podium. From there, one donor at a time was escorted to the podium and delivered a brief speech. The first donor stepped to the microphone.

Lili felt dizzy. She nudged Atharv and showed him the message. His face went pale. He whispered into her ear. "Let's pretend we need to go to the bathroom. Don't show this to Robert, he will freak out and run out of the stadium."

Lili nodded. Atharv leaned over to Robert and whispered something in his ear as well. Robert nodded. Fortunately, the red carpet was clear now. They were sitting almost at the back of the audience. Hopefully not too many people would notice if the three of them left at the same time. They got up. A SUEC employee came rushing to them, asking them to wait for the break. Atharv told him that they all had a sudden stomach problem and needed a bathroom urgently. The young man glanced at them with skepticism, but then let them pass by. What else was he going to do? They slowly walked to the bathrooms beside the café at the other end of the visitors' terrace. Lili thanked the stars that SUEC had mixed gender bathrooms. That would facilitate their conspiracy. They all went in. A woman was washing her hands at the sink. She looked at them with raised eyebrows and left without saying a word. Lili checked the different stalls. There was nobody else and presumably there were no cameras in the restroom either. She looked at the text message again. She had a million questions. She hit the audio button to call Annya back. But there was only an answering machine.

Lili showed Robert the text message as well. He clutched his hands over his mouth. "Oh my God! A bomb? Why did you bring me to *a toilet?* I cannot imagine a worse place to be during a bomb explosion! We should run away as quickly as possible!"

Atharv put his arm around Robert. "We wanted to discuss with you what we should do next."

Robert threw his arms in the air. "What is there to discuss? Let's run!"

"What about all the other people?"

"Well, did you not listen to the instructions on the plane? Secure your own oxygen first! Once we are in a safe place, we can ask the security team to evacuate everyone else."

"If that is a false alarm, we will all lose our jobs!"

"We could inform one of the FBI agents."

"But they are undercover. We do not know who the FBI agents are. If we inform the wrong person, we create mass hysteria. Or worse, it could be somebody who works together with the terrorist."

"How about Agent Weber?"

"He is sitting in the middle of the audience. First, it will take some time to get to him. He cannot walk. If he hears about the threat, he will evacuate everyone, and the symposium will be over! And then, imagine if it was a false alarm!"

Lili thought, *I wished I could inform Terrel.* But Terrel had just disappeared in the woods, perhaps chasing the same problem. Yes, they could also inform Agent Weber. But since the unpleasant encounter in the dean's office, she did not trust him anymore.

Lili sighed. "I think we have to find out if this is a true threat or false alarm. If we have to find the bomb, perhaps we can defuse it."

Robert stared at her. "Are you out of your mind? If you want to kill yourself, that's up to you. But keep Atharv and me out of it!"

Atharv looked at her. "First, we do not know where the bomb is. And let's say we find it; how would we defuse it?"

Lili opened the web browser on her phone and googled. "How to defuse a bomb." She showed the results to Atharv. *The only way to defuse a bomb is to disarm all its modules before its countdown timer expires.*

She looked at him. "Aren't you a computer specialist?"

Atharv shock his head. "Well, I am afraid, my training did not include bomb circuits. I have no idea how to defuse a bomb."

Lili opened the weblink to a twenty-page manual. She scrolled through it while Atharv and Robert looked over her shoulder.

Atharv pointed to a specific paragraph. "Some bombs record strikes. If the defuser makes a mistake, the bomb will record a strike which will be displayed on the indicator above the countdown timer. The time will begin to count down faster when a strike has been recorded."

Robert said. "We are clearly not qualified to deal with this. There are many kinds of bomb and we do not know, which part of this manual might apply or not. We will only make it worse!"

Atharv nodded. "I agree. Let's inform the FBI. Agent Weber was sitting just a few seats down from us."

Robert raised his hands. "I don't know. What if this is a false alarm and the whole point of this text message is to introduce chaos to a once-in-a lifetime event? We do not want to interrupt the celebration. The donors could withdraw their donations at the last minute."

Lili said. "How about a compromise? We look for the bomb first. If we do find it, we can inform Agent Weber and the FBI can take it from there."

Robert shook his head. "I cannot go back there. I just can't."

Atharv embraced him. "I know you cannot stand uncertainties, Rob. I will go with Lili. If we find the bomb, we will let you know how much time is left on the timer. If there is enough time, you can inform Agent Weber."

Robert nodded, tears running down his cheeks. "Please be

careful. I love you, Atharv!" They kissed passionately.

Lili sent a text message to Mark. *I love you!*

A text came right back. *Whatever you are thinking about doing – don't do it!*

They stepped out of the restroom. Atharv stayed back for a moment and then emerged with a package under his arm.

Lili looked at it with great interest. It had a label. Aluminized Fire Blanket.

"Where did you get that?"

"We have these at different locations throughout campus in case a fire breaks out."

"I hope we won't need it! If the bomb goes off, the blast is probably the life-limiting problem, not so much the fire."

Atharv smirked. "It may be useful. You will see."

Lili shrugged. They walked around the café and Robert took a seat on one of the benches at the entrance to the promenade. In case of an emergency, he could take shelter behind the limestone building of the café. Or he could quickly run down the promenade.

One of the SUEC employees on the terrace looked down on them. Was this an FBI agent? Atharv and Lili walked down the promenade, pretending to leave. When the man looked in a different direction, they quickly jumped into the forest and made their way back up to the terrace under the cover of the woods.

Atharv whispered. "Where should we look first?"

Lili said. "I believe the bomb must be somewhere under the terrace. It cannot be on either side. It would not be effective if it detonated in the woods here. The octagon building is reinforced with steel. A bomb in the building would likely not impact the terrace much. Above the terrace is only air. So, there is no place to hide anything. It must be under the terrace!"

Lili looked around. The terrace was built on the slope of the hill. About two thirds rested on the hillside, while one third protruded towards the valley. The floor of the terrace was composed of redwood planks. The protruding part was secured by multiple steel pillars. As they came closer, she saw seven humanoid robots walking around the base of the terrace. Lili had not noticed them earlier. The robots walked around the steel pillars underneath the outer perimeter of the terrace, invisible from the platform. Their heads continuously rotated around, their laser eyes scanning the surrounding area.

Lili gasped. "Fascinating!"

Atharv smiled proudly. "The newest invention of the SUEC Robo-Tech team! These are essentially walking surveillance cameras. Since they continuously move around, they have essentially no blind spots. I helped to design and train the artificial intelligence algorithm that operates them."

"How can we get past them?"

"That's where the fire blanket will come in!" Atharv unfolded the blanket. "Artificial intelligence really is a misnomer. These robots are one hundred per cent artificial, zero per cent intelligent. They do not have common sense."

He waved at her. "Would you please come here and stand really close to me."

Lili raised her eyebrows in humorous protest. "Is this an inappropriate advance?"

Atharv laughed. "No offence intended. We need to play a steel pillar. The robots are trained to recognize living subjects. They will ignore anything that looks like the pillars under the deck."

Lili looked at the unfolded aluminum blanket. What a brilliant idea! They held their arms up in the air and wrapped the aluminum blanket around them. Atharv held the front of the fake pillar, and Lili held the back. Atharv created two small holes, through which he could observe the scene.

"What now?" Lili asked.

"Now we slowly walk towards the deck. When one of the robots looks at us, we stand perfectly still. When they look in a different direction, we move forwards to the deck."

"Okay! I am ready!"

They slowly walked towards the terrace. The robots continued to move around the perimeter of the terrace, apparently unthreatened by the approaching fake silver column.

Atharv suddenly stopped. He whispered. "Do not move!" One of the robots glared at them, the laser eyes scanning their silver cover up and down. He came closer. They stood perfectly still.

"What happens if he recognizes us as humans?"

"He will inform the security guards. They will first use the built-in camera to see what is going on. As soon as they see our aluminum cover, they will be here in seconds, and we will likely get arrested."

"Okay, let's avoid that!"

"Trying my best!"

The robot came closer, now slowly circling around them. Lili held her breath. They heard a metallic clink. The head of the robot moved around and focused on a human at the base of the terrace. It was Robert! He had watched them from above and thrown a pinecone at the head of the robot. He waved, in part at the robot and in part at us. The robot turned around and moved towards Robert. They rushed towards the deck and disappeared in the darkness underneath. Now, they only had to cover their backs to disguise themselves from the patrolling robots. They moved side by side and draped the fire blanket over their backs. Then, they systematically searched the area underneath the terrace. While hearing the ongoing speeches of the donors above them, they looked at the debris-covered floor, turned around every stone and carefully examined the undersurface of the terrace. Nothing.

Lili wondered. "Perhaps it was a false alarm after all?"

Atharv shook his head. "Let's not give up too early. If you were Boris, where would you put a bomb?"

"Somewhere here under the terrace. Preferably underneath the terrace panels, to achieve a maximum effect. Perhaps close to the podium."

"And what if you consider that people like us will look for it?"

"Or the robots? If I knew of the blind spot that you just exploited, then I would probably wrap it in aluminum foil and place it on the column."

"That's it! Let's check the steel columns!"

They walked from column to column, inspecting them closely, especially at their connection with the terrace. And bingo! They found a small box wrapped in aluminum foil, taped to one of the columns in the posterior part of the terrace.

Atharv pulled the aluminum foil off. "We found it!"

Lili came closer and inspected it as well. "Do you think we can move it without triggering an explosion?"

"I don't know. It looks like some homemade construction. I cannot imagine that it has a motion sensor. But to be sure, I think we should hand this over to the FBI."

"Can you see the timer?"

Atharv turned his iPhone on and inspected the box carefully. "I cannot see a timer anywhere."

"Then it must be on the side that faces the deck. We need to know how much time we have. Otherwise, we get the FBI, and the box explodes in the meantime!" Lili pulled on the box. It came off. Accidentally. Lili was so surprised that she dropped it. Atharv suppressed a cry. The box fell into the dirt at their feet. They both jumped back and ducked behind a pillar. But nothing happened. Lili slowly approached the box again and saw the timer now. 00.11.

Lili gasped. "Eleven minutes!"

Atharv looked at her. "There is not enough time to call the FBI! It will take them at least five minutes to get here!"

Lili tried to think. "There is no motion sensor. So, we can carry the box away. There is a lake on the other side of the hill. If we run really fast, I think we could throw it into the water before it explodes."

Atharv looked at her with skepticism. "What if you fall or someone tries to intervene?"

"Then, you can grab the box and continue to run to the lake. It is behind the peak of the hill there." Lili pointed to the peak of the hill in front of them.

Atharv nodded. "I think we can do it. And we can avoid a mass evacuation. If we inform the FBI, the symposium is over, and the donors will be very upset. Robert will appreciate if we prevent that. This event today means the world to him!"

Lili grabbed the box, turned around and — froze. One of the robots was standing behind them, examining them with their laser eyes. A red light was flashing at the robot's temple. Atharv reached into his pocket, produced a small instrument and held it against the robot. Lili heard a sizzling sound. The robot fell to the ground.

Lili looked at the little instrument in Atharv's hand. "What was that?"

"A taser. The robot started to send out an alarm and I had to stop that."

"How did you get a taser through the security check?"

"Remember, I live on campus. So, I did not have to pass the metal detector at the entrance."

"But they had another metal detector at the entrance gate to the terrace?"

"Yes, but we entered through the octagon building and employee gate at the back end of the terrace. Robert told me about the brain chip theft, and I wanted to be able to defend us, if needed."

"Wow! Why did you not use the taser right away, when we were trying to get here?"

"Then, the security guards would be here right now. They do check their robots constantly. They will receive a message now that one of the robots is out. But they will not get any video footage of what is going on. When they arrive, we will be on the top of the hill. But we really do not have time for long discussions, Lili. See, the timer is down to ten minutes!"

"Of course!" Lili grabbed the box with the bomb, ran into the woods besides the terrace and up the hill. Atharv followed closely.

- 53 -
Boris
THE SHOWDOWN

Thursday, May 26, 2032, 10.30 am.

Boris waited under the cover of the trees on the hillside above the terrace. He saw the dean inviting the donors to the stage. The trumpets played a fanfare as the twelve billionaires formed a half circle behind the podium. One by one, the donors stepped on the podium and delivered brief speeches. Dean Bennett stood behind the donors. Boris sent him a text. *There is a bomb under the terrace.* He saw how the dean gazed onto the screen of his iPhone. His eyes widened. He looked around. The symposium went on. He gazed towards Angus Weber. The FBI agent was watching the presenting donors without any sign of concern or urgency. The dean looked at the text message again. Then, he slowly turned around and casually walked into the woods behind him.

Boris chuckled. The dean reacted exactly as he had predicted. He watched him coming closer. The heavy man walked up the hill as quickly as his stocky legs would take him. He was breathing heavily, like a chunky steam locomotive. The dean passed the trees behind which Boris was hiding. Boris stepped on the path behind him and pointed his gun at the back of the dean's head. When he went to pull the trigger, he noticed something from the corner of the eye. A slight movement. Then, he heard a familiar voice. "Stop immediately or I shoot."

Both Boris and the dean froze.

Dean Bennett turned around. He saw Boris behind him and had also recognized Annya's voice. He raised his hands and said loudly. "Dr. Segond, I am so glad you came to rescue me!"

Annya's voice had a threatening undertone. "I said, do not

move!"

The dean raised both arms.

Boris slowly turned towards the left, where the voice had come from. *Where was she exactly? He saw another movement behind a redwood tree about three meters away.* He stepped towards the trees. A gun shot hit the forest floor beside his left foot. He flinched and stopped.

"Anastasia! Is this how you greet your husband?"

"You have hurt enough people, Boris! Drop the gun!"

Boris tried to glance towards his ex-wife. Anastasia was still the same woman he had married twenty years ago. Her voice had toughened up a bit. But she had scruples. She would not kill anybody.

"Don't ruin your life, Anastasia! You are not a killer!"

"You ruined my life a long time ago, Boris."

"You betrayed me, my love. That had to have consequences!"

"You cannot just shoot someone because they break up with you!"

Dean Bennett looked nervously from Boris to Annya. He cleared his throat. "We do not have the time for couples' drama. There is a bomb under the terrace!"

Boris looked at the dean. "Did I allow you to interrupt us?" He raised his gun and shot. A dull sound filled the air and the dean dropped to the ground. Boris looked at Annya. "What were you saying, honey?"

Annya stared at him. Boris used the moment of surprise. He jumped forward and threw his entire body into hers. Annya fell backwards, throwing both hands in the air. The gun flew through the air. Annya hit the forest floor. Boris stepped towards her, lifted his left foot and stomped on her. Annya held both hands in front of her to protect her body. Boris's shoe hit Annya's left hand. She moaned in pain. Boris stood over her. They looked at each other. Boris raised the gun in his hand and pointed it at her chest. "I do not know how I missed your pretty head the first time. But this time, I will finish this chapter once and for all! Goodbye, Anastasia!"

Annya closed her eyes.

Suddenly, a growling furball shot out of the woods and a set of frightening, sharp teeth gripped into the flesh of Boris's right forearm. He screamed and dropped the gun. *What was that? A wolf attack?* Boris tried to suppress the pain and looked at the creature that attacked him.

No, it was not a wolf. It was the goldendoodle from the Perez home!

Annya sat up and rolled away from the scene. Her gun was only a few meters away. She grabbed it with her uninjured right hand.

A Black man emerged from the forest. Terrel Wright! Boris smashed his left fist into the nose of the dog. The dog howled and let go of his arm. With his tail between his legs, the dog cowered behind a fallen tree trunk. Boris turned around, just in time to deflect a punch from Terrel. The two men got into a fistfight. At first, it looked like Terrel would easily overwhelm Boris. The FBI agent threw him to the ground. Boris winced as he hit a tree stump. But he quickly jerked around, grabbed Terrel's ankles and threw him to the ground as well. Boris jumped towards his gun, fetched it, twirled around, and pointed the gun on Terrel.

Annya locked eyes with Boris as she pointed the gun at him. He smiled at her briefly, then looked at Terrel. Another gunshot filled the air. Boris felt a sharp pain in his chest. *I did love her!* he thought before he lost consciousness.

- 54 -
Robert
THE FINALE

Thursday, May 26, 2032, 10.45 am.

Robert Hill anxiously observed Atharv and Lili from the base of the terrace. They were wrapping themselves into an aluminum blanket and the surveillance robot thought they were a walking steel pillar. If the situation had not been so grim, this would have been hilarious. But then the robot seemed to develop an interest in them. Robert fetched a pinecone from the ground and threw it at the head of the walking tin box. The robot turned around, inspecting Robert. Lili and Atharv disappeared under the terrace. For what seemed like an eternity, nothing happened. Robert wondered what would be worse. If Atharv died while trying to defuse the bomb or if he were blown up on the terrace and arrived in heaven without Atharv. He clenched his fists. Neither one of these was an acceptable option. He and Atharv would live together or die together!

Robert's cell phone buzzed. He saw an incoming text message from Dean Bennett. *Robert, I have an emergency. Can you please provide closing remarks after the last donor and invite everyone to the buffet? Thank you! Ben Bennett.*

Robert shook his head. Unbelievable! Perhaps the dean had also heard about the bomb threat, was trying to save himself and threw him under the bus! Robert looked up to the ceremony on the terrace, searching for Bennett. The donors were all on the stage and stepping on the podium one-by-one, to give a speech. Behind them, the dean slowly stepped backwards, away from the audience. As he reached the forest at the back end of the terrace, the dean turned around and disappeared between the trees.

Robert heard a dull sound below him. He looked down the

terrace. One of the robots fell face-first onto the forest floor. *What had happened?* He saw Lili and Atharv appear underneath the terrace, run towards the forest and disappear between the trees. *Was Lili carrying a box? Was that the bomb?* Robert's heart jumped. If Atharv died, he would die with him!

A few seconds after the two had disappeared in the woods, two security guards came down the terrace. One of them stepped towards Robert.

"Hello Dr. Hill, did you notice any unusual activity here?"

"Hello Andy, great to see you! No, I did not see anything unusual. Except one of your androids stumbled and fell to the ground. See, here." He pointed to the robot underneath him.

The security guard looked at the robot with raised eyebrows. "That is unusual. We trained these robots to get up again if they fall."

"Perhaps some type of electrical circuit failure."

"We will have a look. Thanks for your help!" The security guards walked down the stairs towards the base of the terrace. They went to the robot and inspected him closely. Then, they picked it up by its arms and legs and transported the robot away. *Like a dead body*, Robert thought.

A dull sound filled the air. *Was that a gunshot?* Robert looked to the forest, trying to see anything. But he only saw the majestic redwood trees swaying in the wind. Another dull sound. Robert could hardly contain his anxiety. He prayed. *Atharv, wherever you are, I hope you are okay!*

He stepped back on the terrace, thinking perhaps he could see more from there. The last donor had just stepped onto the podium and was addressing the crowd. The organizers had cleverly arranged the speakers such that they started with the first of the five-billion-dollar donors, followed by the two-billion-dollar donors and ended with the second five-billion-dollar donor. Journalists and audience members were taking photos and videos of their speeches.

Robert straightened his suit. He would bring this event to an appropriate conclusion! He walked down the red carpet, up the stairs, onto the stage. Several of the donors looked him up and down, trying to understand his social value. A few audience members took a photo of him. The last donor had finished his speech and stepped off the podium. There was a brief silence. Robert stepped up to the microphone. All eyes were on him.

"Dear colleagues, friends, folks, y'all, you all, and everyone!"

The audience gave him roaring applause.

"My name is Professor Robert Hill. I am in charge of technological innovations at SUEC. First, I would like to thank our donors for paving the path to the future of technological innovations. Your donations matter! I also want to thank the researchers, clinicians, trainees and staff on our teams. Your hard work is the engine of our success!

Imagine this. The average researcher spends fifty to seventy-five per cent of their time writing research grant applications, not doing research! Thousands of brilliant minds are locked down in hamster wheels of grant applications. At SUEC, we will reboot this broken system! Researchers should do what they do best. Innovating the field with hands on research! At SUEC, we will actively create an environment where the world's greatest minds can thrive. Thanks to our generous donors here, our researchers will not waste their time trying to raise funds for their work. Administrators should do that. We will select the greatest minds around the world and provide them with everything they need so that they can generate as many innovations as possible! SUEC will actively build our future! And let me conclude with one of my favorite quotes from the late Albert Einstein. "The true sign of intelligence is not knowledge but imagination!"

As Robert Hill concluded his speech, the air behind him exploded. A huge water fountain, as high as a skyscraper, shot into the sky behind him. Robert flinched slightly and looked over his shoulder. *Was that the bomb?* The water fountain diverged into a cascade of water drops that rained down around him and settled on the redwood hills, creating a picture of millions of multicolored sparkles against the dark-blue California sky. The audience was in awe. At first there was silence. Then, the spectators jumped to their feet and provided Robert Hill with roaring applause. He smiled. *The people thought that the water cascade was part of the symposium entertainment! Why not take the credit for it?* Robert slightly bowed. "And now, please join me for the celebration!"

The trumpets played another fanfare. Donors and spectators got up from their seats, chatting excitedly about the "waterworks" (as opposed to "fireworks") as they walked towards the splendid buffet at the right and left end of the terrace. It had been a unique event indeed with plenty of social currency for its guests. Robert Hill stepped down from the podium, walked onto the terrace and shook hands. People tried to get to him for a little chat or selfie. Several journalists approached him for an interview. He was suddenly the most sought-after celebrity at the symposium. Nobody seemed to wonder where Dean Bennett had gone. Robert Hill looked around anxiously. *Where were Atharv and Lili?* As a scientist, Robert was not exactly a spiritual man. But now, he sent a pledge to heaven. *If anyone is up there, please let Atharv come back to me!*

About half an hour later, a group of people appeared under the redwood trees. FBI agent Terrel Wright, providing support for Annya Segond, followed by Lili, Atharv and a goldendoodle. Annya had draped her right arm around Terrel's shoulder. Her trousers were dirty, and her left hand was severely swollen. Lili held the goldendoodle on a leash and patted his head. Atharv walked beside her, his gaze scanning the area around the terrace. Robert jumped into the air and waved with both arms. "Atharv, I am here!" He ran towards Atharv and embraced him. "I am so happy that you are safe, Atharv!"

Terrel and Annya walked towards Angus and spoke with him for a moment. Angus talked into his phone. A group of security guards and FBI agents appeared from the octagon building and walked into the forest. Two of them carried body bags.

- 55 -
Angus
THE FUTURE

Friday, October 8, 2032, 10.00 am.

Angus Weber walked down the aisle of the neurology ward at SUEC hospital. He opened the door to one of the patient rooms. Ex-FBI agent Corinne Dumas, his previous partner, walked up and down the room in front of the window, supported by a young man in a white lab coat with a tag saying Physiotherapist.

"Hello Corinne, how is it going today? It looks like you are making remarkable progress!"

Corinne beamed at him. "Hello Angus, I can move my legs just fine! And importantly, I can *feel* them. My muscles are gaining strength quickly. We want to try stairs tomorrow. And as soon as I can handle the stairs, I can go home! I will leave the wheelchair here; I don't need it anymore! I am so excited!"

The door opened again, and Robert Hill stepped into the room. "Oh, it seems that I am coming at exactly the right moment. Great to see you both here!" He looked at Corinne. "And our patient is making tremendous progress!"

Corinne laughed. "Thank you so much, Dean Hill! I will be forever grateful that you allowed me to alpha test this amazing new chip!"

"Well, you might want to thank Agent Weber. He rescued this chip, and he had some very convincing arguments for offering it to you."

Angus Weber chuckled. "The details will remain our secret, Robert!"

Robert Hill nodded. "Of course. I am just delighted that we found a safe and highly impactful application for our chip. We changed the name from brain-computer interface to brain-spinal cord interface.

By implanting it over the spinal cord in paralyzed people, we can re-stimulate injured nerves in the spinal cord. At the same time, the chip is far away from the brain so that it cannot cause side effects on the default mode network. Thank you for taking the risk and agreeing to be our first patient on the trial, Corinne! You are doing millions of people with spinal cord paralysis a great service!"

"Thank *you*, Dean Hill! It did not feel like I took a risk at all. What did I have to lose? My spinal cord was already damaged. A chip could not make it worse than it already was. There was just a great opportunity to walk again. And it worked!"

Angus looked at Robert. "How is your new job as the dean of SUEC? Do you enjoy it?"

"Well, I feel incredibly fortunate to be able to shape the next decades to come. That is extremely exciting. I do sometimes miss my hands on, bench research though. I cannot let go of being personally involved. That also brings me here. There is nothing more satisfying than translating new discoveries into innovations that make a difference in our patients' lives."

Angus nodded. "I am so glad that SUEC finally received an ethical dean whose focus is on research, not politics!"

"I heard that Ben Bennett's trial ended yesterday. What was the result?"

"Well, he did get some prison time. But it was positively received by the jurors that he cooperated with the FBI towards the end of the brain chip case. He got the shortest possible sentence. But he is barred from any employment at a government entity for the rest of his life."

"I feel sorry for him. As long as I can remember, he was always diligent and responsible. But the situation before the donation morally overwhelmed him."

"Yes, we should always remember that taking the path of integrity is not a one-time decision. We are finding ourselves at new moral intersections every day and can easily drift into the wrong direction, especially in high stakes situations."

Robert asked. "What about Susan Pellegrini? She was a minor when she stole the brain chips from my lab. I did not press charges. It seemed to me that fate already punished her. Her boyfriend was killed."

"Well, when a felony has been committed, especially when it

threatens our national security, we do not need a formal complaint to press charges. Susan was subjected to a youth diversion plan. The details are confidential."

"I see. I hope she will be okay. She has a lot to process."

"Yes indeed. Some bad choices can have severe consequences. As far as I understand, her mother and Amir Nielsson are taking good care of her. So, she does have emotional support."

Robert nodded. "I am glad to hear that."

Angus turned to Corinne. "My apologies, we are taken away by business talk. But you are most important here. I cannot tell you how happy I am to see you're walking!"

Corinne smiled. "I am very happy about this as well! Please remember. If this girl had not stolen the brain chips and self-implanted one, it would have taken much longer to understand the side effects on the brain. You would not have been involved, an alternate use for paraplegia would not have come up and I would have never gotten into this trial. Cause and effect in our world are not linear. Sometimes, bad things can lead to positive outcomes."

Angus nodded. "Perhaps that is true."

Robert checked his watch. "I'm sorry, but I have to leave. Another donor appointment. I have to keep our researchers fluent with resources!"

Corinne waved at him. "Thank you for coming by Dean Hill. I know you deeply care about every one of us!"

Angus waved him goodbye as well. Then he turned back to Corinne. "I see that you are busy with your physiotherapy. I want to briefly check on a colleague. I will be back in a few minutes and then we can go to lunch together, okay?"

"Of course, see you soon!"

Angus walked down to the Emergency Room. He found Stella Pellegrini at the entrance desk. "Hello Mrs. Pellegrini, are you working here now?

"Hello, Agent Weber! Yes, Aiko and I switched roles. She is now permanently serving the entrance desk at the SUEC building, and I am now receptionist of the ER. We both needed a change."

"I can certainly understand that. How are your hand and leg doing?"

"Oh, the fractures healed just fine. I am as good as new! And I assume your leg healed as well? You are walking as if nothing happened!"

"Yes, the surgeons at the SFGH did a great job! Listen, I was hoping to see Annya. Is she around by any chance?"

"Yes, of course! You might find her in the radiology reading room. You remember the way there, right?"

"Yes, I do! It was good to see you!" Angus walked past the entrance desk to the radiology area. He stepped into the reading room and indeed found Annya there, discussing a radiograph with Lili. Annya turned around and looked at him in surprise. "Hello Angus, great to see you! What brings us the honor of your visit? I hope there is not new trouble coming our way?"

"Hello Annya — or should I say Anastasia? Great to see you, too! I just wanted to check on you. How are you doing?"

"I prefer to stay with Annya. That is the name of the person who divorced a professional killer and started a new life after being shot. I am doing perfectly well, thank you!"

"How is your hand doing?"

"It healed perfectly well. It was a dislocation of the lunate bone of the hand. You can see the radiograph right here."

Annya typed her name into the PACS system. A radiograph came up and she showed Angus the injury.

"As you can see on the frontal radiograph here, the lunate bone overlaps the adjacent capitate bone and has a triangular shape." Annya outlined the lunate bone with a white line. She looked at Lili. "Hi Lili, can you explain the additional findings of the lunate dislocation?

Lili looked at the radiograph. "Sure, the rotation of the lunate bone on the frontal radiograph is also called a "piece of pie" appearance. On the oblique view, the radiograph in the middle here, you can see this triangular rotation of the bone and in addition, an increased gap between the lunate and triquetrum bone." She pointed out the enlarged joint space. "On the lateral view, the right image here, the lunate bone is rotated anteriorly, which some people also call the spilled teacup appearance. Importantly, the lunate does not articulate with the capitate or radius."

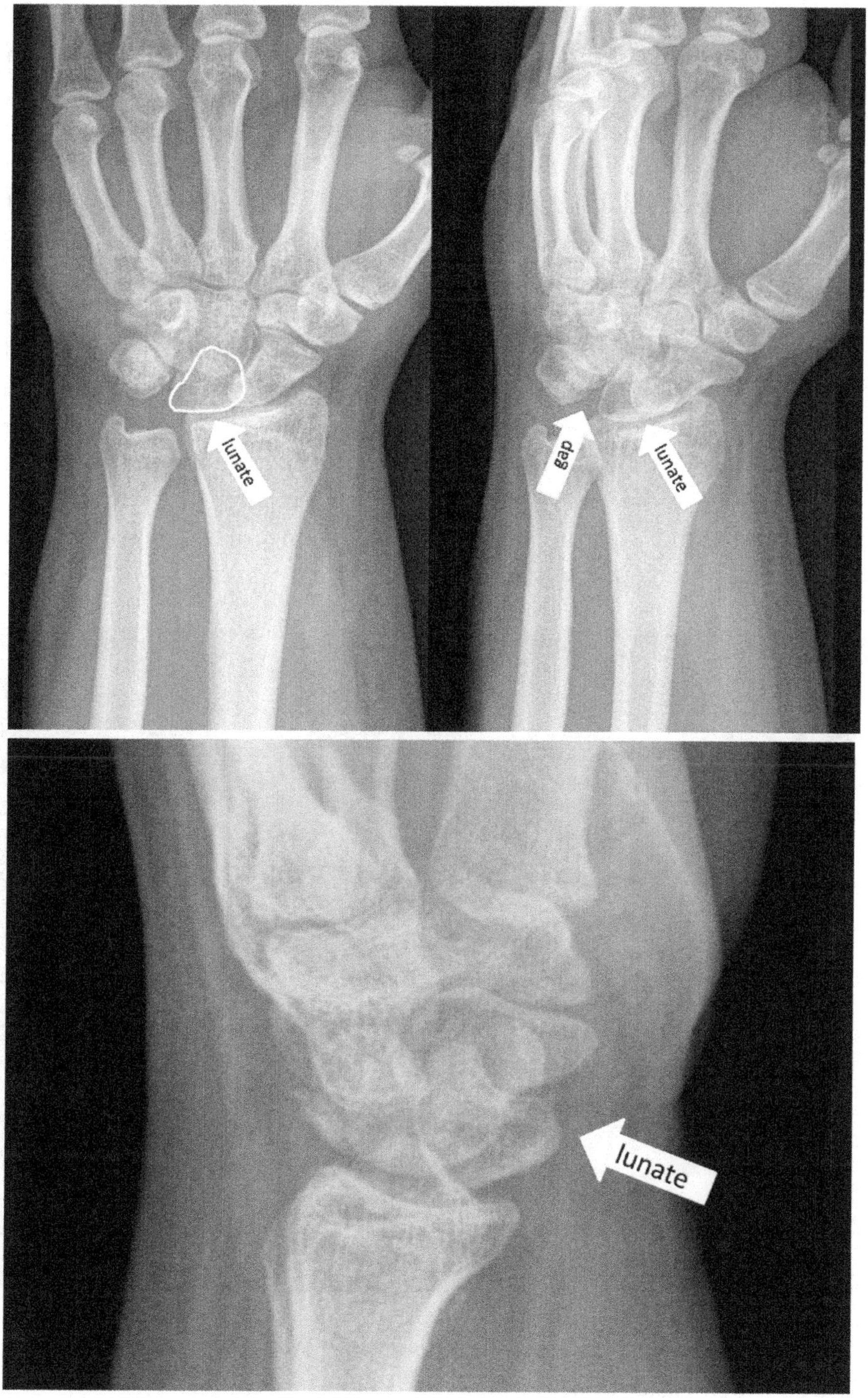
lunate
gap
lunate
lunate

Angus looked at it with squinted eyes. "Ouch, that hurts when looking at it. It must've been painful."

"Well, it needed to be fixed with a surgery. But it healed well."

"I am glad to hear that."

Annya turned to Lili. "Lili, I did not understand why this was not a perilunate dislocation? Can you explain this to me?"

"Of course!" Lili brought up another case from my teaching files. "See this radiograph here. The frontal radiograph also shows a "piece of pie" appearance, consistent with a rotated lunate bone." I pointed at the abnormal bone. "On the lateral radiograph, you can see that the lunate bone remains aligned with the radius." She pointed to the lunate bone. "However, the capitate bone does not sit in the cup of the lunate. Importantly, more than half of the perilunate dislocations are associated with a fracture of the scaphoid bone. This is also the case here." She pointed at the abnormality.

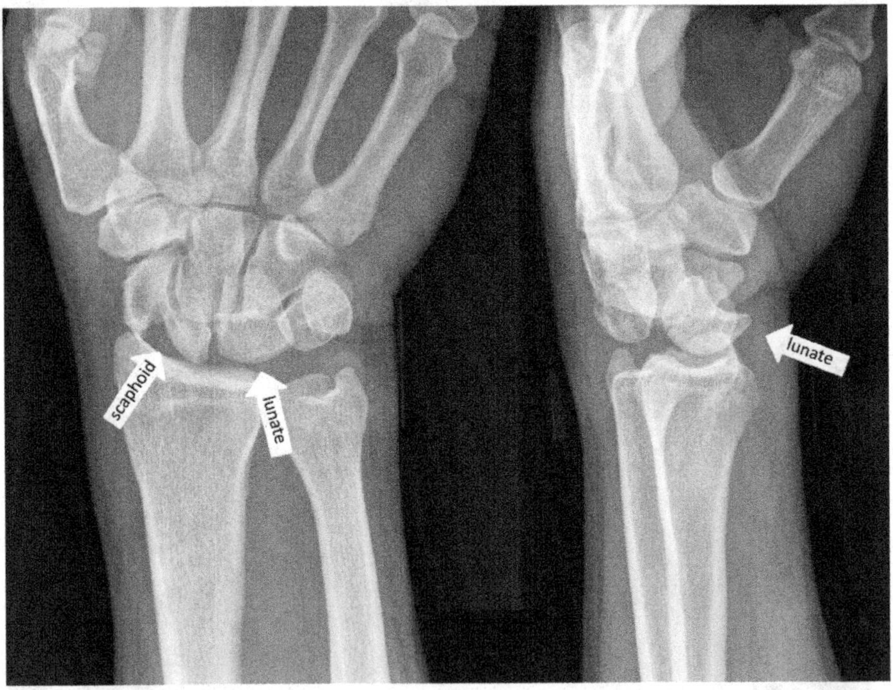

"Thank you for explaining this to us," Annya said. "The findings are so much easier to see, when you point at them."

"That's my job!" Lili smiled at her, then turned to Angus. "Did you bring Agent Wright as well?"

"No, he is busy with a new case. He has been promoted to Assistant Special Agent-in-Charge. In a few years — or perhaps sooner — he will be Special Agent-in-Charge."

"Wow, that is impressive! Good for him! He deserves it!"

Angus nodded. "Yes, he is outstanding." Then, he looked at the pile of radiographs in Lili's queue on the PACS computer. "Looks like you are very busy again."

"Yes, it is one of these sunny days, where everyone is out and about. Many people fall and break a bone. I am so glad to work with Annya. Nobody is as efficient and knowledgeable as she is." Lili lowered her voice. "And I cannot even begin to imagine how she also worked as a CIA agent on the side. As if being an ER physician wasn't a full-time job."

Annya chuckled. "I was of interest to the CIA because of my Russian background, which enabled me to intercept information that could be a threat to the United States. My job was simple. Get to know everything about potential security threats to SUEC. I walked around the hospital and campus, observed people, read internal documents, kept careful files and forwarded these if needed. It was a great job, which gave me a sense of purpose and service to my country. I wanted to make sure that nobody would have to experience the trauma that I had endured as the wife of a terrorist."

Angus nodded. "The CIA agents are the true heroes of the underground world of espionage. They keep us all safe!"

Lili sighed. "Fortunately, Annya decided to close this chapter. She is now one hundred per cent physician and not working for the CIA anymore!"

Angus and Annya exchanged a quick look. "Of course, the CIA time is over."

Or maybe not. Annya thought.

***

Susan and Amir were hiking up Mount Tamalpais in the Marin hills. They had parked at the Mountain Home, passed a nearby fire station and hiked up the Matt Davis trail, which provided great views of the

San Francisco Bay. They then headed into a forest, following a path lined with pine trees, redwood trees, oak trees and eucalyptus trees. The path led along a creek with a small stream. Amir saw a hawk circling in the dark blue sky above them. They finally reached West Point Inn, a small guesthouse, where they sat down at a picnic table. Susan took in the spectacular views of the Pacific Ocean, the surrounding Marin hills, the San Francisco Peninsula and the San Pablo Bay. She sighed. It was peaceful up here.

Amir handed her water bottle.

"Thank you!" she said.

"Would you like a sandwich?" he asked.

Susan shook her head.

Amir put his arm around her. "Beautiful view."

Susan sighed. "Yes, it is beautiful."

"What's on your mind?"

"Kaleo's funeral was five months ago."

"I understand. It is a difficult road if a beloved family member is dead. My parents died more than twenty years ago, and I still miss them dearly."

"Yes, I miss my father as well. But with Kaleo, it is different. He died because of something I did."

"You did not kill Kaleo. Boris did."

"Yes and no. I cannot stop thinking about *what if*? What if we had not broken into that lab that day? What if we had not stolen the brain chips? What if I had listened to you and given the chips back? What if I had not implanted that chip? What if Kaleo had brought five brain chips to the cabin?"

"We cannot change the past. We can only change the future. Life does not come with instructions. We make mistakes – sometimes these are small. At other times, we mess up big time. The important part is to learn from the past and do better in the future."

Susan nodded, tears welling in her eyes.

Amir stroke the back of her head. "I am so glad that the feds gave you a second chance. After you have completed your youth diversion plan next summer, you will go to college!"

"Yes, I want make things better from here. I always wanted to become a physician. But I guess that won't be possible any more with my criminal record."

"Let's see what happens. Perhaps a medical school will take a chance on you. I think you would be a phenomenal physician. You have a good heart, Susan!"

"Thank you for being my friend, Amir!"

Susan leaned her head against Amir's shoulder. They saw the fog coming in from the north, adding a gentle haze to the green hills in front of them.

ACKNOWLEDGMENTS

It has been always peculiar to me how protagonists in action movies engage in multiple fights and seem to come out without any injury. Considering what we healthcare providers see in the ER every day, this is completely unrealistic. Indeed, a whole industry of stuntmen and stuntwomen has evolved to simulate injury-free fights and action scenes, while every other reasonable person would be in shambles. So, while some readers might find it unusual that many of the characters in this book encountered a bone fracture, I would argue that this is the most realistic cast to date for the portrayed situations. And of course, I wrote this novel to teach bone fractures in an engaging, more interesting way than the format of a standard textbook. Whether you are a medical trainee, staff or physician, I hope that this novel will help you remember common and eponymous bone fractures, as outlined in this story.

Of course, a book such as this does not happen in a vacuum. I am grateful for many people who helped me along the way. To everyone who contributed to this book directly or indirectly. Thank you!

I would like to specifically thank my team members, trainees and colleagues for providing inspiration and insights for this story. I would also like to thank Berthold Schroeter for contributing the graphical sketches of the Smith fracture and the Jones fracture. Many thanks to Elisabeth Daldrup, Hendrik Daldrup and Dr. Thomas Link for providing important insights on critical turning points of the story. And a big thanks to my colleagues from the Pegasus Medical Writing Group at Stanford for taking the time to read the first chapters and offering their critical feedback. I am also grateful to Nancy Heafey and Lauren Schoenthaler for providing important input and feedback regarding the use of de-identified medical images in the context of a detective story.

Last but not least, I would like to thank copy editor Gillian Rodgerson for bringing this book into the best possible shape! I am extremely grateful for Gillian's high quality, timely and professional work!

A NOTE FOR THE READER

Thank you for reading an authorized copy of this book. Monasteria Press LLC is a startup company, which is subsidized by its entrepreneurial founders. By purchasing our publications, you are supporting our authors and allowing Monasteria Press to continue to publish new books for future readers.

If you would like to read additional books from Monasteria Press, you can find our newest publications on our website: monasteria-press.com

In case you liked the story about the stolen brain chip, please consider submitting a review about the book on Amazon, Barnes & Noble, Powells, Goodreads or Twitter. Reviews are very important. They help to spread the word about great books and can make an author's day. A great review is also a wonderful reward for the hard work, long weekends and sleepless nights that the author invested to share their story. Our team would also love to hear your insights and opinions. Who do you think was the superman or superwoman in this story? What do *you* think about new brain-computer interfaces? Please share your thoughts on social media or in a blog. Please remember to not give away the entire plot and allow other readers the courtesy of having some surprises.

Thank you for your interest and support!
We hope to welcome you back soon!

Your Monasteria Press Team

BOOKS BY ELISABETH LINK

Who Killed Nia Johnes?
A Tale for Healthcare Professionals

Elisabeth Link, MD
Monasteria Press 2022

A page-turning mystery novel about a promising young scientist who is killed in a network of intrigue and nefarious academic schemes. The story revolves around a fictional university in the hills above Redwood City, CA, known as Silicon Valley University of Evolutionary Computation (SUEC). A young researcher, Dr. Nia Johnes, uncovers unsettling research activities at SUEC and is shot by a mysterious killer. The seemingly idyllic university community is turned upside down as FBI special agent Terrel Wright, CIA operative Dr. Annya Segond and radiologist Dr. Lili Pham work together to solve the mystery behind Nia's death. What are the experiments on human in vitro fertilization (IVF) that SUEC leaders would prefer to keep quiet? Are the unexplained infections that are plaguing the campus somehow connected? Terrel, Annya and Lili must fight to save their lives and their careers as they race to prevent further deaths and uncover the shocking truth behind who killed Nia Johnes.

Paperback ISBN 978-1-7372582-9-2
Hardback ISBN 978-1-958277-90-4
eBook ISBN 978-1-958277-99-7

BOOKS BY ELISABETH LINK

The Claim

Elisabeth Link, MD
Monasteria Press 2023

An elite university. An abduction. An FBI investigation.
On October 8, 2033, a young medical insurance agent, Dr. Frieda Ending, was dragged into a van and disappeared without a trace. FBI special agent Angus Weber and CIA operative Dr. Annya Segond launch an investigation that leads them to the hospital of Silicon Valley University of Evolutionary Computation (SUEC) in Redwood City, California, where all pending medical insurance claims for children with cancer were suddenly approved. Who is behind this? Is Frieda a victim or a villain? The only witness is the parrot Caramba who keeps his beak shut. As Annya and Angus delve deeper into the investigation, they uncover a trail of greed and betrayal that leads them closer to the truth, and finally, a shocking revelation.
The Claim is an insightful and gripping medical mystery novel, which exposes fundamental problems of profit-based medical insurance systems. The game out there is rigged, and everybody knows it.

Coming soon:

Paperback ISBN 978-1-958277-05-8
Hardback ISBN 978-1-958277-07-2
eBook ISBN 978-1-958277-06-5

Made in the USA
Monee, IL
05 November 2026

67381950R00223